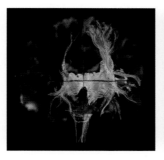
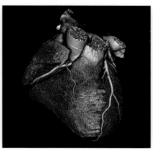
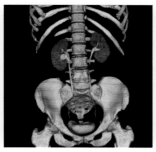
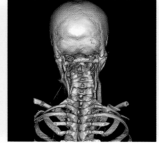
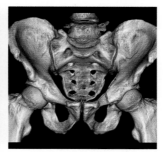

Weir & Abrahams'

Imaging Atlas *of*
Human Anatomy

Fifth Edition

Editors:

Jonathan D. Spratt
BA, MB, BChir, MA(Cantab), FRCS(Eng), FRCS(Glasg), FRCR
Clinical Director of Radiology, Sunderland City Hospitals, UK
Former Examiner in Anatomy, Royal College of Radiologists
and Royal College of Surgeons of England
Visiting Professor of Anatomy
St George's University, Grenada, West Indies

Lonie R. Salkowski
MD, MS, PhD
Professor
Department of Radiology
University of Wisconsin School of Medicine and Public Health
Madison, WI, USA

Marios Loukas
MD, PhD
Professor
Department of Anatomical Sciences
Dean of Basic Sciences, School of Medicine
St George's University
Grenada, West Indies

Tom Turmezei
BMBCh(Oxon), MA(Cantab), MPhil(Cantab), FRCR
Radiology Fellow
Royal National Orthopaedic Hospital
Stanmore, UK

Consultant Editors:

Jamie Weir
MBBS, DMRD, FRCP(Ed), FRANZCR(Hon), FRCR
Emeritus Professor of Radiology
University of Aberdeen
Aberdeen, UK

Peter H. Abrahams
MBBS, FRCS(Ed), FRCR, DO(Hon), FHEA
Professor Emeritus of Clinical Anatomy
Warwick Medical School, Warwick, UK
Professor of Clinical Anatomy
St George's University, Grenada, West Indies
Consultant to LKC Medical School NTU Singapore
National Teaching Fellow 2011, UK
Life Fellow, Girton College, Cambridge, UK
Examiner, MRCS, Royal Colleges of Surgeons (UK)
Family Practitioner, Brent, London, UK

ELSEVIER

ELSEVIER

Notices

Knowledge and best practice in this field are constantly changing. As new research and experience broaden our understanding, changes in research methods, professional practices, or medical treatment may become necessary.

Practitioners and researchers must always rely on their own experience and knowledge in evaluating and using any information, methods, compounds, or experiments described herein. In using such information or methods they should be mindful of their own safety and the safety of others, including parties for whom they have a professional responsibility.

With respect to any drug or pharmaceutical products identified, readers are advised to check the most current information provided (i) on procedures featured or (ii) by the manufacturer of each product to be administered, to verify the recommended dose or formula, the method and duration of administration, and contraindications. It is the responsibility of practitioners, relying on their own experience and knowledge of their patients, to make diagnoses, to determine dosages and the best treatment for each individual patient, and to take all appropriate safety precautions.

To the fullest extent of the law, neither the Publisher nor the authors, contributors, or editors assume any liability for any injury and/or damage to persons or property as a matter of products liability, negligence or otherwise, or from any use or operation of any methods, products, instructions, or ideas contained in the material herein.

ISBN: 978-0-7234-3826-7

     978-0-7234-3822-9

     978-0-7234-3823-6

     978-0-7234-3825-0

     978-0-7234-3824-3

ELSEVIER your source for books, journals and multimedia in the health sciences

www.elsevierhealth.com

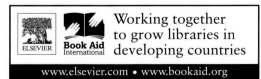

Working together to grow libraries in developing countries

www.elsevier.com • www.bookaid.org

The publisher's policy is to use paper manufactured from sustainable forests

Printed in China

Last digit is the print number: 9 8 7 6 5 4 3 2 1

Weir & Abrahams

Imaging Atlas *of*
Human Anatomy

Content Strategist: *Jeremy Bowes*
Content Development Specialist: *Sharon Nash*
Project Manager: *Joanna Souch*
Design: *Christian Bilbow*
Illustration Manager: *Karen Giacomucci*
e-Product Content Development Specialist: *Kim Benson*
Marketing Manager: *Melissa Darling*

Contents

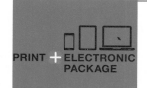

PRINT + ELECTRONIC PACKAGE

Guide to accompanying enhanced electronic content

We believe that the printed book remains an important medium for self-driven education and exploration. However, the advance of medical imaging so far into the digital age marks an impressive and inescapable progression. This field change arose from momentum in the teleradiology revolution of the 1990s, coming to fruition in clinical practice at the start of the 21st century, around the time our 3rd edition was released. There are inherent strengths and weaknesses to viewing images in digital space, while the means to do this are constantly evolving. Therefore we have included a gamut of enhanced electronic material to accompany all the other developments in this 5th edition, incorporating new dynamic, interactive and navigable image sets.

You will be able to move through **radiograph slidelines** from all common sites around the body, revealing important anatomical structures, features and spaces. We have created labelled **image stacks** that allow you to review cross-sectional imaging as if using an imaging workstation. This facility will enhance the appreciation of relationships between neighbouring structures that is the key to a deeper understanding in such clinical applications as staging cancers and appreciating pathological involvement of structures that may not be well seen on single images but can be followed on serial images in block sets, for example, nerves. There is a test-yourself facility included in the new **multi-tier labelling slideshows** that caters to beginner and expert levels of understanding. We have also included exciting new and labelled **ultrasound videos**. In this edition we have focused on the upper and lower limbs, showing dynamic anatomy in the context of ultrasound probe position (insets). These videos can be watched as they come, but also work well by taking control of the slider to move back and forth as you interpret the motions.

The enhanced content includes many **single best answer questions** allied to each chapter (apart from functional imaging), which if not directly based on aspects of imaging, emphasize the importance of understanding anatomy for good clinical practice. Additional emphasis has also been placed on recognising that 'normal' anatomy is in reality a spectrum of variance. Accordingly we have set out common and clinically important **anatomical variant lists** at the end of certain chapters that are hoped to inspire self-directed research and observational prowess and provide an awareness that at least 20% of human bodies have at least one clinically important anatomical variant. We would be delighted to hear from our readers if they felt that important variants had been overlooked.* We've also provided access to **selected pages from the 4th edition** to enhance understanding of key topics. Finally, we are pleased to re-introduce a set of excellent **pathology tutorials** that lead you through the relationship between normal anatomy and altered, abnormal anatomy that is the discipline of pathology. Based around nine key concepts, these tutorials close the circle that encompasses anatomy, imaging and pathology.

A substantial motivation behind this developing new ancillary electronic content has been to reflect current standards in clinical practice, but we have been equally motivated by our recognition of the importance that digital imaging has in anatomy education for all healthcare professionals. We hope that this will enhance your own experiences accordingly.

To access this wealth of electronic material, please see the instructions on the inside front cover. Also, please look out for this icon throughout the book indicating where there is directly related electronic content – as well as electronic content summary boxes at the end of each chapter.

---

*Send your ideas to IAHA@elsevier.com

Preface to the fifth edition

There is increasing importance placed on the interpretation of radiological anatomy in a world that has seen considerable changes in medical student training programmes over the last decade, in particular the reduction in cadaver dissection and didactic anatomical teaching.

We have updated and revised this atlas, by the addition of new images and techniques, to reflect these trends. The 'author' team has also changed to reflect the world-wide expertise that this atlas requires. Professor Marios Loukas from St George's University, Grenada, and Dr. Tom Turmezei from Cambridge, UK, have brought their own extensive knowledge of radiological anatomy to enhance this new addition.

The general format for this fifth edition remains the same, but the layout of the chapters on the brain and the head and neck have been altered to reflect the increased resolution and the greater flexibility of anatomical demonstration offered by newer techniques.* We have retained approximately 20% of the images from the last edition, mainly those that show basic anatomy by older methods, for example radiography, lymphography and some angiography. Further anatomical images and video run-throughs are also available to view on the web as well as 34 tutorials that will provide a comprehensive review of radiological pathology. These tutorials are based on nine 'concepts', as follows:

1. 'things pushed'
2. 'things pulled'
3. 'things added'
4. 'things missing'
5. 'things larger than normal'
6. 'things smaller than normal'
7. 'things that have an abnormal structure, either locally or diffusely'
8. 'things that have an abnormal shape, either locally or generally' and
9. 'things you cannot see despite knowing they are present pathologically, that is, you are either using the wrong imaging technique or you will never see any abnormality because the disease is only microscopic and has not induced any visible anatomical (or physiological) change'.

Further explanations together with numerous case examples to demonstrate these 'concepts' are also on the website. We believe the ongoing reliance placed by clinicians on the imaging of pathological processes will be facilitated by this novel and exciting approach, and the addition of pathology combined with this extensively revised radiological anatomy text will enhance the understanding of imaging to the benefit of you, the reader, and your patients.

Jamie Weir, Peter Abrahams, Jonathan Spratt, Lonie Salkowski, Marios Loukas and Tom Turmezei

January 2017

*Where the MRI weighting is not given, assume T1 weighting ("anatomical weighting") with bright fat, intermediate muscle signal and low fluid signal.

Preface to the first edition

Imaging methods used to display normal human anatomy have improved dramatically over the last few decades. The ability to demonstrate the soft tissues by using the modern technologies of magnetic resonance imaging, X-ray computed tomography, and ultrasound has greatly facilitated our understanding of the link between anatomy as shown in the dissecting room and that necessary for clinical practice. This atlas has been produced because of the new technology and the fundamental changes that are occurring in the teaching of anatomy. It enables the preclinical medical student to relate to basic anatomy while, at the same time, providing a comprehensive study guide for the clinical interpretation of imaging, applicable for all undergraduate and postgraduate levels.

Several distinguished authors, experts in their fields of imaging, have contributed to this book, which has benefitted from editorial integration to ensure balance and cohesion. The atlas is designed to complement and supplement the *McMinn's Clinical Atlas of Human Anatomy* 6th edition.

Duplication of images occurs only where it is necessary to demonstrate anatomical points of interest or difficulty. Similarly, examples of different imaging modalities of the same anatomical region are only included if they contribute to a better understanding of the region shown. Radiographs that show important landmarks in limb ossification centre development, together with examples of some common congenital anomalies, are also documented. In certain sections, notably MR and CT, the legends may cover more than one page, so that a specific structure can be followed in continuity through various levels and planes.

Human anatomy does not alter, but our methods of demonstrating it have changed significantly. Modern imaging allows certain structures and their relationships to be seen for the first time, and this has aided us in their interpretation. Knowledge and understanding of radiological anatomy are fundamental to all those involved in patient care, from the nurse and the paramedic to medical students and clinicians.

Jamie Weir and Peter H Abrahams
February 1992

Acknowledgements

Thank you to Dr Alison Murray, who has kindly granted permission for use of images used in the online pathology tutorials. The two images in the Introduction, the body MRA and the MR tractography, were kindly supplied by Toshiba Medical Systems. Thank you to Jeremy Bowes and Sharon Nash from Elsevier for their courteous patience in production and to Miss Elizabeth Matunda for her stamina during an 8-hour 'MRI modelling' session for the upper and lower limb sections on New Years' Eve 2014–15 at Spire Washington Hospital.

We would like to thank Scott Nagle, PhD, MD, Sean Fain, PhD, and Robert Cadman, PhD for supplying imaging and sharing knowledge of lung perfusion and ventilation techniques in MR imaging. We would also like to thank Aaron Field, MD, PhD, Vivek Prabhakaran MD, PhD, and Tammy Heydle, RT for supplying and developing images to demonstrate the range and ability of MR functional techniques of the brain.

For proof reading and reviewing we are most grateful for the eagle eyes of many ex-students and radiological colleagues ie professors and doctors from 3 continents who have tried to reduce the errors of over 12000 labels! i.e. J Cleary, RML Warren, B Dhesi, SJ Fawcett, A Vohrah, J Chambers, R Wellings, J Roebuck, S Greenwood, B Hankinson, M Khan, T Peachy as well as the team from Perth Fiona Stanley Hospital, viz. L Celliers, M Chandratilleke, O Chin, D McKay, J Runciman, R Sekhon, M van Wyk and Nor Fariza Abu Hassan.

The editors would also like to thank Dr James Tanner and Dr Timothy Sadler, radiology trainees in Cambridge, for their invaluable contribution to the acquisition of new ultrasound images, both for the book and the ancillary e-material.

Tom Turmezei would also like to express his thanks to Addenbrooke's Hospital, Cambridge, UK, as his host institution while preparing this new edition.

Dedication

To our students – past, present and future

Introduction – The role of imaging in teaching and diagnosis: technical aspects and applications

The role of imaging in anatomical education

Imaging has become an increasingly important component in the field of medical anatomy instruction since the 1960s, and in most academic curricula today it has been integrated as a part of anatomical education, albeit taught using a very wide variety of strategies with considerable variation in the time allocation, content and delivery. Medical students unanimously agree that early radiology exposure is beneficial not only to their anatomical education but to their careers, with early exposure to multi-modality imaging techniques being particularly beneficial. In particular, clinical imaging tutorials have been shown scientifically to enhance anatomy education, and self-guided radiology tutorials, such as those accompanying this book, are becoming an increasingly promising learning solution in a flexible environment throughout the entirety of medical school, into junior doctor training and beyond, especially given the overall trend of decreasing time in anatomy instruction under the increasing envelope of vertical integration.

Most publications conclude that imaging enhances the quality and efficiency of instruction in human anatomy and that a relative standardisation could be useful in improving the teaching of imaging anatomy and could facilitate its assessment, thus reinforcing its effectiveness. Although more medical schools around the world are using medical imaging to teach anatomy, some regions, such as the US, show a decline in the proportion of imaging taught by radiologists. Radiology as a specialty must overcome several challenges for it to become more involved in anatomy education, including teaching incentives and protected academic time.

Recent technical advances in diagnostic radiology, such as multi-planar imaging, virtual endoscopy and functional, molecular and spectroscopic magnetic resonance imaging (MRI), as described later in this Preface, offer new ways in which to use imaging for teaching. This coupled with the broad dissemination of picture archiving and communications systems is making such revelatory images readily available to medical schools, providing new opportunities for the incorporation of diagnostic imaging into the undergraduate medical curriculum, in which current reforms on a background of the establishment of new medical schools in the UK further underline the prospects for an expanding role for imaging in medical education.

Plain radiography and legal responsibilities of diagnostic radiation exposure

A 'plain film' is an X-ray radiograph taken without the use of a barium- or iodine-based contrast agent. In an X-ray tube, thermionic emission from a heated cathode generates electrons which are accelerated through kilovoltage to collide with a rotating tungsten target, creating X-rays that pass through the body, today captured by a digital detector rather than photographic film. Four densities are demonstrated: gas (shown in black), fat (dark grey), soft tissue/fluid (light grey) and bone/enamel/calcification (white).

At diagnostic energies, X-ray photons interact with atomic electrons of tissues either through the photoelectric effect at lower energies with total photonic absorption (with the emergence of a highly energetic electron) or via Compton scatter at higher X-ray energies – the freeing of a lower energy outer electron and a deflected less energetic X-ray photon. These emergent electrons create highly reactive ions that alter chemical bonds in tissue, inducing cancer with a latent period of years or decades after exposure.

X-rays were discovered by the German Wilhelm Roentgen in 1895, gaining him the first Nobel Prize for Physics in 1901. In 1896 Major John Hall-Edwards made the first use of X-rays diagnostically at Birmingham General Hospital when he radiographed a needle stuck in a colleague's hand. A month later he took the first radiograph to direct a surgical operation. His left arm was amputated in 1908 due to X-ray dermatitis.

Today in the UK the Ionising Radiation (Medical Exposure) Regulations define the legal standards and aims of the justification process for analysis of the risk/benefit ratio to patient radiation exposure, whether X-rays generating plain films, contrast studies or computed tomography (CT) or particulate radiation generating nuclear medicine or antimatter generating positron emission tomography (PET) images. The criminal law states the referrer is responsible for the provision of sufficient clinical information to enable justification, involving consideration of the appropriateness of each and every request, optimisation of the imaging strategy, analysis of risk versus benefit, understanding of the immediate and cumulative radiation effects, consideration of age-specific issues (e.g. seeking alternative non-ionising radiation procedures in children and younger adults), the urgency of the exposure (e.g. in potential or actual pregnancy), the efficacy of imaging in different clinical situations and appropriate delegation. The referrer has a legal responsibility to ensure the completeness and accuracy of data relating to the patient's condition and to be kept fully informed about patient history, the presenting complaint and relevant physical signs, past history and previous imaging. If an inappropriate exposure occurs, legally termed a 'radiation incident', this must be reported by law to the local Radiation Protection Advisor and then to the Department of Health in London.

The diagnostic value of plain films is greatly enhanced with full, legible and accurate clinical information. It is best practice to record immediate interpretation of plain films in the medical notes, and legally compulsory if there are no arrangements for formal reporting.

Angiography/interventional radiology

Angiographic imaging began in 1927 by Egas Moniz, a physician and neurologist, with the introduction of contrast X-ray cerebral angiography. In 1949 he was awarded the Nobel Prize for his work. The field of angiography however was revolutionised with the advent of the Seldinger technique in 1953, in which no sharp needles remained inside the vascular lumen during imaging.

Although the field of angiography began with X-ray and fluoroscopic imaging of blood vessels and organs of the body by injecting radio-opaque contrast agents into the blood, it has evolved to so much more. Many of the procedures performed by angiography can be diagnostic; as newer techniques arose, it has allowed for the advent of minimally invasive procedures performed with image guidance and thus the name change of the discipline to 'interventional radiology' (or vascular and interventional radiology).

Angiograms are typically performed by gaining access to the blood vessels; whether this is through the femoral artery, femoral vein or jugular vein depends on the area of interest to be imaged. Angiograms can be obtained of the brain as cerebral angiograms, of the heart as coronary angiograms, of the lungs as pulmonary angiograms and so on. Imaging of the arterial and venous circulation of the arms and legs can demonstrate peripheral vascular disease. Once vascular access is made, then catheters are directed to the specific location to be imaged in the body by the use of guide wires. Contrast agents are injected through these catheters to visualise the vessels or the organ with X-ray imaging.

In addition to diagnostic imaging, treatment and/or interventions can often be performed through similar catheter-based examinations. Such procedures might involve angioplasties where a balloon mechanism is placed across an area of narrowing, or stenosis, in a vessel or lumen.

With controlled inflation of the balloon, the area of narrowing can be widened. Often to keep these areas from narrowing again, stents can be placed within the lumen of the vessel or even in the trachea or oesophagus.

Imaging in diagnostic or interventional procedures can be still images or motion (cine) images. The technique often used is called 'digital subtraction angiography'. In this type of imaging, images are taken at 2–30 frames per second to allow imaging of the flow of blood through vessels. A preliminary image of the area is taken before the contrast is injected. This 'mask' image is then electronically subtracted from all the images, leaving behind only the vessels filled with contrast. This technique requires the patient to remain motionless for optimal subtraction.

Angiograms can be performed of the heart to visualise the size and contractility of the chambers and anatomy of the coronary vessels. The thorax can also be studied to evaluate the pulmonary arteries and veins for vascular malformations, blood clots and possible origins of hemoptysis. The neck is often imaged to visualise the vessels that supply the brain as they arise from the aortic arch to the cerebral vessels, in the investigation of atherosclerotic disease, vascular malformations and tumoural blood supplies. Renal artery imaging can elucidate the cause of hypertension in selected patients, as can imaging of the mesenteric vessels discover the origin of gastrointestinal bleeding or mesenteric angina.

In addition to angiograms and venograms, the field of interventional radiology also performs such procedures as coil-embolisation of aneurysms and vascular malformations, balloon angioplasty and stent placement, chemoembolisation directly into tumours, drainage catheter insertions, embolisations (e.g. uterine artery for treatment of fibroids), thrombolysis to dissolve blood clots, tissue biopsy (percutaneous or transvascular), radiofrequency (RF) ablation and cryoablation of tumours, line insertions for specialised vascular access, inferior vena cava filter placements, vertebroplasty, nephrostomy placement, gastrostomy tube placement for feeding, dialysis access, transjugular intrahepatic porto-systemic shunt (TIPS) placement, biliary interventions and, most recently, endovenous laser ablation of varicose veins.

Computed tomography

The limitation of all plain radiographic techniques is the two-dimensional representation of three-dimensional structures: the linear attenuation coefficient of all the tissues in the path of the X-ray beam form the image.

CT obtains a series of different angular X-ray projections that are processed by a computer to give a section of specified thickness. The CT image comprises a regular matrix of volumetric elements (voxels). All of the tissues contained within the voxel attenuate the X-ray projections and result in a mean attenuation value for the voxel. This value is compared with the attenuation value of water and is displayed on the Hounsfield scale. Water by definition has an attenuation of 0 Hounsfield units (HU); air typically has an HU number of −1000; fat is approximately −100 HU; soft tissues are in the range +20 to +70 HU; and bone >+400 HU.

Modern multi-slice helical CT scanners can obtain images of the whole body in as little as a few seconds, allowing dynamic imaging of arteries and veins at different times after the injection of intravenous contrast agents. The continuous acquisition of data from a helical CT scanning allows reconstruction of an image in any plane (multi-planar reconstruction [MPR]), commonly sagittal and coronal and axial. This orthogonal imaging greatly improves the understanding of the three-dimensional aspects of pathological radiological anatomy.

No specific preparation is required for most CT examinations of the brain, spine or musculoskeletal system. Studies of the chest, abdomen and pelvis usually and those of the brain with complex histories require intravenous contrast medium that contains iodine, defining vascular relationships and discerning normal and pathological soft tissues to a greater extent. Opacification of the bowel in CT studies of the abdomen and pelvis can be accomplished by oral ingestion of a water-soluble contrast medium from 24 hours prior to the examination to show the colon, combined with further oral intake 0–60 minutes prior to the scan, for outlining the stomach and small bowel. This is much less frequently performed with the latest generation of scanners that exquisitely differentiate different enhancing layers within the bowel wall. Occasionally, direct insertion of rectal contrast to show the distal large bowel may be required.

Generally all studies are performed with the patient supine, and images are obtained in the transverse or axial plain. Modern CT scanners allow up to 25 degrees of gantry angulation, which is particularly valuable in spinal imaging. Occasionally, direct coronal images are obtained in the investigation of cranial and maxillofacial abnormalities; in these cases the patient lies prone with the neck extended and the gantry appropriately angled, but this technique has largely been superseded by the orthogonal imaging described above.

Magnetic resonance imaging

MRI produces images by first magnetising the patient in the bore of a powerful magnet and then broadcasting short pulses of RF energy at 46.3 MHz, the resonance frequency of mobile protons (hydrogen nuclei) found in the fat, protein and water of body soft tissues and bone marrow. Resonance of magnetically aligned spinning hydrogen nuclei protons occurs due to their behaviour akin to tiny bar magnets, aligning either with or against the magnetic field, producing a small net magnetic vector. This temporary energy store within altered resonated nuclear states is rapidly given up as radio waves, 'RF echoes', which enable the density and location of these single-proton hydrogen nuclei to be exactly correlated using complex mathematical algorithms (Fourier transformation) into an image matrix.

RF energy from various types of coil, some built into the scanner and some attachable to specific body parts, generates a second magnetic field, perpendicular to the static magnetic field, which rotates or 'flips' the protons away from the static magnetic field. Once the RF pulse is switched off, the protons flip back (relax) to their original position of equilibrium, emitting the RF energy they had acquired into the antenna around the patient, which is then amplified, digitised and, finally, spatially encoded by the array processor.

MRI systems are graded according to the strength of the magnetic field they produce. Routine high-field systems are those capable of producing a magnetic field strength of 3–8 T (Tesla) using a superconducting electromagnet immersed in liquid helium. Open magnets for claustrophobic patients and limb scanners use permanent magnets between 0.2 and 0.75 T. For comparison, the earth's magnetic field varies from 30 to 60 uT. MRI does not present any recognised biological hazard. Patients who have any form of pacemaker or implanted electro-inductive device, ferromagnetic intracranial aneurysm slips, certain types of cardiac valve replacement and intra-ocular metallic foreign bodies must never be examined due to high risk of death or blindness. Many extra-cranial vascular clips and orthopaedic prostheses are now 'MRI friendly', but these may cause local artefacts, although newer sequences exist to reduce artefact. Loose metal items, 'MR unfriendly' anaesthetic equipment and credit cards must be excluded from the examination room. Pillows containing metallic coiled springs have been known to near suffocate patients and heavy floor buffing equipment has been found wedged in the magnet bore due to suboptimally informed domestic staff!

T1-weighted images best accentuate fat and other soft tissues, nicknamed the 'anatomy weighting' amongst radiologists who publish or teach anatomy. Fluid is low signal. T2-weighted images reveal fluid as high signal as well as fat. Fat suppression sequences using T2 fat saturation (T2FS) or short tau inversion recovery (STIR) are very sensitive in highlighting soft tissue or bone marrow oedema that almost invariably accompanies pathological states such as inflammation or tumour. Contrast-enhanced images with gadolinium, when essentially used with T1 fat saturation (T1FS) sequences, also exquisitely directly highlight hypervascularity, particularly that associated with tumours and inflammation, especially in pathologies causing neuraxial breakdown of the blood–brain barrier. Metallic artefact reduction sequences (MARS) are superior in imaging periprosthetic soft tissues after joint replacement or other orthopaedic metalwork implantation.

High-field-strength magnets of course give significant improvement in spatial resolution and contrast. MR images have been acquired at 8 T of the microvasculature of the live human brain allowing close comparison with histology. This has significant implications in the treatment of reperfusion injury and research into the physiology of solid tumours and angiogenesis. There is every reason to believe that continued efforts to push the envelope of high-field-strength applications will open new vistas in what appears to be a never-ending array of potential clinical applications.

New methods of analysing normal and pathologic brain anatomy are now at the forefront of research, namely MR spectroscopy (MRS), functional MRI (fMRI), diffusion tensor imaging (DTI) and high angular resolution diffusion imaging (HARDI) for MR tractography (MRT; see below) and molecular MRI (mMRI), the latter taking on a new direction since the description of the human genome. MRS assesses function within the living brain.

MRS capitalises on the fact that protons residing in differing chemical environments possess slightly different resonant properties (chemical shift). For a given volume of brain the distribution of these proton resonances can be displayed as a spectrum. Discernible peaks can be seen for certain neurotransmitters: *N*-acetylaspartate varies in multiple sclerosis, stroke and schizophrenia, while choline and lactate levels have been used to evaluate certain brain tumours.

fMRI depends on the fact that haemoglobin is diamagnetic when oxygenated but paramagnetic when deoxygenated. These different signals can be weighted to the smaller vessels, and hence closer to the active neurons, by using larger magnetic fields. mMRI uses biomarkers that interact chemically with their surroundings and alter the image according to molecular changes occurring within the area of interest, potentially enabling early detection and treatment of disease and basic pharmaceutical development; this also allows for quantitative testing.

Magnetic resonance tractography (MRT) is a three-dimensional modelling technique used to visually represent neural tracts using data collected by diffusion tensor imaging and more recently HARDI, with results presented in two- and three-dimensional images (**fig**).

In addition to the long tracts that connect the brain to the rest of the body, there are complicated neural networks formed by short connections among different cortical and subcortical regions, their existence revealed by histochemistry and post-mortem biological techniques. Central nervous system tracts are not identifiable by direct examination, CT or conventional MRI scans, explaining the paucity of their description in neuroanatomy atlases and the poor understanding of their functions.

MRI sequences look at the symmetry of brain water diffusion. Bundles of fibre tracts make the water diffuse asymmetrically in a 'tensor', the major axis parallel to the direction of the fibres. There is a direct relationship between the number of fibres and the degree of anisotropy. DTI assumes that the direction of least restriction corresponds to the direction of white matter tracts. Diffusion MRI was introduced in 1985, with the more recent evolution of the technique into DTI, where the relative mobility of the water molecules from the origin is modelled as an ellipsoid rather than a sphere, allowing full characterisation of molecular diffusion in the three dimensions of space and formation of tractograms. Barriers cause uneven anisotropic diffusion, and in white matter the principal barrier is the myelin axonal sheath. Bundles of axons provide a barrier to perpendicular diffusion and a path for parallel diffusion along the orientation of the fibres. Anisotropic diffusion is expected to be increased overall in areas of high mature axonal order and conditions where barriers such as the myelin or the structure of the axon itself are disrupted, such as trauma; tumours and inflammation reduce anisotropy and yield DTI data used to seed various tractographic assessments of the brain, including development of arcuate and superior longitudinal fasciculi and corona radiata. Data sets may be rotated continuously into various planes to better appreciate the structure, and colour can be assigned based on the dominant direction of the fibres. A leading clinical application of MRT is in the presurgical mapping of eloquent regions. Intra-operative electrical stimulation (IES) provides a clinical gold standard for the existence of functional motor pathways that can be used to determine the accuracy and sensitivity of fibre tracking algorithms.

DTI will not accurately describe the microstructure in complex white matter voxels that contain more than one fibre population, due to intersecting tracts or to partial volume averaging of adjacent pathways with different fibre orientations, such as in the centrum semiovale, where major white matter tracts such as the pyramidal tract, the superior longitudinal fasciculus and the corpus callosum intersect. This has hindered preoperative mapping of the pyramidal tract in brain tumour patients.

More recently, HARDI has more accurately delineated pathways within complex regions of white matter. The q-ball reconstruction of HARDI data provides an orientation distribution function (ODF) that can be used to determine the orientations of multiple fibre populations contributing to a voxel's diffusion MR signal, mapping fibre trajectories through regions of complex tissue architecture in a clinically feasible time frame.

Ultrasound

Uniquely, ultrasound images do not depend on the use of electromagnetic wave forms. It is the properties of high-frequency sound waves (longitudinal waves) and their interaction with biological tissues that go to form these 'echograms'.

A sound wave of appropriate frequency (diagnostic range 3.5–20 MHz) is produced by piezo-electric principles, namely that certain crystals can change their shape and produce a voltage potential, and vice versa. As the beam passes through tissues, two important effects determine image production: attenuation and reflection. Attenuation is caused by the loss of energy due to absorption, reflection and refraction in soft tissues with resulting reduction in signal intensity. Reflection of sound waves within the range of the receiver produces the image, the echotexture of which is dependent upon tiny differences in acoustic impedance between different tissues. Blood flow and velocity can be measured (using the Doppler principle) in duplex mode.

Techniques such as harmonic imaging and the use of ultrasound contrast agents (stabilised microbubbles) have enabled non-invasive determination of myocardial perfusion to be recently discovered. These contrast agents clearly improve the detection of metastases in the liver and spleen. Ultrasound is the most common medical imaging technique for producing elastograms, in which stiffness or strain images of soft tissue are used to detect or classify tumours. Cancer is 5–28 times stiffer than the background of normal soft tissue. When a mechanical compression or vibration is applied, the tumour deforms less than the surrounding tissue. Elastography can be used for example to measure the stiffness of the liver in vivo or in the detection of breast or thyroid tumours. A correlation between liver elasticity and the cirrhosis score has been shown.

Real-time nature ultrasound video loops have been included on the web in various chapters throughout this landmark 41st edition of *Gray's Anatomy*. Interpretation of the anatomy and pathology from static ultrasound images is more difficult than that from other imaging modalities, as the technique is highly operator-dependent and provides unique information on tissue structure and form not obtained from other imaging techniques.

Nuclear medicine

Historically the field of nuclear medicine began in 1946 when radioactive iodine was administered as an 'atomic cocktail' to treat thyroid cancer. Since that time, nuclear medicine has advanced and was recognized in the early 1970s as a diagnostic subspeciality.

Nuclear medicine, unlike diagnostic radiology which creates an image by passing energy through the body from an external source, creates an image by measuring the radiation emitted from tracers taken internally. Overall the radiation dosages are comparable to CT and vary depending on the examination.

Nuclear medicine also differs from most other imaging modalities in that the tests demonstrate the physiological function of a specific area of the body. In some instances this physiological information can be fused with more anatomical imaging of CT or MRI, thus combining the strengths of anatomy and function for diagnosis.

Rather than a contrast medium for imaging, nuclear medicine uses pharmaceuticals that have been labelled with a radionuclide (radiopharmaceuticals) which are administered to patients by intravenous injection, ingestion or inhalation. The method of administration depends on the type of examination and the organ or organ process to be imaged. The emitted radiation is detected and imaged with specialised equipment such as gamma cameras, PET, and single photon emission computed tomography (SPECT). Radiation in certain tests can be measured from parts of the body by the use of probes, or samples can be taken from patients and measured in counters.

The premise of nuclear medicine imaging involves functional biology; thereby not only can studies be done to image a disease process but they can also be used to treat diseases. Radiopharmaceuticals that are used for imaging emit a gamma ray (γ) and those used for treatment emit a beta (β) particle. Gamma rays are of higher energy to pass through the body and be detected by a detection camera, whereas beta particles travel only short distances and emit their radiation dose to the target organ. For example, technetium-99m or iodine-123 may be used to detect thyroid disease, but certain thyroid diseases or thyroid cancer may be treated solely or in part by treatment with iodine-131. The difference in the agent used depends on the type and energy levels of the radiation particle that the radioisotope emits.

Radionuclides, or the radioactive particles, used in nuclear medicine are often chemically bound to a complex called a tracer so that when administered it acts in a characteristic way in the body. The way the body handles this tracer can differ in disease or pathologic processes and thus demonstrate images different from normal in disease states. For example, the tracer used in bone imaging is methylene- diphosphonate (MDP). MDP is bound to technetium-99m for bone imaging. MDP attaches to hydroxyapatite in the bone. If there is a physiological change in the bone from a fracture, metastatic bone disease or arthritic change, there will be an increase in bone activity and thus more accumulation of the tracer in this region compared with the normal bone. This will result in a focal 'hot spot' of the radiopharmaceutical on a bone scan.

Technetium-99m is the major workhorse radioisotope of nuclear medicine. It can be eluted from a molybdenum/technetium generator stored within a nuclear medicine department, allowing for easy access. It has a short half-life (6 hours), which allows for ease of medical imaging and disposal. Its pharmacological properties allow it to be easily bound to various tracers and it emits gamma rays that are of suitable energy for medical imaging.

In addition to technetium-99m, the most common intravenous radionuclides used in nuclear medicine are iodine-123 and 131, thallium-201, gallium-67, 18-fluorodeoxyglucose (FDG) and indium-111 labelled leukocytes. The most common gaseous/aerosol radionuclides used are xenon-133, krypton-81m, technetium-99m (Technegas) and technetium-99m diethylene-triamine-pentaacetate (DTPA).

The images obtained from nuclear medicine imaging can be in the form of one or many images. Image sets can be represented as time-sequence imaging (e.g. cine), such as dynamic imaging or cardiac gated sequences, or by spatial sequence imaging where the gamma camera is moved relative to the patient, such as in SPECT imaging. Spatial sequence imaging allows the images to be presented as a slice-stack of images, much like CT or MRI images are displayed. Spatial sequence imaging can also be fused with concomitant CT or MR imaging to provide combined physiologic and anatomical imaging. Time and spatial sequence imaging offer a unique perspective on and information about physiological processes in the body.

A PET scan is a specialised type of nuclear medicine imaging that measures important body functions, such as blood flow, oxygen use and glucose metabolism, to evaluate how well organs and tissues are functioning. PET imaging involves short-lived radioactive tracer isotopes that emit an 'anti-electron' – actual antimatter! These radioisotopes are chemically incorporated into biologically active molecules, most commonly the sugar FDG. An hour after injection, FDG becomes concentrated into the tissues of interest, and imaging occurs as the isotope undergoes positron emission decay. The positron travels only a few millimetres and annihilates with an electron, producing a pair of gamma photons moving in opposite directions. The PET scan detectors process only those photon pairs that are detected simultaneously (coincident detection). These data are then processed to create an image of tissue activity with respect to that particular isotope. These images can then be fused with CT or even MR images.

A limitation of PET imaging is the short half-life of the isotopes. Thus close access to a cyclotron for generation of the isotopes plays an important role in the feasible location of a PET scanner. Typical isotopes used in medical imaging and their half-lives are: carbon-11 (~20 minutes), nitrogen-13 (~10 minutes), oxygen-13 (~2 minutes) and fluorine-18 (~110 minutes).

1 Brain and cranial nerves

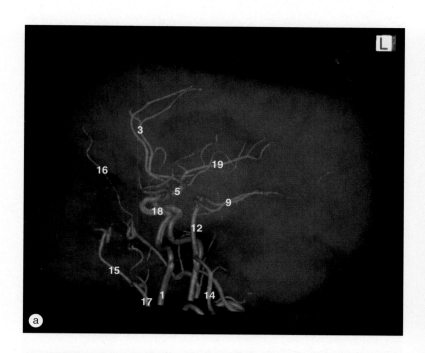

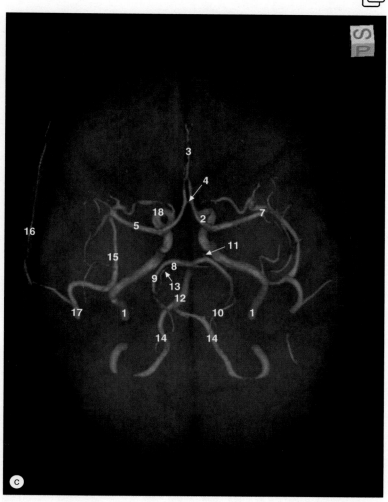

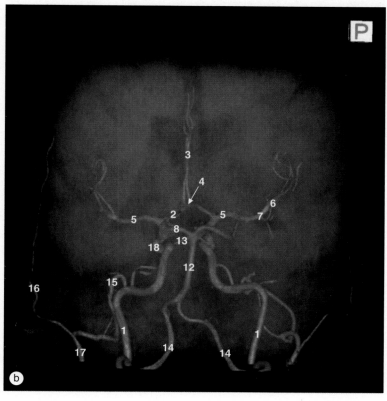

Brain, 3D CT angiogram. (a) Lateral. (b) Occipitomental. (c) Circle of Willis.

For labels see page 4.

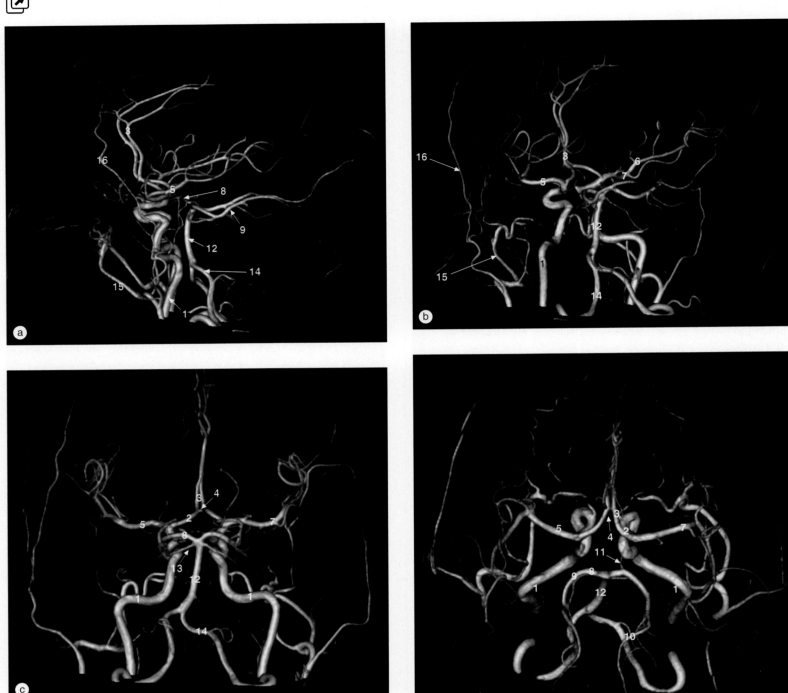

Brain, 3D CT angiogram. (a) Lateral. (b) Sagittal (posterolateral).
(c) Occipitomental. (d) Circle of Willis.

For labels see page 4.

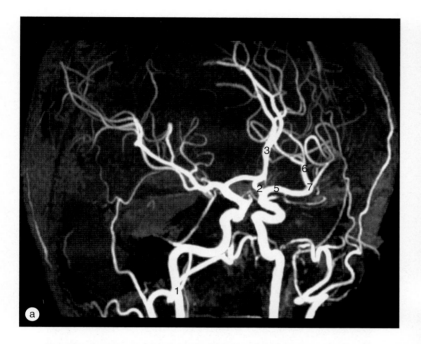

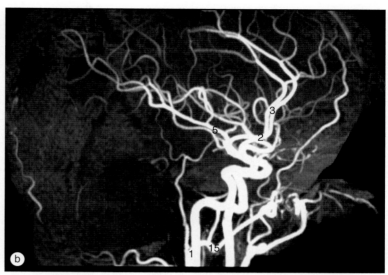

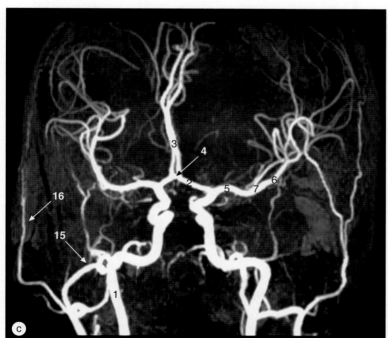

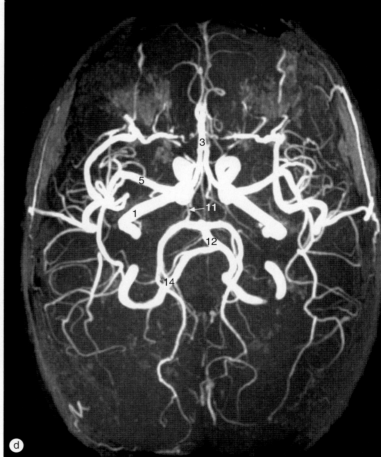

Brain, MR angiogram. (a) Sagittal rotation view. (b) Lateral view.
(c) Coronal view. (d) Axial view.

For labels see page 4.

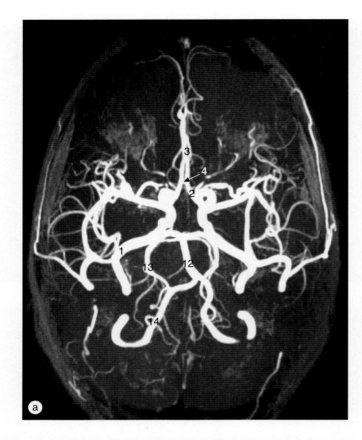

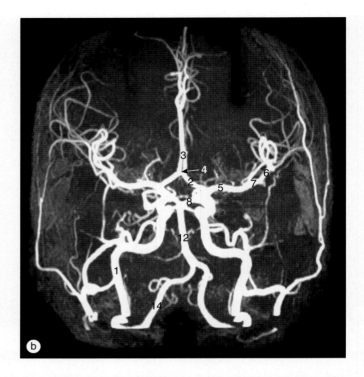

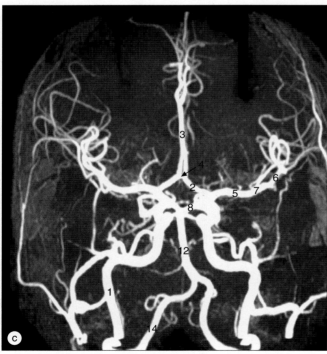

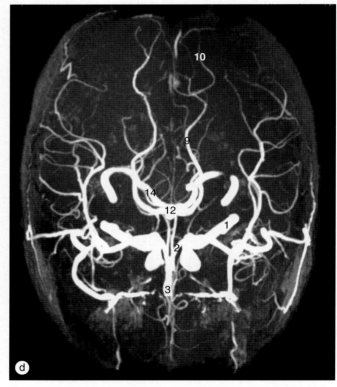

Brain, MR angiogram. **(a)** Axial. **(b)** Frontal. **(c)** Frontal. **(d)** Cranial.

1. Internal carotid artery
2. Horizontal (A1) anterior cerebral artery (ACA) segment
3. Vertical (A2) ACA segment
4. Anterior communicating artery
5. Horizontal (M1) middle cerebral artery (MCA) segment
6. Insular (M2) MCA segment
7. MCA genu (bifurcation)
8. Precommunicating (P1) posterior cerebral artery (PCA) segment
9. Ambient (P2) PCA segment
10. Quadrigeminal (P3) PCA segment
11. Posterior communicating artery
12. Basilar artery
13. Superior cerebellar artery
14. Vertebral artery
15. Maxillary artery
16. Superficial temporal artery
17. External carotid artery
18. Carotid siphon
19. Superior and inferior terminal branches of middle cerebral artery

Numbers 1–19 are common to pages 1–4.

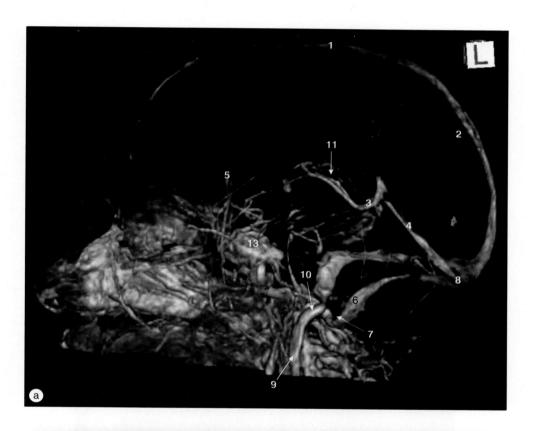

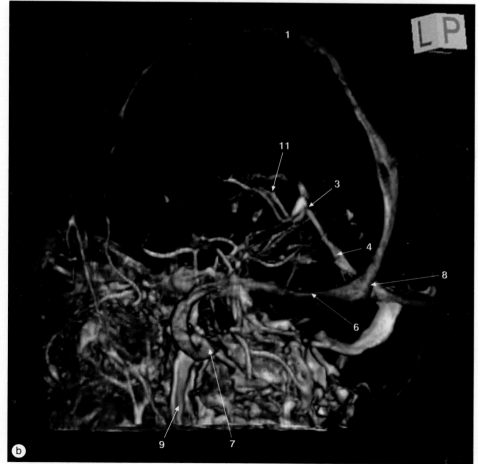

3D CT venograms. **(a)** Left lateral view. **(b)** Posterolateral.

For labels see page 6.

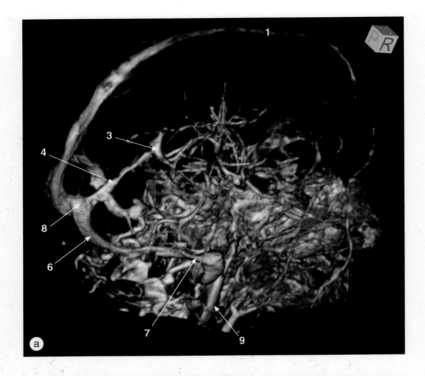

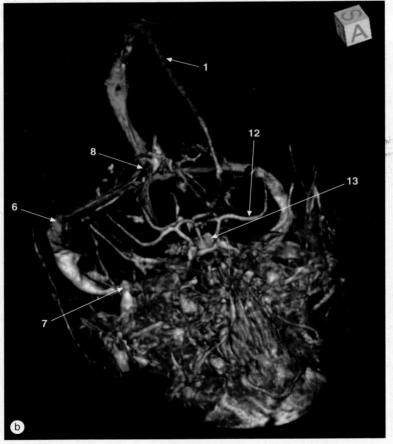

3D CT venograms. (a) Right posterolateral. (b) Antero-posterior.

1. Superior sagittal sinus
2. Bridging vein
3. Internal cerebral vein (of Galen)
4. Straight sinus
5. Sphenoparietal sinus

6. Transverse sinus
7. Sigmoid sinus
8. Sinus confluence (torcular Herophili)
9. Internal jugular vein
10. Jugular bulb

11. Internal cerebral vein
12. Superior petrosal sinus
13. Cavernous sinus

Numbers 1–13 are common to pages 5–6.

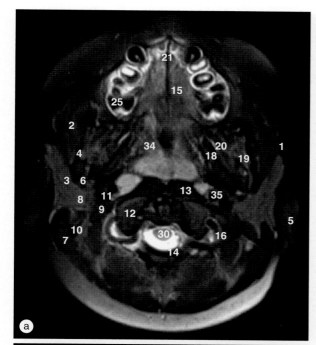

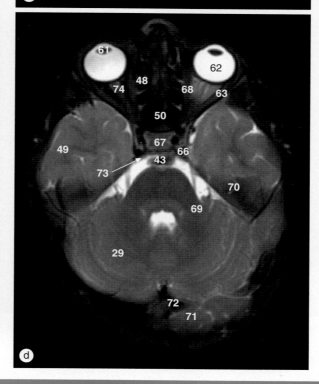

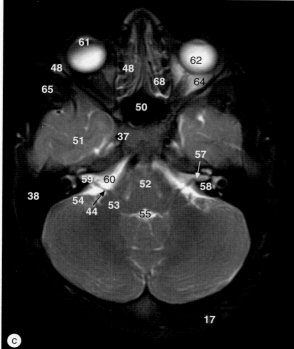

Brain, axial T2-weighted MR images, from inferior to superior.

1. Parotid duct
2. Masseter muscle
3. Parotid gland (superficial lobe)
4. Ramus of mandible
5. Pinna of ear
6. Retromandibular vein
7. Sternocleidomastoid muscle
8. Parotid gland (deep lobe)
9. Internal jugular vein
10. Mastoid process
11. Internal carotid artery
12. Occipital condyle
13. Longus capitis muscle
14. Foramen magnum
15. Hard palate
16. Vertebral artery
17. Occipital emissary vein
18. Medial pterygoid muscle
19. Lateral pterygoid muscle
20. Lateral pterygoid plate
21. Incisive foramen
22. Inferior turbinate
23. Nasal septum
24. Medulla oblongata
25. Tooth bony socket
26. Cerebellar tonsil
27. Coronoid process of mandible
28. Temporalis muscle
29. Folia of cerebellar hemisphere
30. Spinal cord
31. Nasolacrimal duct
32. Zygomatic arch

33. Head of mandible
34. Medial pterygoid plate
35. Contents of jugular foramen
36. Petrous temporal bone
37. Internal carotid artery
38. Mastoid air cells
39. Maxillary sinus (antrum)
40. Cochlea
41. Posterior semicircular canal
42. Clivus
43. Basilar artery
44. Labyrinthine artery
45. Inferior cerebellar vermis
46. Inion (internal occipital protuberance)
47. Foramen of Luschka

48. Ethmoid air cells
49. Middle temporal gyrus
50. Sphenoid sinus
51. Temporal lobe
52. Pons
53. Middle cerebellar peduncle
54. Flocculonodular lobe of cerebellum
55. Fourth ventricle
56. Cisterna magna
57. Facial nerve (seventh cranial nerve)
58. Vestibulocochlear nerve (eighth cranial nerve)
59. Internal auditory meatus
60. Cerebellopontine angle
61. Lens

62. Vitreous humour
63. Lateral rectus muscle
64. Retro-orbital fat
65. Temporalis muscle
66. Internal carotid artery (cavernous part)
67. Body of sphenoid
68. Medial rectus muscle
69. Superior cerebellar peduncle
70. Superior semicircular canal
71. Calcarine cortex of occipital lobe
72. Torcular Herophili (confluence of venous sinuses)
73. Petroclinoid ligament
74. Optic nerve (second cranial nerve)

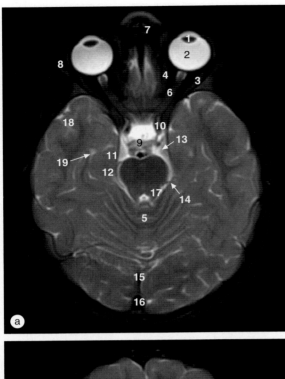

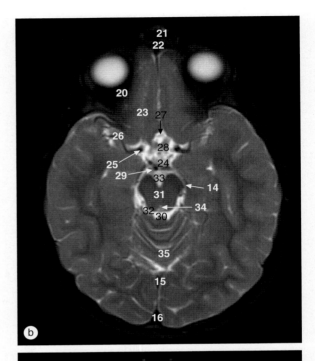

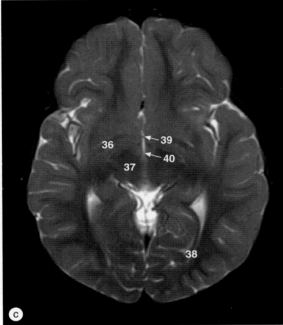

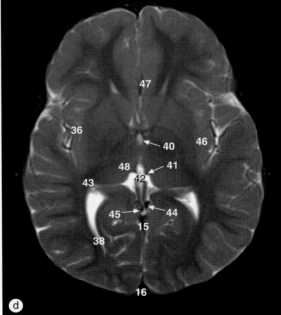

Brain, axial T2-weighted MR images, from inferior to superior.

1. Lens
2. Vitreous humour
3. Lateral rectus muscle
4. Medial rectus muscle
5. Superior cerebellar vermis
6. Optic nerve (second cranial nerve)
7. Infundibulum of frontal sinus
8. Lacrimal gland
9. Pituitary gland
10. Internal carotid artery (supraclinoid part)
11. Uncus of temporal lobe
12. Hippocampus
13. Ambient cistern
14. Posterior cerebral artery
15. Straight sinus
16. Superior sagittal sinus
17. Inferior colliculus
18. Sylvian fissure (lateral sulcus)
19. Temporal horn of lateral ventricle
20. Superior rectus muscle
21. Frontal sinus
22. Crista galli
23. Olfactory nerve (first cranial nerve)
24. Suprasellar cistern
25. Bifurcation of internal carotid artery
26. Middle cerebral artery
27. Anterior communicating artery
28. Optic chiasma
29. Basilar artery bifurcation
30. Quadrigeminal cistern
31. Midbrain (mesencephalon)
32. Superior colliculus
33. Interpeduncular cistern
34. Aqueduct of Sylvius
35. Folia of cerebellum
36. Insular gyri
37. Cerebral peduncle
38. Occipital horn of lateral ventricle
39. Anterior commissure
40. Third ventricle
41. Posterior commissure
42. Pineal gland
43. Trigone of lateral ventricle
44. Basal vein (of Rosenthal)
45. Internal cerebral vein (of Galen)
46. Claustrum
47. Anterior cerebral artery
48. Thalamus

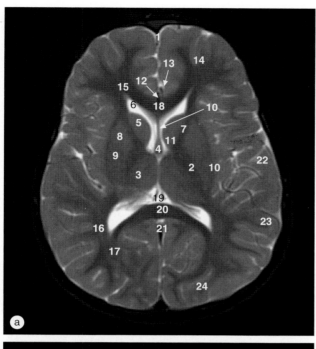

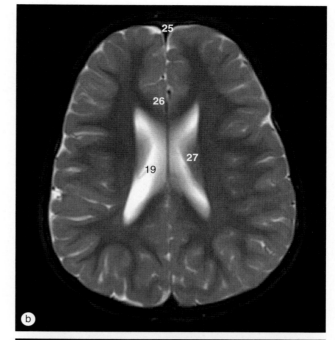

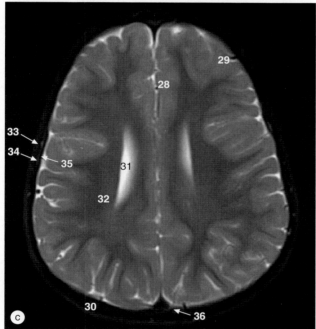

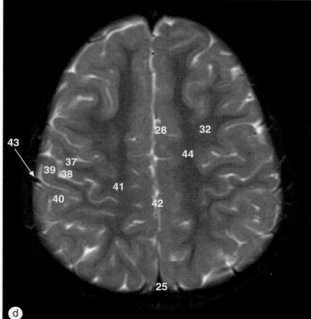

Brain, axial T2-weighted MR images, from inferior to superior.

1. Interhemispheric fissure	16. Optic radiation	31. Body (atrium) of lateral ventricle
2. Posterior limb of internal capsule	17. Forceps major	32. Corona radiata
3. Thalamus	18. Genu of corpus callosum	33. Outer table of calvarium
4. Posterior commissure	19. Choroidal vessels	34. Diploë
5. Head of caudate nucleus	20. Splenium of corpus callosum	35. Inner table of calvarium
6. Frontal horn of lateral ventricle	21. Inferior sagittal sinus	36. Arachnoid granulation
7. Anterior limb of internal capsule	22. Temporal lobe	37. Precentral gyrus
8. Globus pallidus	23. Parietal lobe	38. Central sulcus (of Rolando)
9. Putamen	24. Occipital lobe	39. Postcentral gyrus
10. External capsule	25. Superior sagittal sinus	40. Grey matter
11. Body of caudate nucleus	26. Cingulate gyrus	41. White matter
12. Callosomarginal artery	27. Choroid plexus	42. Falx cerebri
13. Frontopolar artery	28. Anterior cerebral artery	43. Middle cerebral artery (second order
14. Frontal lobe	29. Cortical vein	branch)
15. Forceps minor	30. Calvarium of skull	44. Centrum semiovale

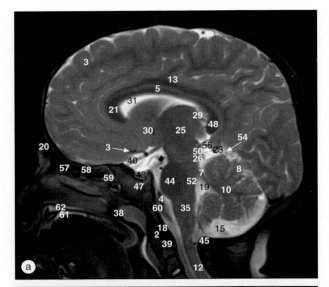

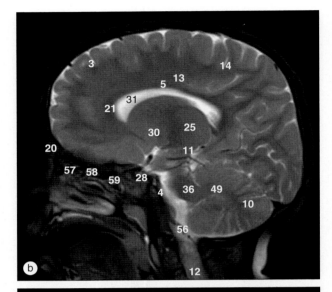

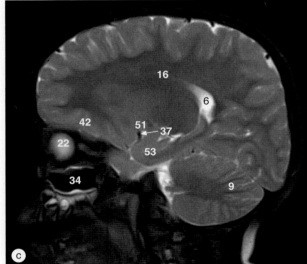

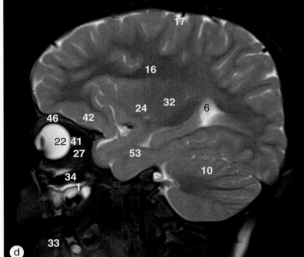

Brain, sagittal T2-weighted MR images.

1. Alveolar ridge
2. Anterior arch of atlas (first cervical vertebra)
3. Anterior cerebral artery
4. Basilar artery
5. Body of corpus callosum
6. Body of lateral ventricle
7. Superior medullary velum
8. Cerebellar folia
9. Cerebellar hemisphere
10. Cerebellum
11. Cerebral peduncle
12. Cervical spinal cord
13. Cingulate gyrus
14. Cingulate sulcus
15. Cisterna magna (cerebellomedullary cistern)
16. Corona radiata
17. Cortical vein
18. Foramen magnum
19. Fourth ventricle
20. Bulbus oculi

21. Genu of corpus callosum
22. Globe
23. Great cerebral vein (of Galen)
24. Head of caudate nucleus
25. Massa intermedia of thalamus
26. Inferior colliculus
27. Inferior rectus muscle
28. Internal carotid artery (in cavernous sinus)
29. Internal cerebral vein
30. Interventricular foramen of Monro
31. Lateral ventricle
32. Lentiform nucleus
33. Mandible
34. Maxillary sinus (antrum)
35. Medulla oblongata
36. Middle cerebellar peduncle
37. Middle cerebral artery
38. Nasopharynx
39. Odontoid process (dens)
40. Optic chiasma in suprasellar cistern
41. Optic nerve

42. Orbital cortex of frontal lobe
43. Pituitary gland
44. Pons
45. Posterior arch of atlas
46. Superior rectus
47. Sphenoccipital synchondrosis
48. Splenium of corpus callosum
49. Superior cerebellar peduncle
50. Superior colliculus
51. Sylvian fissure (lateral sulcus)
52. Tegmentum of pons
53. Temporal lobe
54. Tentorium cerebelli
55. Pineal gland
56. Vertebral artery
57. Anterior ethmoidal air cells
58. Middle ethmoidal air cells
59. Posterior ethmoidal air cells
60. Prepontine cistern
61. Hard palate
62. Incisive canal

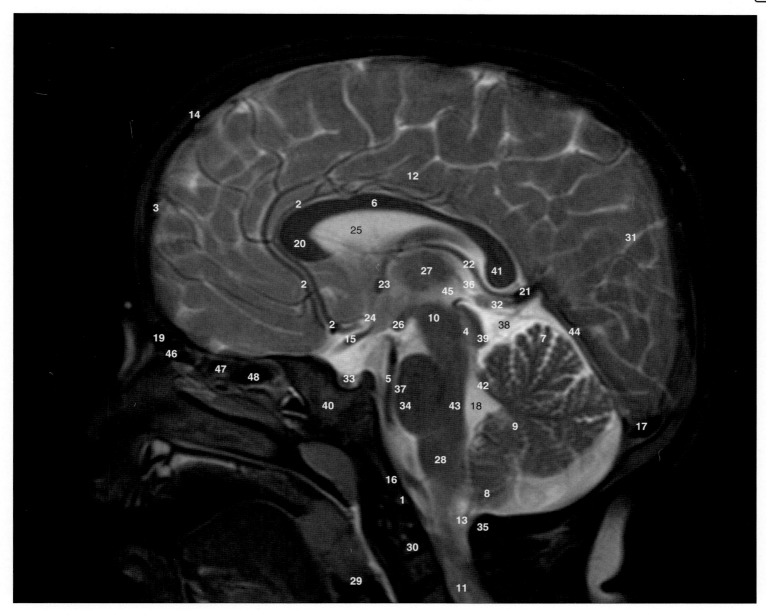

Brain, mid-sagittal T2-weighted MR image.

1. Anterior arch of atlas (first cervical vertebra)
2. Anterior cerebral artery
3. Superior sagittal sinus
4. Aqueduct (of Sylvius)
5. Basilar artery
6. Body of corpus callosum
7. Cerebellar folia
8. Cerebellar tonsil
9. Cerebellum
10. Cerebral peduncle of midbrain
11. Cervical spinal cord
12. Cingulate gyrus
13. Cisterna magna (cerebellomedullary cistern)
14. Diploë of calvarium
15. Optic chiasma

16. Foramen magnum
17. Confluence of venous sinuses (torcular Herophili)
18. Fourth ventricle
19. Frontal sinus
20. Genu of corpus callosum
21. Great cerebral vein (of Galen)
22. Internal cerebral vein
23. Interventricular foramen (of Monro)
24. Lamina terminalis
25. Lateral ventricle
26. Mammillary body
27. Massa intermedia of thalamus
28. Medulla oblongata
29. Nasopharynx
30. Odontoid process (dens)
31. Parieto-occipital fissure

32. Pineal gland
33. Pituitary gland
34. Pons
35. Posterior arch of atlas
36. Posterior commissure
37. Prepontine cistern
38. Quadrigeminal cistern
39. Quadrigeminal plate (tectum) of midbrain
40. Sphenoidal sinus
41. Splenium of corpus callosum
42. Superior medullary velum
43. Tegmentum of pons
44. Tentorium cerebelli
45. Third ventricle
46. Anterior ethmoidal air cells
47. Middle ethmoidal air cells
48. Posterior ethmoidal air cells

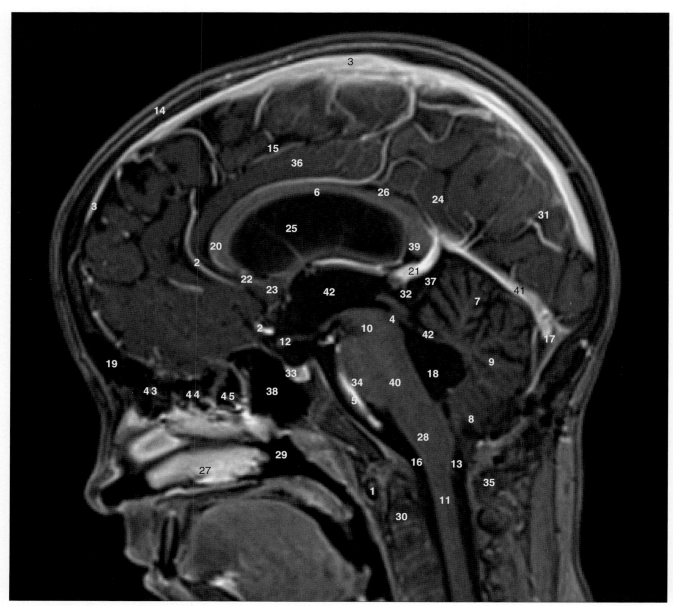

Brain, mid-sagittal T1-weighted MR image, contrast enhanced.

1. Anterior arch of atlas (first cervical vertebra)
2. Anterior cerebral artery
3. Superior sagittal sinus
4. Aqueduct (of Sylvius)
5. Basilar artery
6. Body of corpus callosum
7. Cerebellar folia
8. Cerebellar tonsil
9. Cerebellum
10. Cerebral peduncle of midbrain
11. Cervical spinal cord
12. Optic chiasm
13. Cisterna magna (cerebellomedullary cistern)
14. Diploë of calvarium
15. Cingulate sulcus
16. Foramen magnum
17. Confluence of venous sinuses (torcular Herophili)
18. Fourth ventricle
19. Frontal sinus
20. Genu of corpus callosum
21. Great cerebral vein (of Galen)
22. Rostrum of corpus callosum
23. Anterior commissure
24. Subparietal sulcus
25. Lateral ventricle
26. Pericallosal cistern
27. Inferior nasal concha
28. Medulla oblongata
29. Nasopharynx
30. Odontoid process (dens)
31. Parieto-occipital fissure
32. Pineal gland
33. Pituitary gland
34. Pons
35. Posterior arch of atlas
36. Cingulate gyrus
37. Quadrigeminal cistern
38. Sphenoidal sinus
39. Splenium of corpus callosum
40. Tegmentum of pons
41. Tentorium cerebelli
42. Third ventricle
43. Anterior ethmoidal air cells
44. Middle ethmoidal air cells
45. Posterior ethmoidal air cells

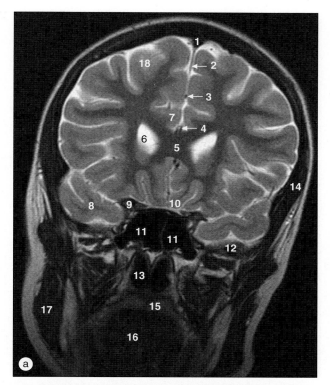

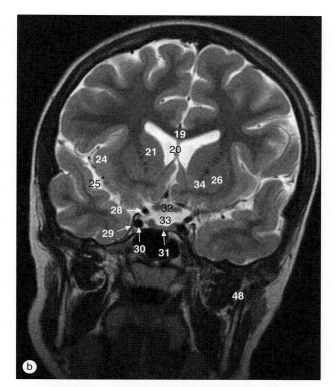

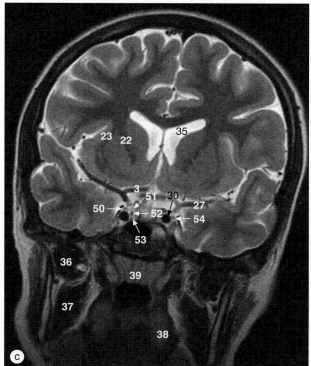

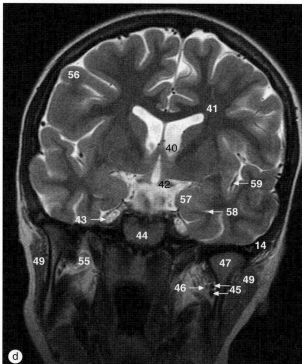

(a)–(p) Brain, coronal T2-weighted MR images, from anterior to posterior.

1. Superior sagittal sinus	**12.** Greater wing of sphenoid	**23.** External capsule
2. Falx cerebri	**13.** Nasopharynx	**24.** Insular gyrus
3. Anterior cerebral artery	**14.** Temporalis muscle	**25.** Sylvian fissure (lateral sulcus)
4. Callosomarginal artery	**15.** Hard palate	**26.** Putamen
5. Genu of corpus callosum	**16.** Oropharynx	**27.** Middle cerebral artery
6. Frontal horn of lateral ventricle	**17.** Masseter muscle	**28.** Supraclinoid part of internal carotid
7. Cingulate gyrus	**18.** Frontal lobe	artery
8. Temporal lobe	**19.** Body of corpus callosum	**29.** Dural lateral wall of cavernous sinus
9. Anterior clinoid process	**20.** Septum pellucidum	**30.** Internal carotid artery
10. Olfactory cortex	**21.** Head of caudate nucleus	**31.** Pituitary gland
11. Sphenoidal sinus	**22.** Anterior limb of internal capsule	**32.** Optic chiasma

Numbers 1–130 are common to pages 13–16.

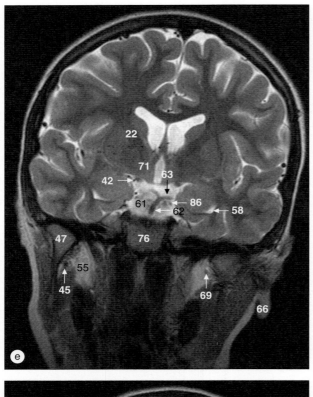

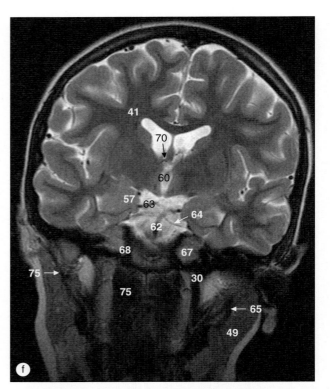

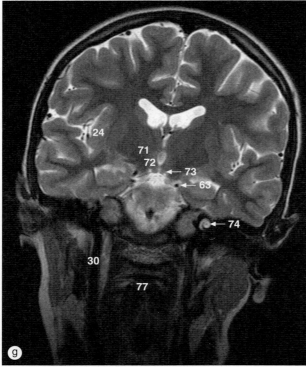

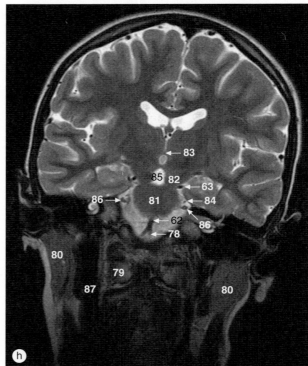

(a)–(p) Brain, coronal T2-weighted MR images, from anterior to posterior.

33. Suprasellar cistern
34. Globus pallidus
35. Body (atrium) of lateral ventricle
36. Lateral pterygoid muscle
37. Medial pterygoid muscle
38. Tongue
39. Soft palate
40. Choroid plexus
41. Corona radiata
42. Optic tract
43. Trigeminal ganglion in Meckel's cave

44. Body of sphenoid
45. Inferior alveolar vessels
46. Inferior alveolar nerve
47. Head of mandible
48. Coronoid process of mandible
49. Parotid gland
50. Oculomotor nerve (third cranial nerve)
51. Trochlear nerve (fourth cranial nerve)
52. Ophthalmic nerve (fifth cranial nerve, first division)

53. Maxillary nerve (fifth cranial nerve, second division)
54. Abducens nerve (sixth cranial nerve)
55. Infratemporal fossa
56. Parietal lobe
57. Hippocampus
58. Temporal horn of lateral ventricle
59. Middle cerebral artery (second order branch)
60. Third ventricle

Numbers 1–130 are common to pages 13–16.

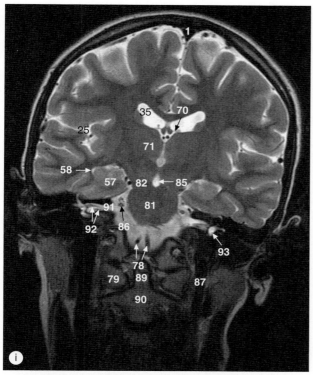

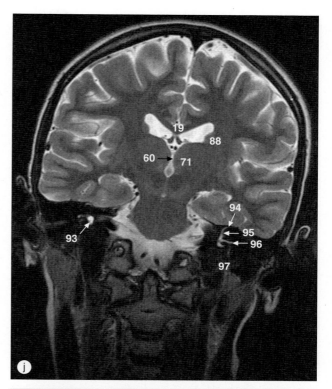

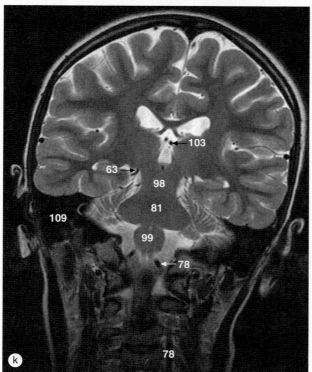

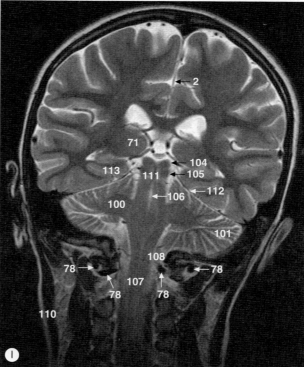

(a)–(p) Brain, coronal T2-weighted MR images, from anterior to posterior.

61. Prepontine cistern	**71.** Thalamus	**81.** Pons
62. Basilar artery	**72.** Hypothalamus	**82.** Cerebral peduncle
63. Posterior cerebral artery	**73.** Mammillary body (of hypothalamus)	**83.** Massa intermedia of thalamus
64. Superior cerebellar artery	**74.** Cochlea	**84.** Abducens nerve (sixth cranial nerve) in ambient cistern
65. Retromandibular vein	**75.** Pharyngobasilar raphe	**85.** Interpeduncular cistern
66. Tragus of external ear	**76.** Basisphenoid	**86.** Trigeminal nerve (fifth cranial nerve)
67. Basiocciput	**77.** Anterior arch of C1	**87.** Internal jugular vein
68. Spheno-occipital synchondrosis	**78.** Vertebral artery	**88.** Body of caudate nucleus
69. Auriculotemporal nerve	**79.** Lateral mass of C1	
70. Foramen of Monro	**80.** Sternocleidomastoid muscle	

89. Odontoid peg of C2	
90. Body of C2	
91. Internal auditory meatus	
92. Facial (seventh) and vestibulocochlear (eighth) nerves	
93. Vestibule of vestibular apparatus	
94. Arcuate eminence of petrous temporal bone	
95. Superior semicircular canal	

Numbers 1–130 are common to pages 13–16.

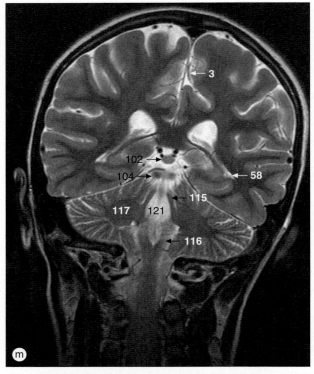

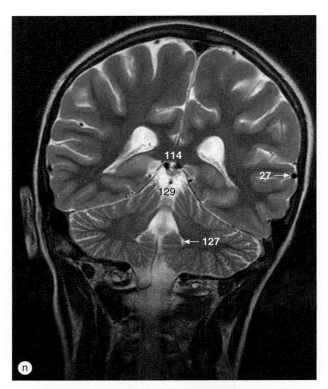

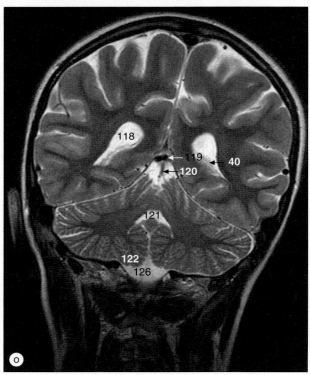

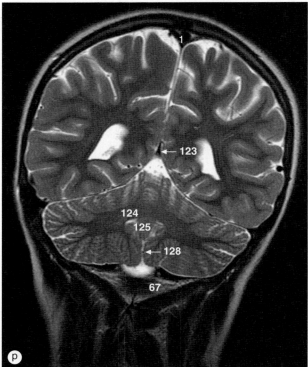

(a)–(p) Brain, coronal T2-weighted MR images, from anterior to posterior.

96. Horizontal (lateral) semicircular canal	**106.** Aqueduct (of Sylvius)	**115.** Superior cerebellar peduncle	**123.** Inferior sagittal sinus
97. Posterior semicircular canal	**107.** Spinal cord	**116.** Inferior cerebellar peduncle	**124.** Dentate nucleus of cerebellum
98. Midbrain (mesencephalon)	**108.** Foramen magnum		**125.** Nodule of cerebellum
99. Medulla oblongata	**109.** Mastoid air cells	**117.** Cerebellar hemisphere	**126.** Cisterna magna
100. Middle cerebellar peduncle	**110.** Trapezius muscle	**118.** Trigone of lateral ventricle	**127.** Lateral foramen (of Luschka)
101. Cerebellar folia	**111.** Tectum (quadrigeminal plate) of midbrain	**119.** Great cerebral vein (of Galen)	**128.** Medial foramen (of Magendie)
102. Pineal gland	**112.** Tentorium cerebelli	**120.** Basal vein (of Rosenthal)	
103. Internal cerebral veins	**113.** Uncus of temporal lobe	**121.** Fourth ventricle	**129.** Quadrigeminal cistern
104. Superior colliculus	**114.** Splenium of corpus callosum	**122.** Cerebellar tonsil	
105. Inferior colliculus			

Numbers 1–130 are common to pages 13–16.

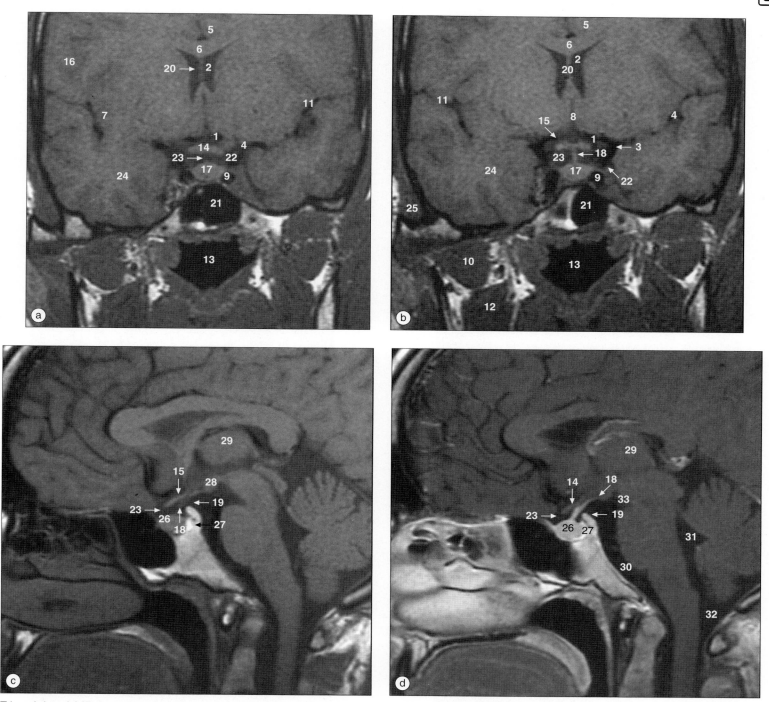

T1-weighted MR images of pituitary fossa (a) and (b) coronal, (c) sagittal, (d) sagittal post gadolinium.

1. Anterior cerebral artery
2. Anterior horn of lateral ventricle
3. Bifurcation of internal carotid artery
4. Branch of middle cerebral artery in lateral sulcus (Sylvian fissure)
5. Cingulate gyrus
6. Corpus callosum
7. Insula
8. Interhemispheric fissure
9. Internal carotid artery in cavernous sinus
10. Lateral pterygoid muscle
11. Lateral sulcus (Sylvian fissure)
12. Medial pterygoid muscle
13. Nasopharynx
14. Optic chiasma
15. Optic tract
16. Parietal lobe of brain
17. Pituitary gland
18. Pituitary stalk
19. Posterior clinoid process
20. Septum pellucidum
21. Sphenoidal sinus
22. Supraclinoid carotid artery
23. Suprasellar cistern
24. Temporal lobe
25. Temporalis muscle
26. Anterior pituitary gland
27. Posterior pituitary gland
28. Mammillary body
29. Thalamus
30. Prepontine cistern
31. Fourth ventricle
32. Cisterna magna
33. Interpeduncular cistern

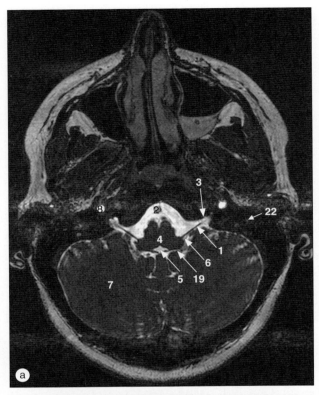

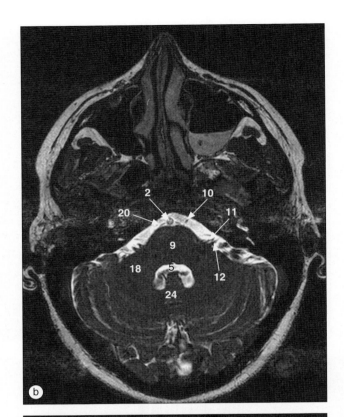

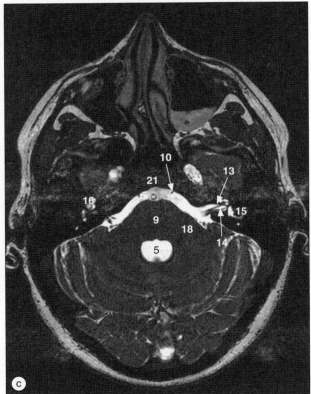

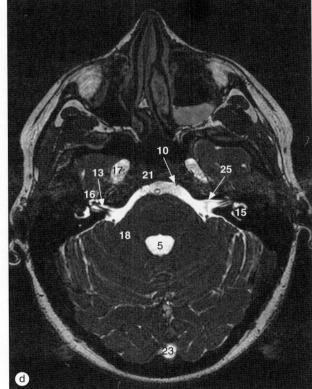

(a)–(h) Axial MR images, from inferior to superior.

1. Glossopharyngeal nerve (CN9)	**5.** Fourth ventricle	**9.** Pons
2. Basilar artery	**6.** Vagus nerve (CN10)	**10.** Abducens nerve (CN6)
3. Jugular foramen	**7.** Cerebellar hemisphere	**11.** Facial nerve (CN7)
4. Medulla	**8.** Internal carotid artery	**12.** Vestibulocochlear nerve (CN8)

Numbers 1–47 are common to pages 18–21.

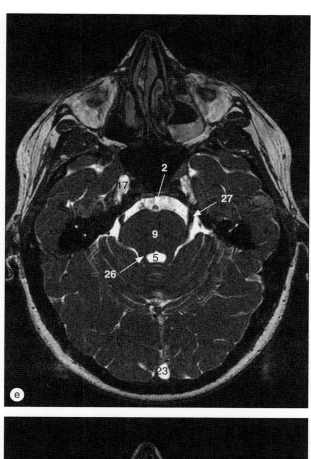

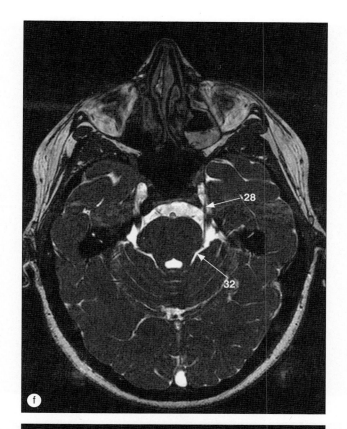

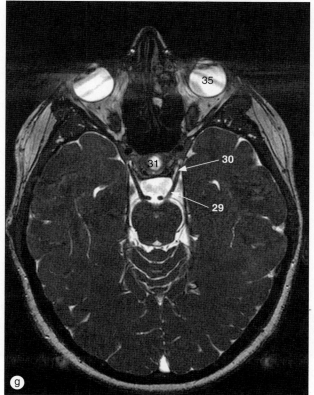

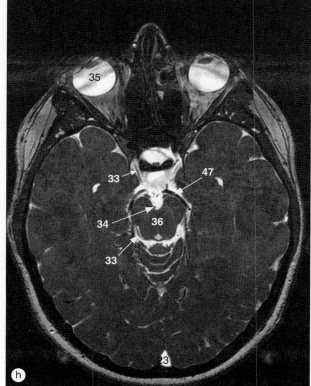

(a)–(h) Axial MR images, from inferior to superior.

Numbers 1–47 are common to pages 18–21.

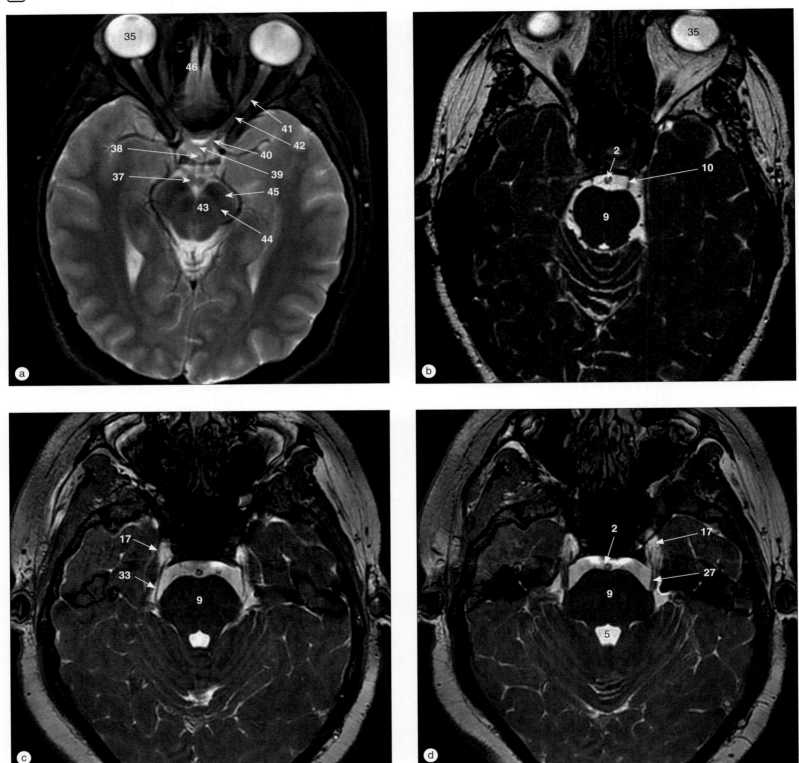

Cranial nerves, MR images of (**a**) olfactory and optic nerves, (**b**) oculomotor nerve, (**c**) trochlear nerve, (**d**) trigeminal nerve, (**e**) and (**f**) abducens, facial and auditory nerves, (**g&h**) glossopharyngeal and vagus nerves.

25. Internal auditory canal	**28.** CN5 enters Meckel's cave	**32.** Ambient cistern
26. Superior cerebellar peduncle	**29.** Oculomotor nerve (CN3)	**33.** Trochlear nerve (CN4)
27. Preganglionic segment of CN5 (trigeminal)	**30.** CN3 in oculomotor cistern	**34.** Interpeduncular cistern
	31. Pituitary	**35.** Globe of eye

Numbers 1–47 are common to pages 18–21.

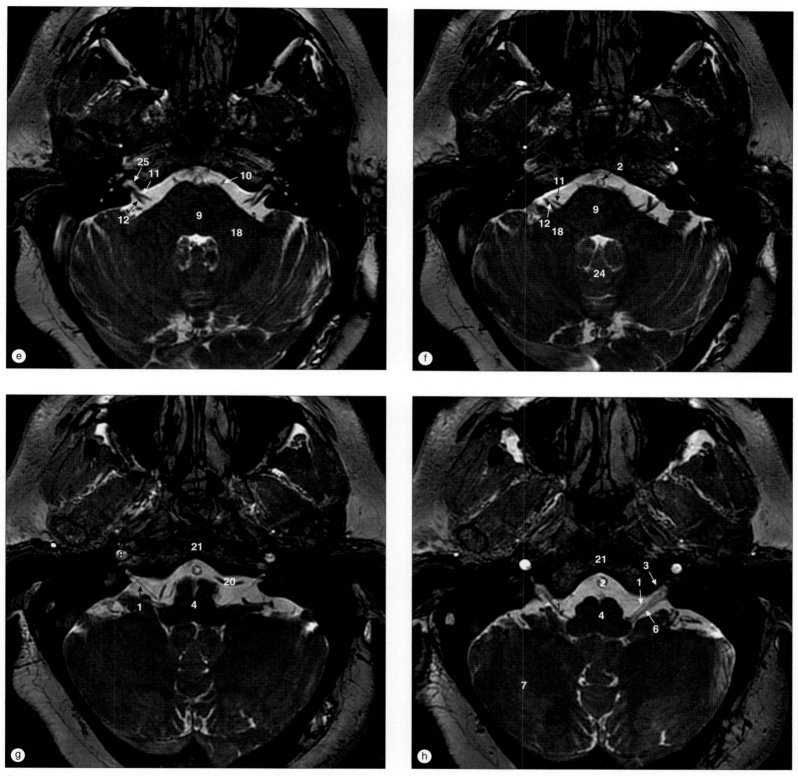

Cranial nerves, MR images of (a) olfactory and optic nerves, (b) oculomotor nerve, (c) trochlear nerve, (d) trigeminal nerve, (e) and (f) abducens, facial and auditory nerves, (g&h) glossopharyngeal and vagus nerves.

36. Midbrain	40. Optic nerve, intracranial portion	44. Substantia nigra
37. Mammillary body	41. Optic nerve, intraocular segment	45. Cerebral peduncle
38. Infundibulum	42. Optic nerve, intracanalicular segment	46. Olfactory tract and bulb (CN1)
39. Optic chiasm	43. Red nucleus of midbrain	47. Posterior cerebral artery

Numbers 1–47 are common to pages 18–21.

Bonus e-materials

Cross-sectional image stack slideshows: Axial CT of the head (unenhanced)

Multi-tier labelling in slideshow/test yourself: Midline sagittal T1-weighted MRI of the brain with intravascular contrast medium

Selected pages from Imaging Atlas 4e

Tutorials: Tutorials 2c, 2d, 2e, 2f

Single best answer (SBA) self-assessment questions

Table of variations

Variant	Frequency	Clinical implications
Chiari I malformation	<0.1%	Severe headaches.
Cerebellar hypoplasia	<0.01%	Developmental delay, hypotonia, ataxia, seizures.
Hydrocephalus	<0.05%	Headaches, vomiting, nausea, papilledema, sleepiness or coma.

2 Skull, orbits, paranasal sinuses and face

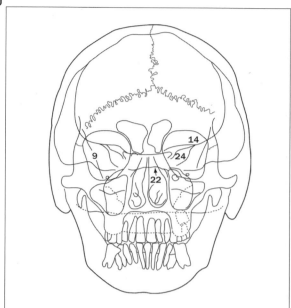

(a) Skull, occipitofrontal radiograph.
(b) Skull, occipitofrontal radiograph demonstrating the foramina rotunda.

1. Basi-occiput
2. Body of sphenoid
3. Crista galli
4. Ethmoidal air cells
5. Floor of maxillary sinus (antrum)
6. Floor of pituitary fossa
7. Foramen rotundum
8. Frontal sinus
9. Greater wing of sphenoid
10. Inferior turbinate
11. Internal acoustic meatus
12. Lambdoid suture
13. Lateral mass of atlas (first cervical vertebra)
14. Lesser wing of sphenoid
15. Mastoid process
16. Middle turbinate
17. Nasal septum
18. Odontoid process (dens) of axis (second cervical vertebra)
19. Petrous part of temporal bone
20. Ramus of mandible
21. Sagittal suture
22. Planum sphenoidale
23. Sphenoid air sinus
24. Superior orbital fissure
25. Temporal surface of greater wing of sphenoid

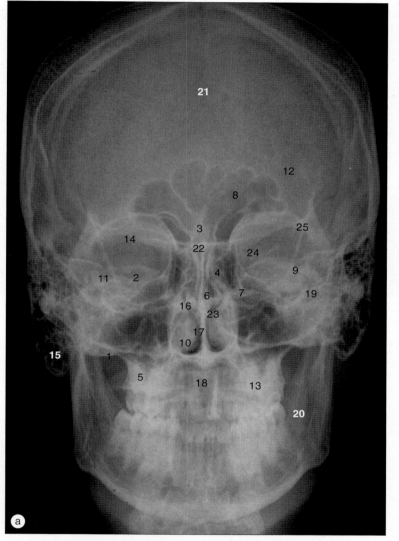

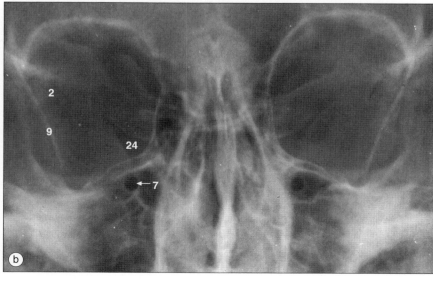

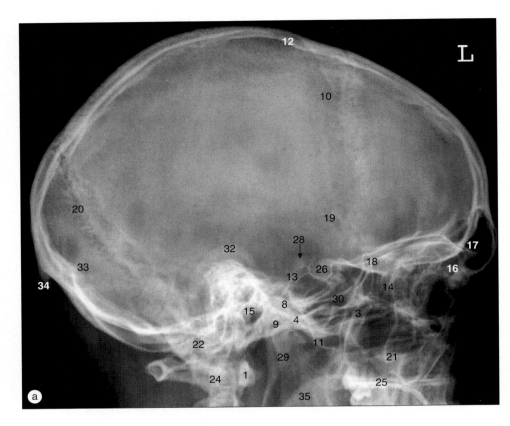

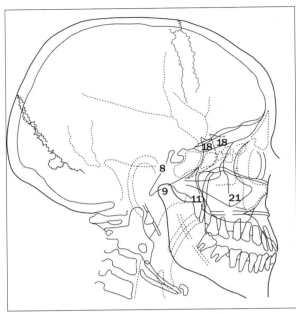

(a) Skull, lateral radiograph.

Pituitary fossa (sella turcica) lateral radiographs, (b) of a 7-year-old child, (c) of a 23-year-old woman.

1. Anterior arch of atlas (first cervical vertebra)
2. Anterior clinoid process
3. Arch of zygoma
4. Articular tubercle for temporomandibular joint
5. Basilar part of occipital bone
6. Basisphenoid/basi-occiput synchondrosis
7. Carotid sulcus
8. Clivus
9. Condyle of mandible
10. Coronal suture
11. Coronoid process of mandible
12. Diploë
13. Dorsum sellae
14. Ethmoidal air cells
15. External acoustic meatus
16. Frontal process of zygoma
17. Frontal sinus
18. Greater wing of sphenoid
19. Grooves for middle meningeal vessels
20. Lambdoid suture
21. Malar process of maxilla
22. Mastoid air cells
23. Middle clinoid process
24. Odontoid process (dens) of axis (second cervical vertebra)
25. Palatine process of maxilla
26. Pituitary fossa (sella turcica)
27. Planum sphenoidale
28. Posterior clinoid process
29. Ramus of mandible
30. Sphenoidal sinus
31. Tuberculum sellae
32. Pinna of ear
33. Inion
34. External occipital protuberance
35. Soft palate

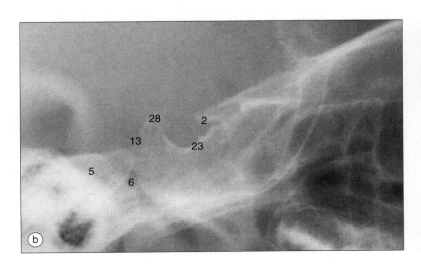

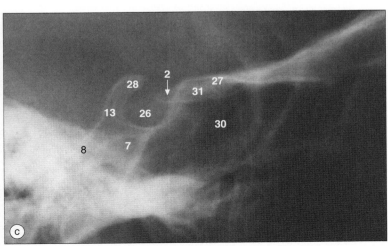

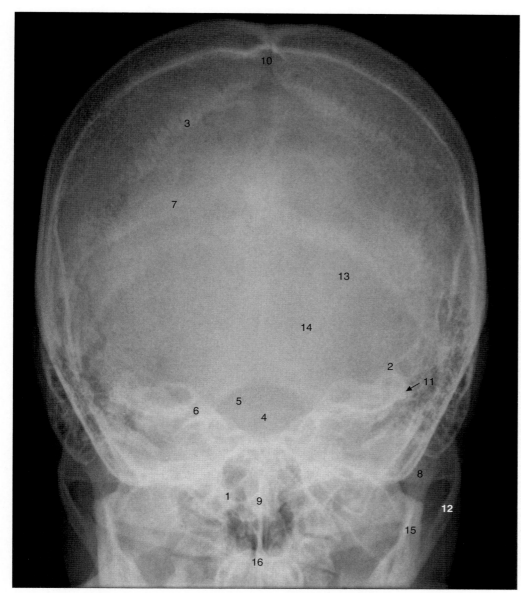

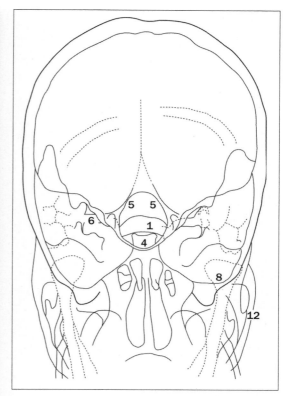

Skull, 30° fronto-occipital (Townes') radiograph. Note the arch of C1 is below the foramen magnum on the radiograph.

1. Arch of atlas (first cervical vertebra)
2. Arcuate eminence of temporal bone
3. Coronal suture
4. Dorsum sellae
5. Foramen magnum
6. Internal acoustic meatus
7. Lambdoid suture
8. Mandibular condyle
9. Odontoid process (dens) of axis (second cervical vertebra)
10. Sagittal suture
11. Superior semicircular canal
12. Zygomatic arch
13. Groove for transverse sinus
14. Squamous occipital bone
15. Mandible
16. Nasal septum

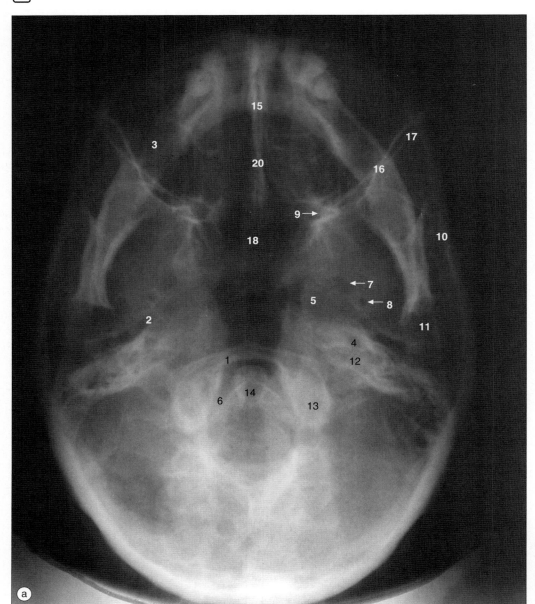

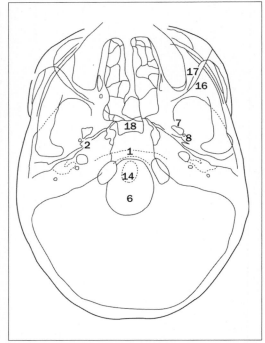

(a) Skull, submentovertical radiograph.
(b) Skull, submentovertical radiograph,
with additional angulation for zygomatic
arches.

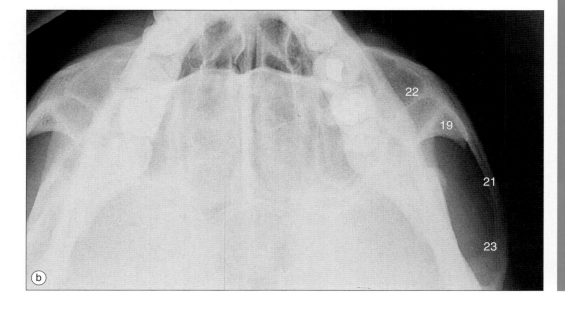

1. Anterior arch of atlas (first cervical
   vertebra)
2. Auditory (Eustachian) tube
3. Body of mandible
4. Carotid canal
5. Foramen lacerum
6. Foramen magnum
7. Foramen ovale
8. Foramen spinosum
9. Greater palatine foramen
10. Greater wing of sphenoid
11. Head of mandible
12. Jugular foramen
13. Occipital condyle
14. Odontoid process (dens) of axis
    (second cervical vertebra)
15. Perpendicular plate of ethmoid
16. Posterior margin of orbit
17. Posterior wall of maxillary sinus
    (antrum)
18. Sphenoidal sinus
19. Temporal process of zygomatic bone
20. Vomer
21. Zygomatic arch
22. Zygomatic bone
23. Zygomatic process of temporal bone

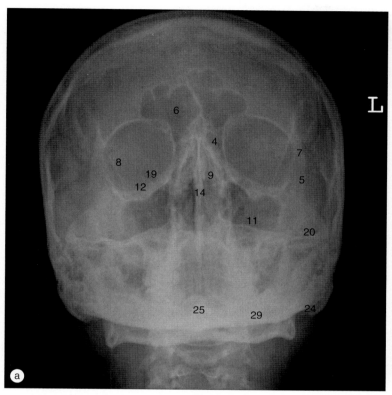

(a) Modified occipitofrontal radiograph.

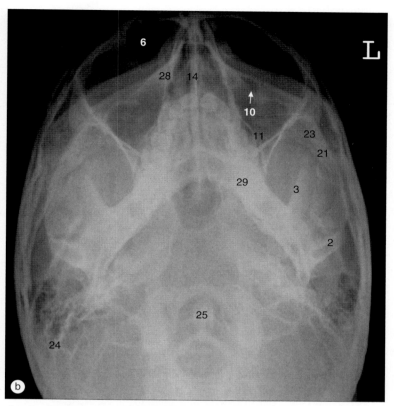

(b) Occipitomental radiograph.

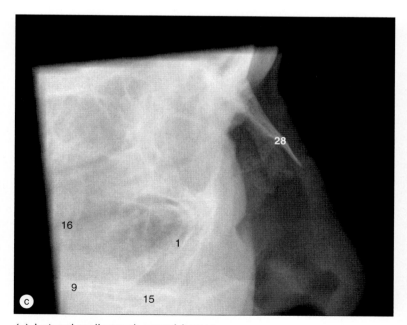

(c) Lateral radiograph nasal bones.

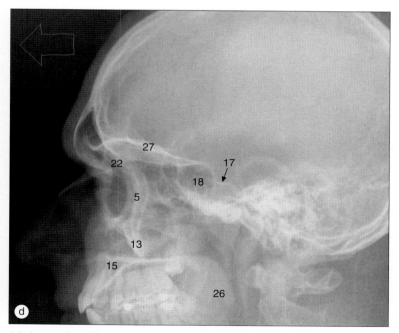

(d) Lateral radiograph sinuses.

1. Anterior wall of maxillary sinus (antrum)
2. Condyle of mandible
3. Coronoid process of mandible
4. Ethmoidal sinuses
5. Frontal process of zygomatic bone
6. Frontal sinuses
7. Frontozygomatic suture
8. Greater wing of sphenoid
9. Horizontal plate of palatine bone
10. Infra-orbital foramen

11. Left maxillary sinus (antrum)
12. Lesser wing of sphenoid
13. Malar process of maxilla
14. Nasal septum
15. Palatine process of maxilla
16. Posterior wall of maxillary sinus (antrum)
17. Sella turcica
18. Sphenoidal sinus
19. Superior orbital fissure
20. Temporal process of zygomatic bone

21. Zygomatic arch
22. Zygomatic process of frontal bone
23. Zygomatic process of temporal bone
24. Mastoid process
25. Odontoid peg
26. Soft palate
27. Floor of anterior cranial fossa
28. Nasal bones
29. Mandible

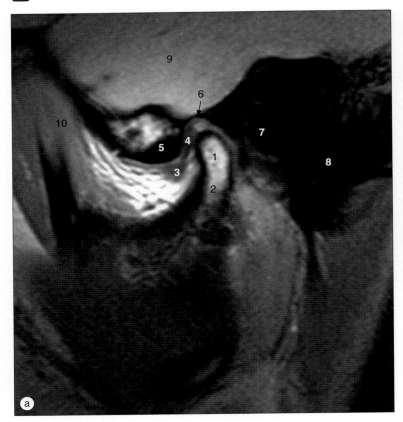

(a) Mouth closed.

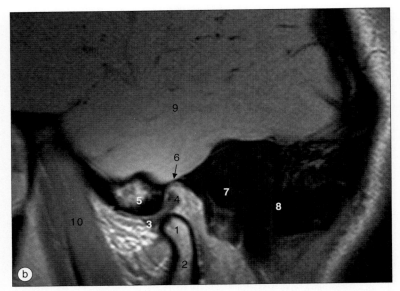

(b) Mouth open, mandibular condyle protracted onto articular eminence.

Temporomandibular joint, sagittal T1w MR images with the subject's face on the left.

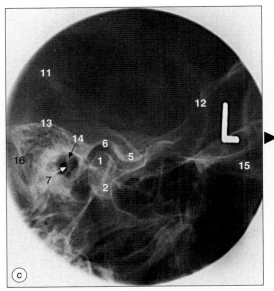

(c) Mouth open.

1. Condylar head
2. Condylar neck
3. Anterior band of disc
4. Posterior band of disc
5. Articular eminence
6. Mandibular fossa
7. External auditory canal
8. Mastoid process of temporal bone
9. Temporal lobe of brain
10. Temporalis muscle
11. Pinna of ear
12. Greater wing of sphenoid
13. Tegmen tympani
14. Malleus
15. Zygomatic process of temporal bone
16. Sinus plate

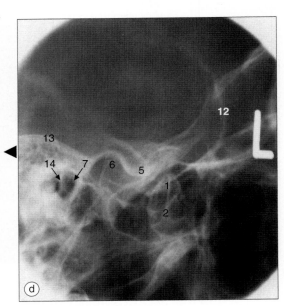

(d) Mouth closed.

Lateral radiographs of the temporomandibular joint with the subject's face on the right.

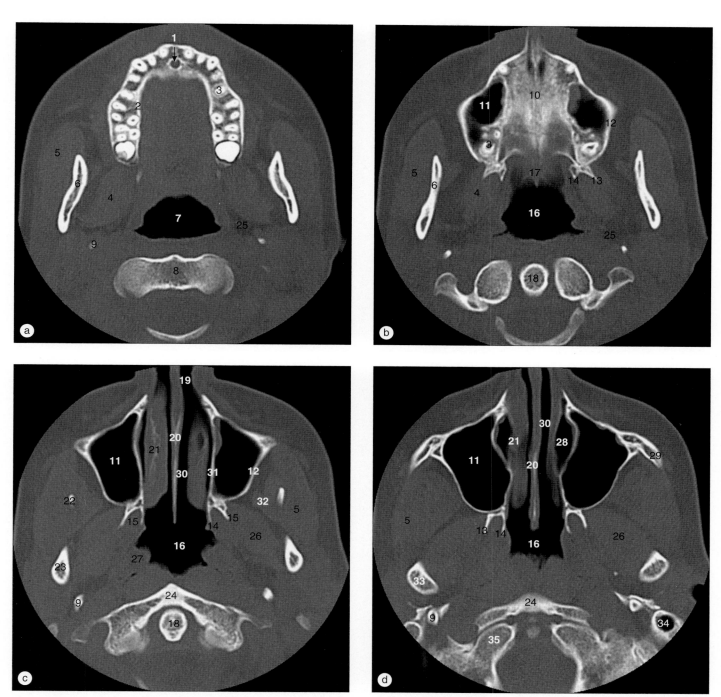

Facial bones and paranasal sinuses, axial CT images demonstrated at the following levels: (**a**) alveolar process of the maxilla, (**b**) hard palate, (**c**) nares, (**d**) maxillary sinus, (**e**) middle turbinate, (**f**) zygomatic arch, (**g**) sphenoid sinus, (**h**) ethmoid sinus.

1. Incisive canal
2. Alveolar rim
3. Alveolar recess
4. Medial pterygoid muscle
5. Masseter muscle
6. Ramus of mandible
7. Oropharynx
8. Body of C2
9. Styloid process
10. Hard palate
11. Maxillary sinus (antrum)
12. Lateral wall of maxillary sinus (antrum)
13. Lateral pterygoid plate

14. Medial pterygoid plate
15. Pterygoid fossa
16. Nasopharynx
17. Vomer
18. Odontoid process (dens)
19. Nares
20. Nasal septum
21. Inferior turbinate
22. Coronoid process of mandible
23. Condylar neck of mandible
24. Anterior arch of C1 (atlas)
25. Parapharyngeal space
26. Lateral pterygoid muscle

27. Torus tubarius
28. Inferior meatus (at location of nasolacrimal opening)
29. Zygoma
30. Nasal cavity
31. Medial wall of maxillary sinus (antrum)
32. Temporalis muscle
33. Condylar head of mandible
34. Mastoid air cells
35. Occipital condyle
36. Middle turbinate
37. Middle meatus

Numbers 1–70 are common to pages 29–30.

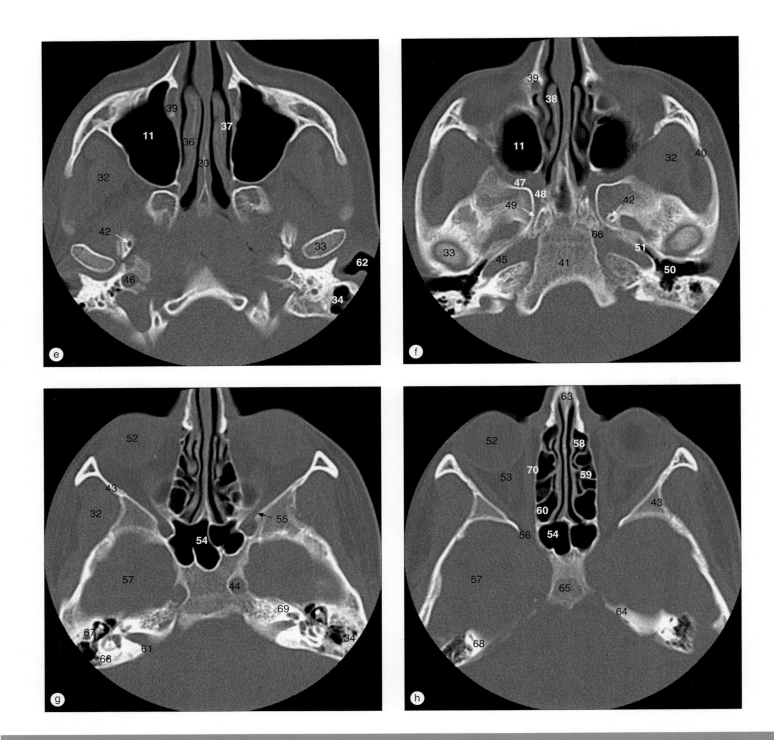

Numbers 1–70 are common to pages 29–30.

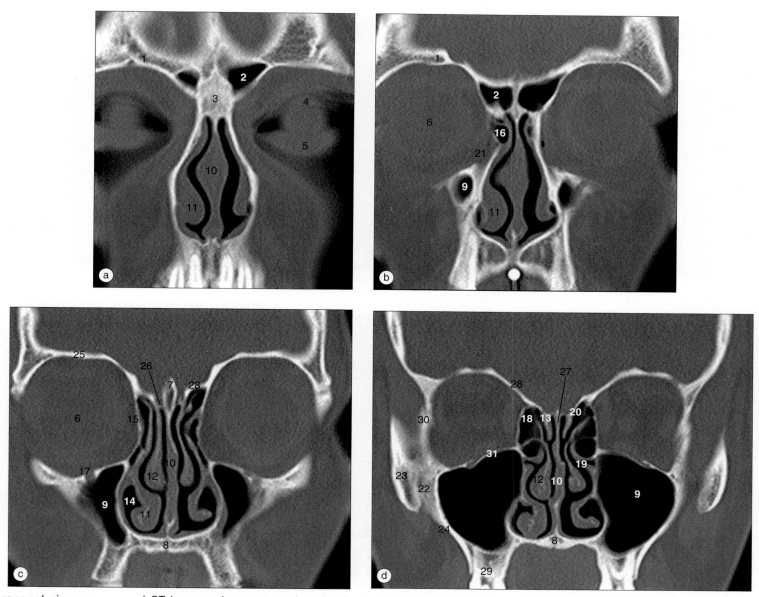

Paranasal sinuses, coronal CT images demonstrated at the following levels: (a) frontal sinuses, (b) nasolacrimal duct, (c) cribriform plate, (d) anterior ethmoids, (e) middle ethmoids, (f) pterygopalatine fossa, (g) sphenoid sinus, (h) nasopharynx.

1. Frontal bone	11. Inferior turbinate (concha)
2. Frontal sinus (antrum)	12. Middle turbinate (concha)
3. Nasal bone	13. Superior turbinate (concha)
4. Upper eyelid	14. Inferior meatus
5. Lower eyelid	15. Lamina papyracea
6. Globe of eye	16. Air in nasolacrimal sac
7. Crista galli	17. Inferior orbital canal
8. Hard palate	18. Anterior ethmoidal air cells
9. Maxillary sinus (antrum)	19. Middle meatus
10. Nasal septum	20. Superior meatus

Numbers 1–52 are common to pages 31–32.

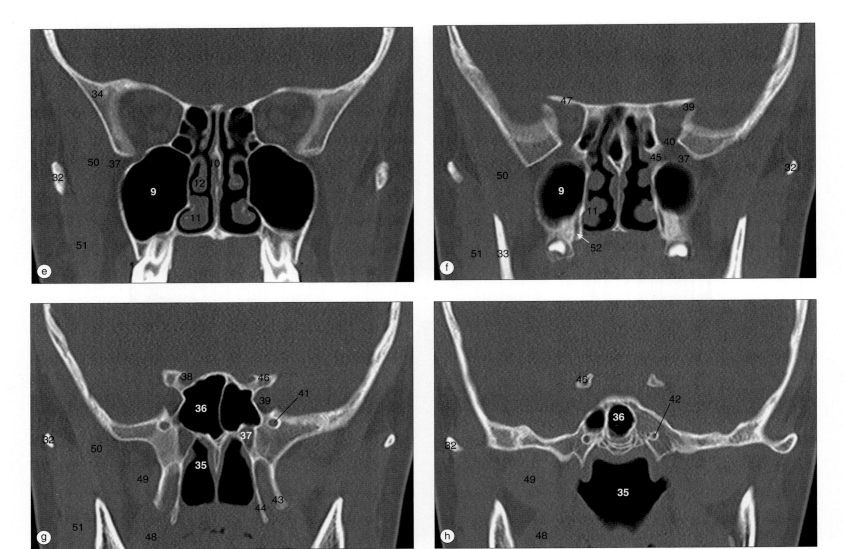

Paranasal sinuses, coronal CT images demonstrated at the following levels: (a) frontal sinuses, (b) nasolacrimal duct, (c) cribriform plate, (d) anterior ethmoids, (e) middle ethmoids, (f) pterygopalatine fossa, (g) sphenoid sinus, (h) nasopharynx.

21. Nasolacrimal duct	32. Zygomatic arch	43. Lateral pterygoid plate
22. Maxilla	33. Ramus of mandible	44. Medial pterygoid plate
23. Zygoma	34. Greater wing of sphenoid	45. Sphenopalatine foramen
24. Lateral wall of maxillary sinus	35. Nasopharynx	46. Anterior clinoid process
25. Orbital roof, frontal bone	36. Sphenoid sinus (antrum)	47. Lesser wing of sphenoid
26. Cribriform plate, ethmoid bone	37. Pterygopalatine fossa	48. Medial pterygoid muscle
27. Perpendicular plate, ethmoid bone	38. Optic canal	49. Lateral pterygoid muscle
28. Fovea ethmoidalis, frontal bone	39. Superior orbital fissure	50. Temporalis muscle
29. Upper alveolar ridge of maxilla	40. Inferior orbital fissure	51. Masseter muscle
30. Lateral orbital wall, zygomatic bone	41. Foramen rotundum	52. Greater palatine foramen
31. Orbital floor, maxillary bone	42. Vidian canal	

Numbers 1–52 are common to pages 31–32.

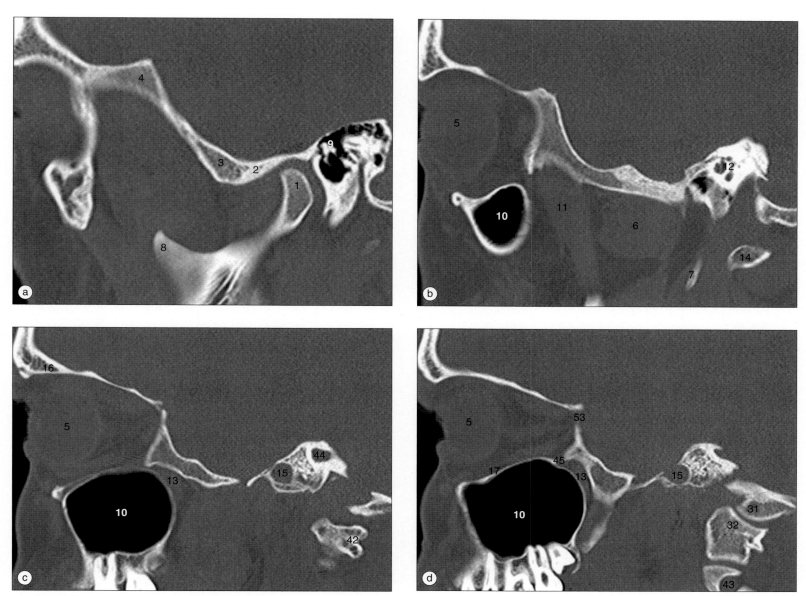

(a)–(h) Paranasal sinuses, sagittal CT images, from lateral to midline.

1. Condyle of mandible	**15.** Internal carotid artery (intrapetrous horizontal part)
2. Articular eminence	**16.** Frontal bone, orbital roof
3. Zygomatic arch	**17.** Maxillary bone, orbital floor
4. Zygoma	**18.** Hard palate
5. Globe of eye	**19.** Soft palate
6. Lateral pterygoid muscle	**20.** Tongue
7. Styloid process	**21.** Oropharynx
8. Coronoid process of mandible	**22.** Nasopharynx
9. Middle ear	**23.** Sphenoid sinus (antrum)
10. Maxillary sinus (antrum)	**24.** Frontal sinus (antrum)
11. Masseter muscle	**25.** Posterior ethmoidal air cells
12. Inner ear	**26.** Anterior ethmoidal air cells
13. Pterygopalatine fossa	**27.** Greater palatine foramen
14. Transverse process of C1	**28.** Inferior turbinate (concha)

Numbers 1–53 are common to pages 33–34.

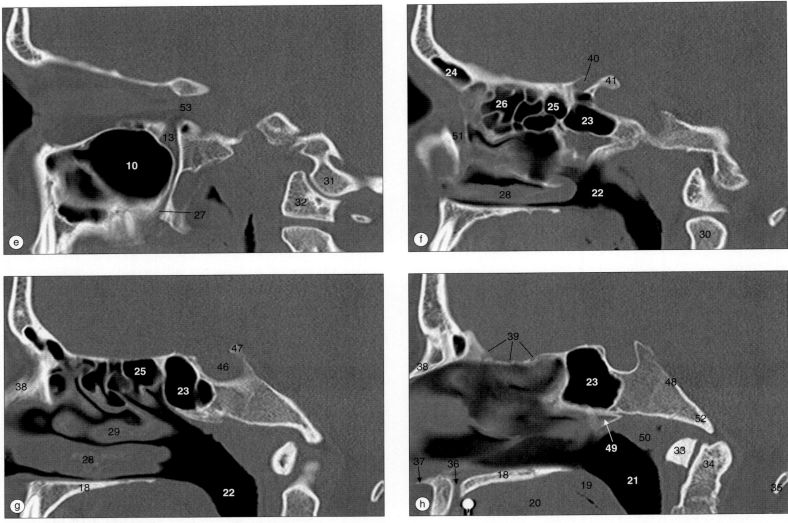

(a)–(h) Paranasal sinuses, sagittal CT images, from lateral to midline.

29. Middle turbinate (concha)
30. Base of C2
31. Occipital condyle
32. Lateral mass of C1
33. Anterior arch of C1
34. Dens (odontoid process)
35. Posterior arch of C1
36. Incisive foramen (contains nasopalatine nerve – V2 sensory branch)
37. Anterior nasal spine of maxilla
38. Nasal bone
39. Cribriform plate
40. Optic canal

41. Anterior clinoid
42. Tubercles of transverse process of C1
43. Transverse foramen of C2
44. Internal auditory canal
45. Inferior orbital fissure
46. Pituitary fossa
47. Dorsum sellae
48. Clivus
49. Vomer
50. Pharyngeal tonsil
51. Nasolacrimal duct
52. Basion
53. Superior orbital fissure

Numbers 1–53 are common to pages 33–34.

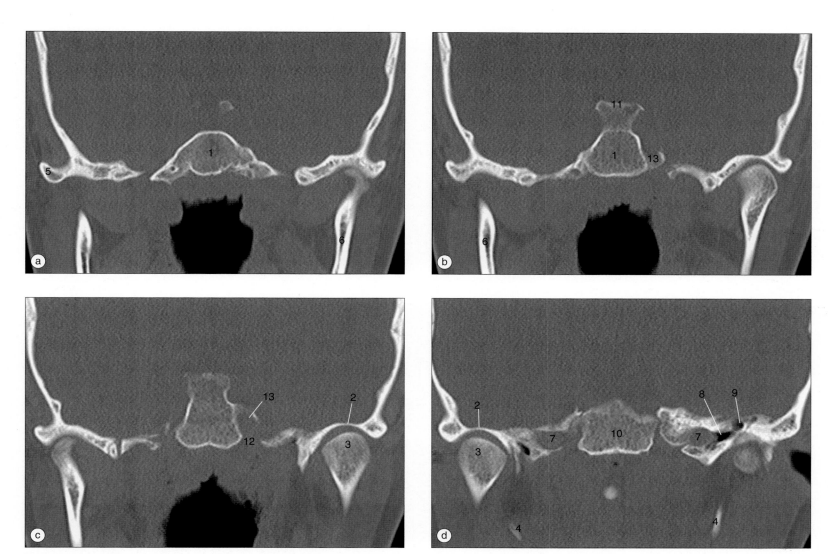

(a)–(h) Coronal CT images, from anterior to posterior.

1. Sphenoid body
2. Condylar fossa of temporomandibular joint
3. Mandibular condyle head
4. Styloid process
5. Zygomatic arch
6. Mandibular ramus
7. Internal carotid artery (intrapetrous horizontal part)
8. Hypotympanum
9. Epitympanum
10. Basi-occiput (lower clivus)
11. Dorsum sellae
12. Foramen lacerum
13. Internal carotid artery (within foramen lacerum)
14. Anterior arch of C1
15. Dens of C2 (odontoid process)
16. Body of C2

Numbers 1–31 are common to pages 35–36.

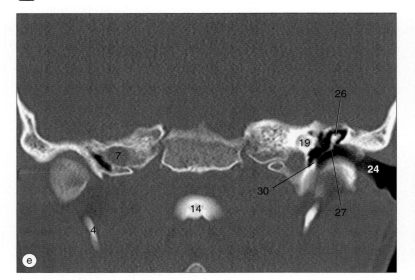

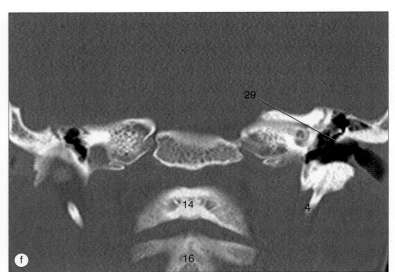

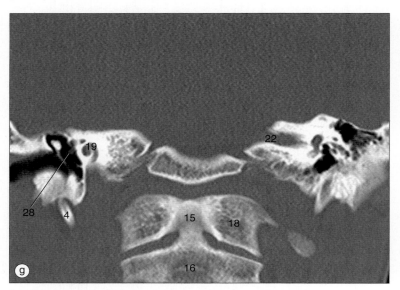

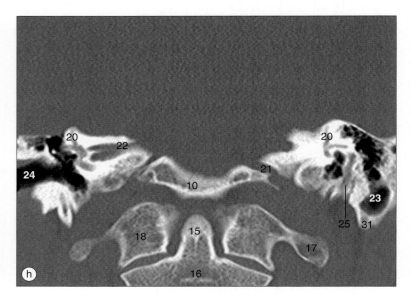

(a)–(h) Coronal CT images, from anterior to posterior.

17. Transverse process of C1	25. Stylomastoid foramen (location of mastoid segment of CN7)
18. Lateral mass of C1	26. Incus
19. Cochlea	27. Malleus
20. Semicircular canal	28. Tendon of tensor tympani muscle
21. Jugular foramen	29. Scutum
22. Internal acoustic canal	30. Tympanic annulus
23. Mastoid air cells	31. Mastoid tip
24. External auditory canal	

Numbers 1–31 are common to pages 35–36.

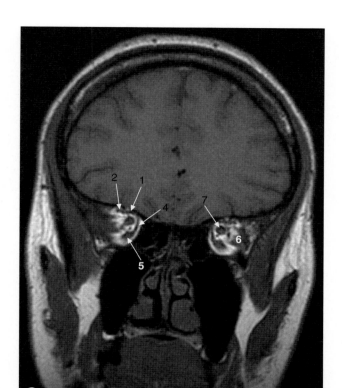

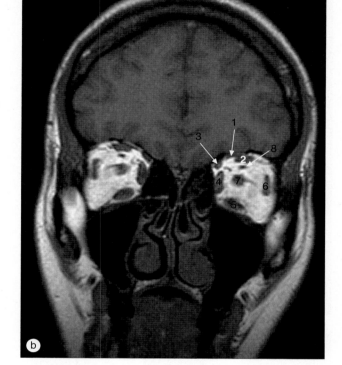

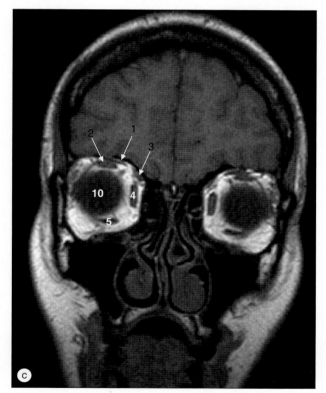

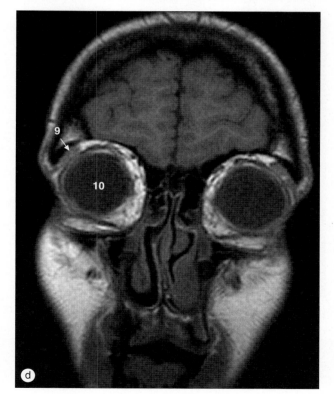

(a)–(d) Coronal MR images, from posterior to anterior.

1. Levator palpebrae superioris muscle
2. Superior rectus muscle
3. Superior oblique muscle
4. Medial rectus muscle
5. Inferior rectus muscle
6. Lateral rectus muscle
7. Optic nerve/sheath complex
8. Superior ophthalmic vein
9. Lacrimal gland
10. Globe of eye

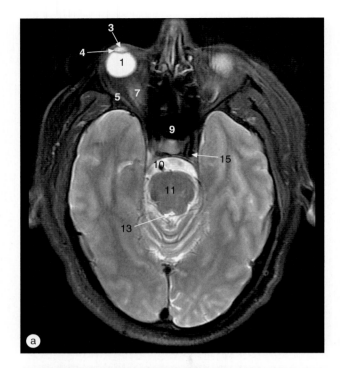

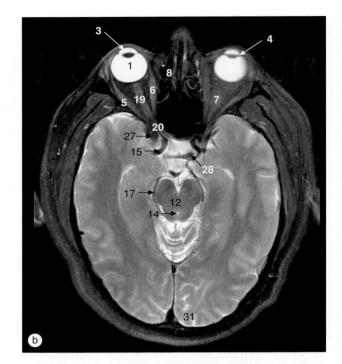

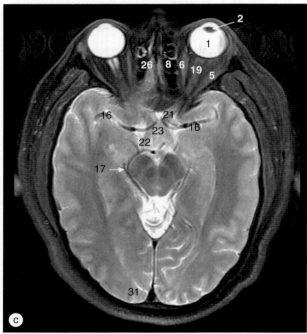

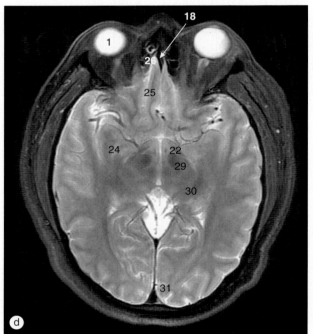

(a)–(d) Orbit, axial MR images, from inferior to superior.

1. Vitreous chamber of globe
2. Lens
3. Anterior chamber of globe
4. Ciliary body
5. Lateral rectus muscle
6. Medial rectus muscle
7. Superior rectus muscle
8. Ethmoidal air cells
9. Sphenoid sinus (antrum)
10. Basilar artery
11. Pons
12. Midbrain
13. Superior recess, fourth ventricle
14. Cerebral aqueduct (of Sylvius)
15. Internal carotid artery
16. Middle cerebral artery
17. Posterior cerebral artery
18. Crista galli
19. Optic nerve (CN2, intraorbital segment)
20. Optic nerve (CN2, intracanalicular segment)
21. Optic nerve (CN2, intracranial segment)
22. Optic tract
23. Optic chiasma
24. Anterior commissure
25. Gyrus rectus
26. Olfactory nerve (CN1)
27. Anterior clinoid process
28. Dorsum sellae
29. Cerebral peduncle
30. Medial and lateral geniculate bodies
31. Visual (calcarine) cortex

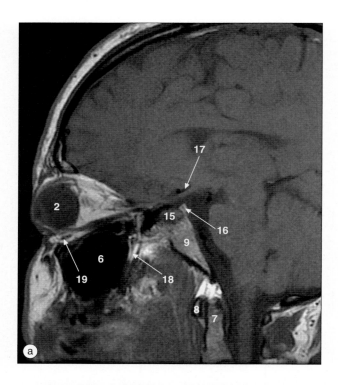

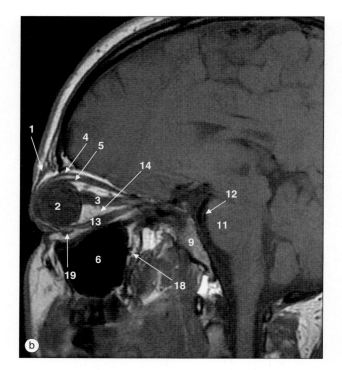

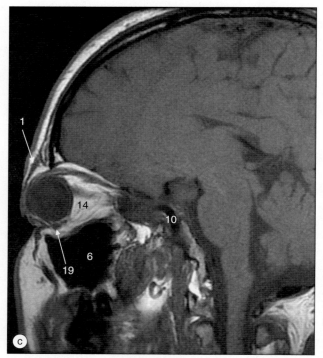

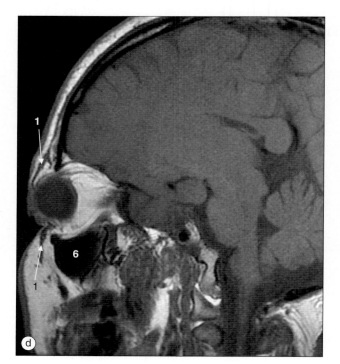

(a)–(d) Orbit, sagittal MR images, from medial to lateral.

1. Orbicularis oculi muscle
2. Globe
3. Optic nerve, intraocular segment
4. Levator palpebrae superioris
5. Superior rectus muscle
6. Maxillary sinus (antrum)
7. Dens (odontoid process)
8. Anterior arch of C1
9. Clivus
10. Internal carotid artery
11. Pons
12. Basilar artery
13. Inferior rectus muscle
14. Retrobulbar fat
15. Pituitary gland
16. Dorsum sellae
17. Optic nerve, intracranial segment
18. Pterygopalatine fossa
19. Inferior oblique muscle

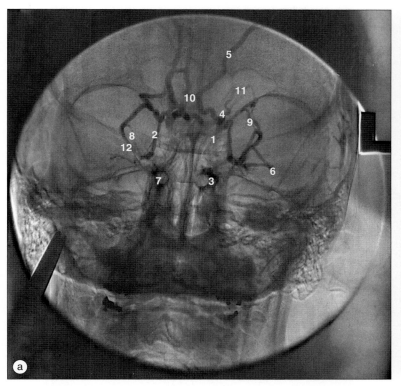

(a) Orbital venogram.

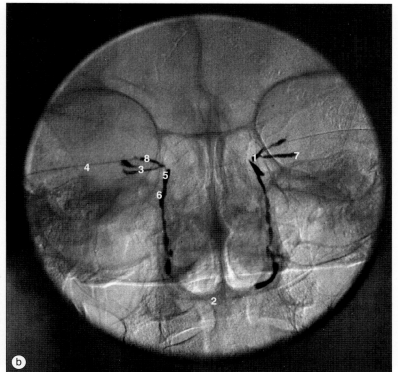

(b) Macrodacryocystogram.

1. Angular veins
2. Anterior collateral vein
3. Cavernous sinus
4. First part of superior ophthalmic vein
5. Frontal veins
6. Inferior ophthalmic vein
7. Internal carotid artery
8. Medial collateral vein
9. Second part of superior ophthalmic vein
10. Superficial connecting vein
11. Supraorbital vein
12. Third part of superior ophthalmic vein

1. Common canaliculus	5. Lacrimal sac
2. Hard palate	6. Nasolacrimal duct
3. Inferior canaliculus	7. Site of lacrimal punctum
4. Lacrimal catheters	8. Superior canaliculus

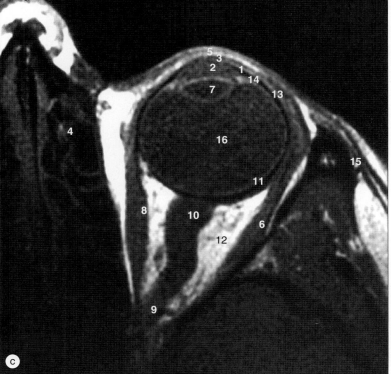

1. Anterior chamber	10. Optic nerve
2. Aqueous humour	11. Retina and choroid
3. Cornea	12. Retroorbital fat
4. Ethmoidal sinuses	13. Sclera
5. Eyelid	14. Suspensory ligament of the lens
6. Lateral rectus muscle	15. Temporalis muscle
7. Lens	16. Vitreous humour
8. Medial rectus muscle	
9. Ophthalmic artery	

(c) Globe, axial MR image.

Bonus e-materials

Slidelines for radiograph features:
Occipitofrontal radiograph of the skull

Selected pages from Imaging Atlas 4e

Tutorials: Tutorials 2a, 2b, 2g, 2h

Single best answer (SBA) self-assessment
questions

Table of variations

Variant	Frequency	Clinical implications
Pneumatised middle turbinate (concha bullosa)	35%	Interferes with transnasal surgery; respiratory epithelium inside prone to obstruction (mucocoele), infection and carcinoma; associated with deviated nasal septum, which increases risk of sinus disease.
Deviated nasal septum	29%	If severe, compresses turbinates, causing inflammation and infection.
Haller cell (infraorbital ethmoid air cell/maxilloethmoidal cell)	20%	If infected, can perforate into orbit; may lead to inadvertent entry into orbit if not appreciated at time of endoscopic surgery; narrows osteomeatal complex if large, causing ipsilateral maxillary antrum obstruction.
Agger nasi cells	16%	If enlarged, can contribute to nasofrontal duct obstruction and chronic frontal sinusitis.
Facial artery hypoplasia	10% (1% vestigial)	Alters planning for microvascular free flap surgery (contralateral facial or ipsilateral transverse facial arteries contribute).
Onodi (sphenoethmoid) air cell	10%	Mistakenly introduced during endoscopic access to the sphenoid sinus, presumably through the most posterior ethmoid air cell, risking damage to optic nerve and ICA. Pathology such as mucocoele, carcinoma and sinusitis may cause early optic nerve involvement.
Wormian bones	10% children	Wormian bones are common and can sometimes be numerous without necessarily pointing to osteogenesis imperfecta, since 10% of the children have at least four. Rickets, hypothyroidism, Down's syndrome, pyknodysostosis and cleidocranial dysplasia are other rarer causes.
Sphenoid sinus variant morphology	5%	Pneumatisation of the sphenoid sinuses can extend into the greater sphenoid wing, resulting in lateral recesses which may be a site of mucosal retention cysts or polyps. Additionally, pneumatisation can also involve the posterior orbital wall, pterygoid processes and lesser sphenoid wing. The pattern of pneumatisation of the sphenoid sinus significantly affects the safe access to the sella; if highly pneumatised, it may distort the anatomic configuration, so in these cases it is extremely important to be aware of the midline when opening the sella to avoid accidental injury to the carotid and optic nerves.
Solitary lucent skull lesions: arachnoid granulation, venous lake, emissary vein, parietal thinning	5%	Mimics multiple myeloma or metastases.
Arrested pneumatisation of skull base	1%	Arrested skull base pneumatisation can be confused with significant skull base disease processes. When encountering a nonexpansile lesion with osteosclerotic borders, internal fat, and curvilinear calcifications in the basisphenoid, pterygoid processes and clivus, radiologists should strongly consider this variant - associated atypical fatty marrow is often seen as contiguous foci across multiple sphenoid subsites. Microcystic components are also typical on MRI.
Olfactory fossa type 3 cribriform plate (8–16 mm deep)	1%	Increased risk of cribriform plate damage during local nasal surgery or orbital decompression. Thinner plate in this variant is more prone to CSF erosion in chronic benign intracranial hypertension.
Accessory parietal and occipital sutures	<1%	Fracture mimics: the parietal and occipital bones are common regions for accessory sutures due to their multiple ossification centers. The parietal bone ossifies from two centers, whilst the occipital bone ossifies from six. An accessory intraparietal or subsagittal suture is rare but can be seen dividing the parietal bone, explained on the basis of incomplete union of the two separate ossification centers. These are usually bilateral and fairly symmetrical.

CSF, *cerebrospinal fluid;* MRI, *magnetic resonance imaging.*

3 Neck

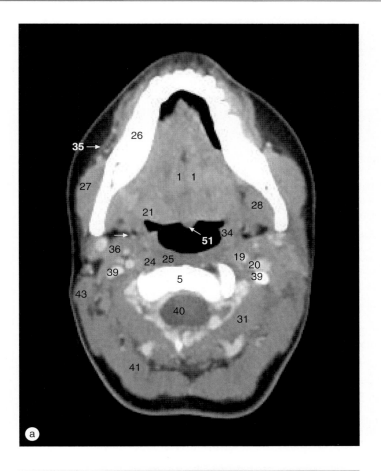

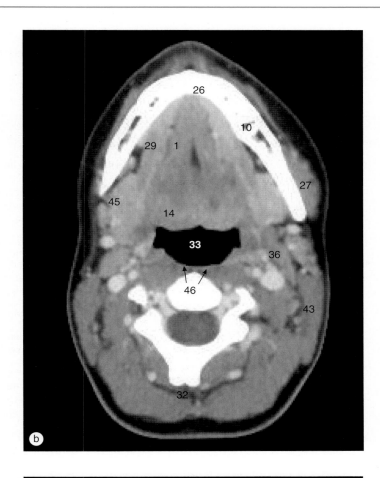

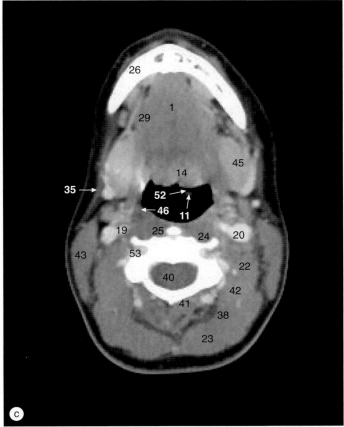

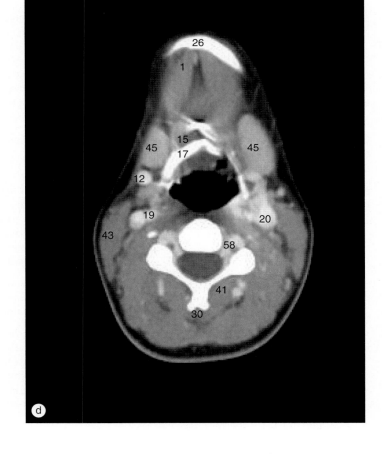

(a)–(h) Neck, axial CT images, from superior to inferior.

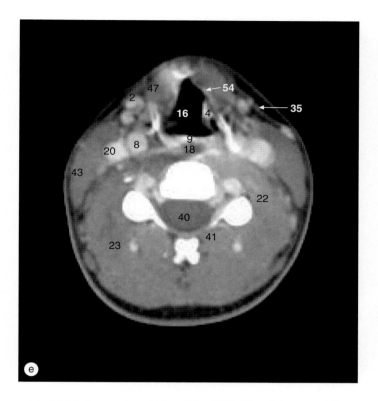

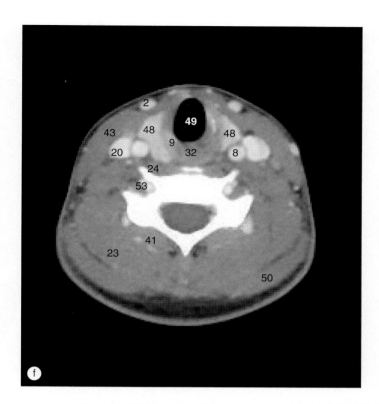

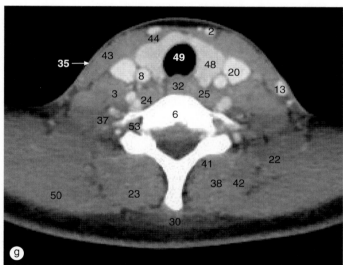

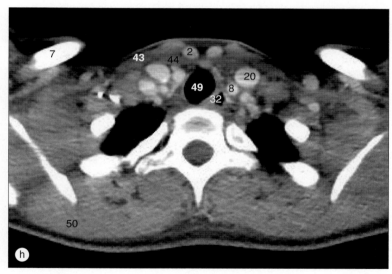

(a)–(h) Neck, axial CT images, from superior to inferior.

1. Anterior belly of digastric muscle
2. Anterior jugular vein
3. Anterior scalene muscle
4. Arytenoid cartilage
5. Body of C2 vertebra
6. Body of C5 vertebra
7. Clavicle
8. Common carotid artery
9. Cricoid cartilage
10. Dental root
11. Epiglottis
12. External carotid artery
13. External jugular vein
14. Genioglossus muscle
15. Geniohyoid muscle
16. Glottis
17. Hyoid
18. Hypopharynx
19. Internal carotid artery

20. Internal jugular vein
21. Levator palati muscle
22. Levator scapulae muscle
23. Longissimus capitis muscle
24. Longus capitis muscle
25. Longus coli muscle
26. Mandible
27. Masseter muscle
28. Medial pterygoid muscle
29. Mylohyoid muscle
30. Nuchal ligament
31. Obliquus capitis inferior muscle
32. Oesophagus
33. Oropharynx
34. Pharyngeal tonsil
35. Platysma muscle
36. Posterior belly of digastric muscle
37. Posterior scalene muscle
38. Semispinalis capitis muscle

39. Styloid process
40. Spinal cord
41. Spinalis capitis muscle
42. Splenius capitis muscle
43. Sternocleidomastoid muscle
44. Sternohyoid muscle
45. Submandibular gland
46. Superior constrictor muscle of pharynx
47. Thyroid cartilage (lamina)
48. Thyroid gland
49. Trachea
50. Trapezius muscle
51. Uvula
52. Vallecula
53. Vertebral vessels (within foramen transversarium)
54. Vocalis muscle

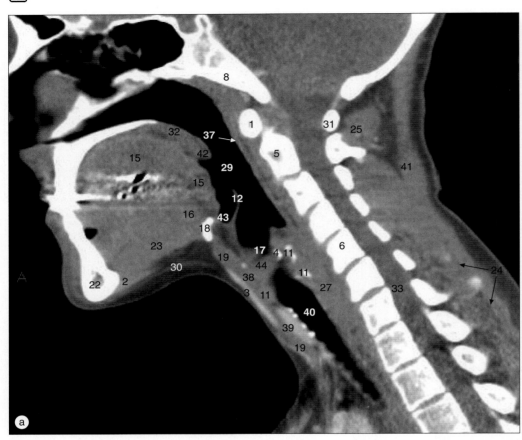

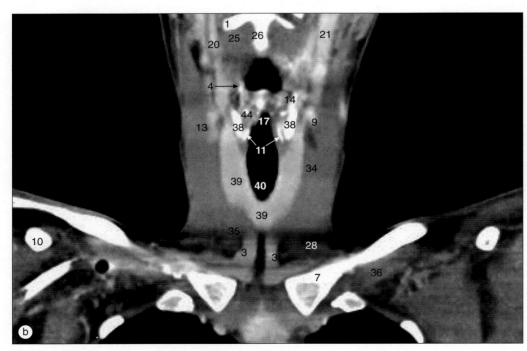

1. Anterior arch of atlas
2. Anterior belly of digastric muscle
3. Anterior jugular vein
4. Arytenoid cartilage
5. Body of C2 vertebra (axis)
6. Body of C5 vertebra
7. Clavicle
8. Clivus
9. Common carotid artery
10. Coracoid process of scapula
11. Cricoid cartilage
12. Epiglottis
13. External carotid artery
14. External jugular vein
15. Genioglossus muscle
16. Geniohyoid muscle
17. Glottis
18. Hyoid
19. Infrahyoid strap muscle
20. Internal carotid artery
21. Internal jugular vein
22. Mandible
23. Mylohyoid muscle
24. Nuchal ligament
25. Obliquus capitis inferior muscle
26. Odontoid process (dens) of C2 (axis)
27. Oesophagus
28. Omohyoid muscle
29. Oropharynx
30. Platysma muscle
31. Posterior arch of atlas
32. Soft palate
33. Spinal cord
34. Sternocleidomastoid muscle
35. Sternohyoid muscle
36. Subclavius muscle
37. Superior constrictor muscle of pharynx
38. Thyroid cartilage (lamina)
39. Thyroid gland
40. Trachea
41. Trapezius muscle
42. Uvula
43. Vallecula
44. Vocalis muscle

Neck, (a) mid-sagittal and (b) midcoronal CT images.

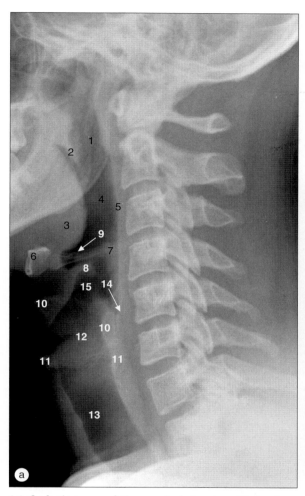

1. Nasopharynx
2. Soft palate
3. Base of tongue
4. Oropharynx
5. Retropharyngeal soft tissues
6. Body of hyoid
7. Greater horn of hyoid
8. Epiglottis
9. Vallecula
10. Thyroid cartilage
11. Cricoid cartilage
12. Laryngeal space
13. Trachea
14. Entrance to oesophagus
15. Hypopharynx

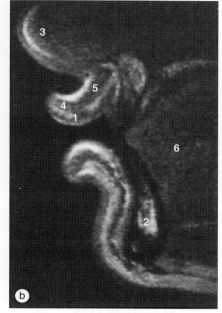

1. Deltoid insertion of levator muscle
2. Mandible
3. Nose
4. Pars marginalis of orbicularis oris muscle
5. Pars peripheralis of orbicularis oris muscle
6. Tongue

(a) Soft tissues of the neck, lateral radiograph.   **(b)** The kiss, sagittal MR image.

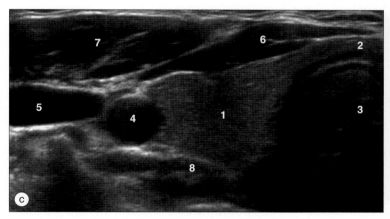

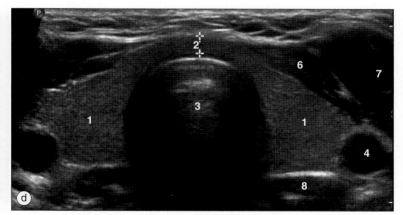

(c) and **(d)** Thyroid ultrasound, transverse image.

1. Thyroid gland lobe
2. Thyroid gland isthmus
3. Trachea
4. Common carotid artery
5. Internal jugular vein
6. Infrahyoid strap muscle
7. Sternocleidomastoid muscle
8. Prevertebral muscle

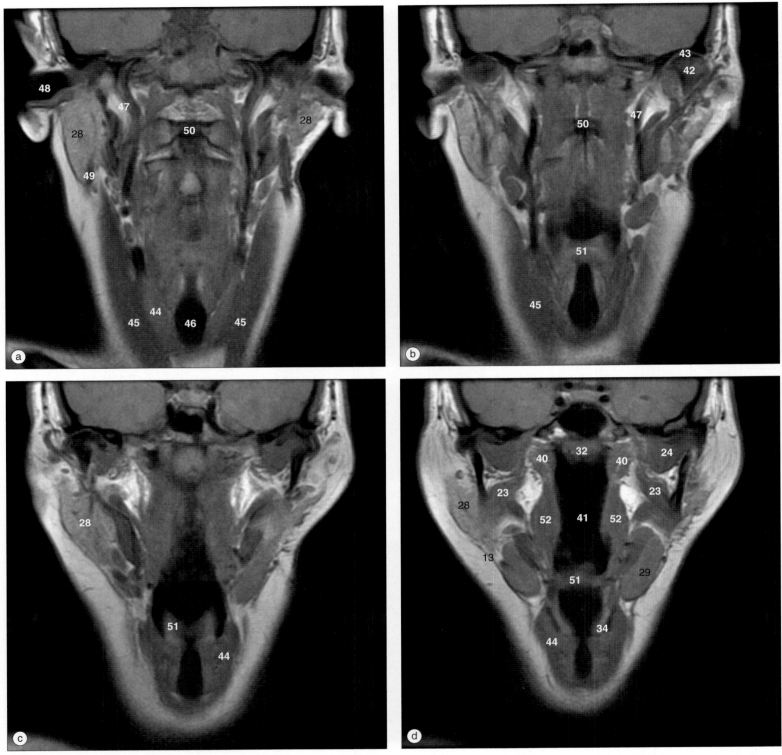

(a)–(l) Pharynx, coronal MR images, from posterior to anterior.

1. Maxillary sinus (antrum)	8. Nasal septum
2. Hard palate	9. Genioglossus muscle
3. Mandible	10. Geniohyoid muscle
4. Alveolar ridge of maxilla	11. Anterior belly of digastric muscle
5. Oral cavity	12. Lingual septum
6. Inferior turbinate	13. Platysma muscle
7. Middle turbinate	14. Hypoglossus muscle

Numbers 1–53 are common to pages 46–48.

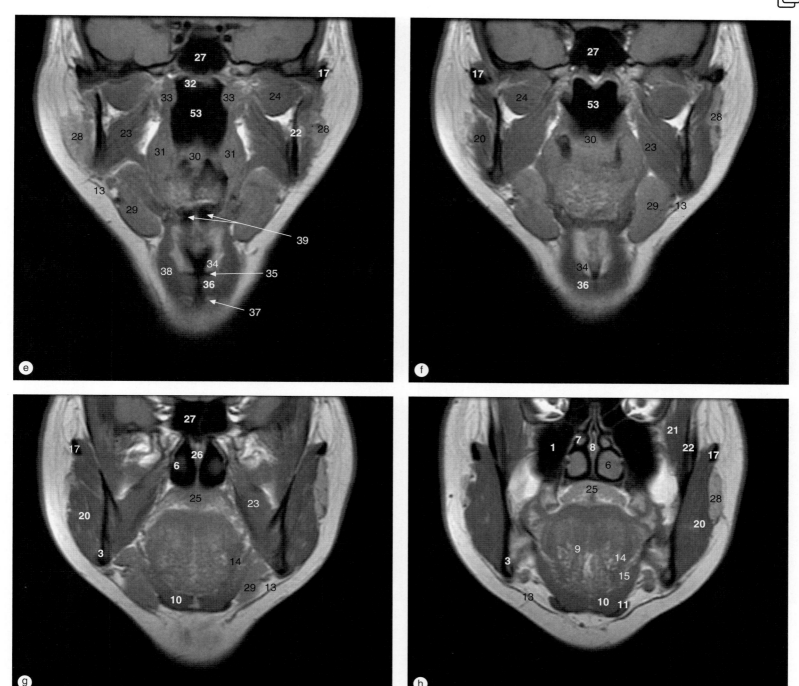

(a)–(l) Pharynx, coronal MR images, from posterior to anterior.

15. Mylohyoid muscle	**24.** Lateral pterygoid muscle
16. Zygomatic bone	**25.** Soft palate
17. Zygomatic arch	**26.** Vomer
18. Transverse muscle of tongue	**27.** Sphenoid sinus (antrum)
19. Longitudinal muscle of tongue	**28.** Parotid gland
20. Masseter muscle	**29.** Submandibular gland
21. Temporal muscle	**30.** Uvula
22. Ramus of mandible	**31.** Palatopharyngeus muscle
23. Medial pterygoid muscle	**32.** Pharyngeal tonsils

Numbers 1–53 are common to pages 46–48.

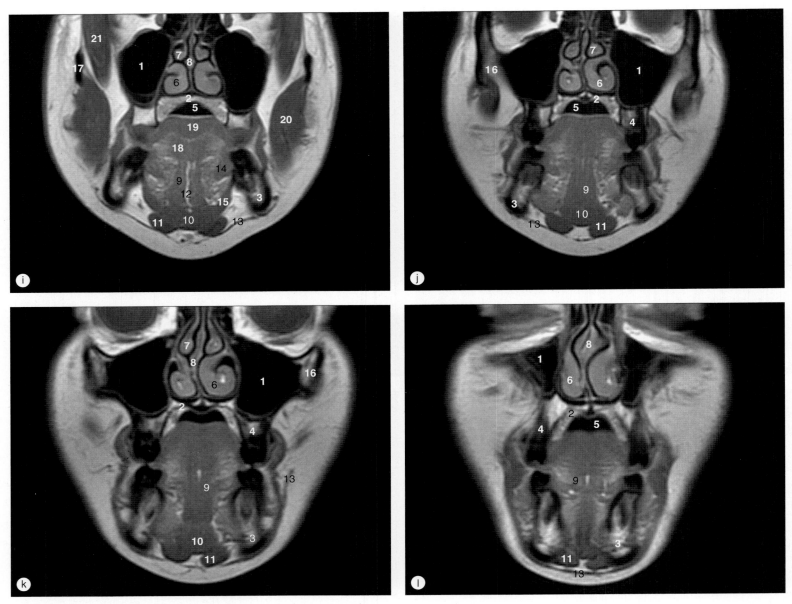

(a)–(I) Pharynx, coronal MR images, from posterior to anterior.

33. Levator veli palatini muscle
34. Vestibular fold
35. Laryngeal ventricle
36. Vocalis muscle
37. Cricoid cartilage
38. Thyrohyoid muscle
39. Vallecula
40. Auditory (Eustachian) tubes
41. Oropharynx
42. Mandibular condyles
43. Temporomandibular joint

44. Thyroid gland
45. Sternocleidomastoid muscle
46. Trachea
47. Internal carotid artery
48. External auditory canal
49. Retromandibular vein
50. Anterior arch of C1
51. Epiglottis
52. Palatine tonsils
53. Nasopharynx

Numbers 1–53 are common to pages 46–48.

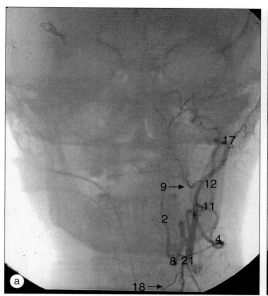

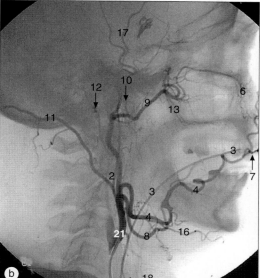

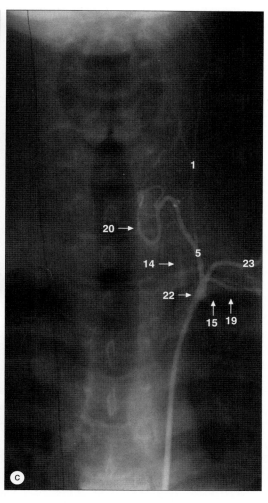

Digitally subtracted arteriograms of the external carotid artery: (a) anteroposterior projection, (b) lateral projection. (c) Thyroid arteriogram.

1. Ascending cervical artery	10. Middle meningeal artery	18. Superior thyroid artery
2. Ascending pharyngeal artery	11. Occipital artery	19. Suprascapular artery
3. Endotracheal tube	12. Posterior auricular artery	20. Thyroid branches of inferior thyroid artery
4. Facial artery	13. Posterior superior alveolar artery	21. Tip of catheter in external carotid artery
5. Inferior thyroid artery	14. Reflux of contrast into vertebral artery	22. Tip of catheter in thyrocervical trunk
6. Infra-orbital artery	15. Subclavian artery	23. Transverse cervical artery
7. Labial branch of facial artery	16. Submental artery	
8. Lingual artery	17. Superficial temporal artery	
9. Maxillary artery		

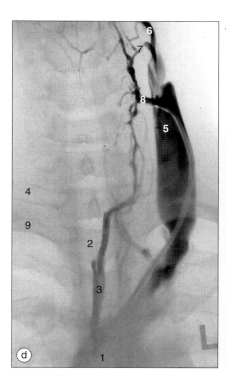

1. Left brachiocephalic vein	5. Internal jugular vein
2. Trachea	6. Lingual vein
3. Inferior thyroid vein	7. Superior thyroid vein
4. Transverse process of C7	8. Tip of catheter in middle thyroid vein
	9. Right first rib

1. Aortic arch	11. Right common carotid artery
2. Brachiocephalic artery	12. Left vertebral artery
3. Left common carotid artery	13. Superior vena cava
4. Left subclavian artery	14. External carotid artery
5. Left internal thoracic artery	15. Internal carotid artery
6. Right internal thoracic artery	16. Basilar artery
7. Right brachiocephalic vein	17. Sigmoid sinus
8. Right lobe of the thyroid gland	18. Internal jugular vein
9. Costocervical trunk	19. Right subclavian vein
10. Right vertebral artery	20. Petrous portion of the internal carotid artery
	21. Right subclavian artery
	22. Jugular bulb

(d) Neck venogram.
(e) Neck vessels, MR angiogram.

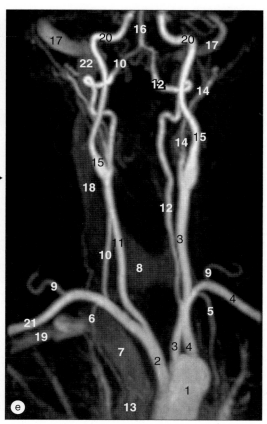

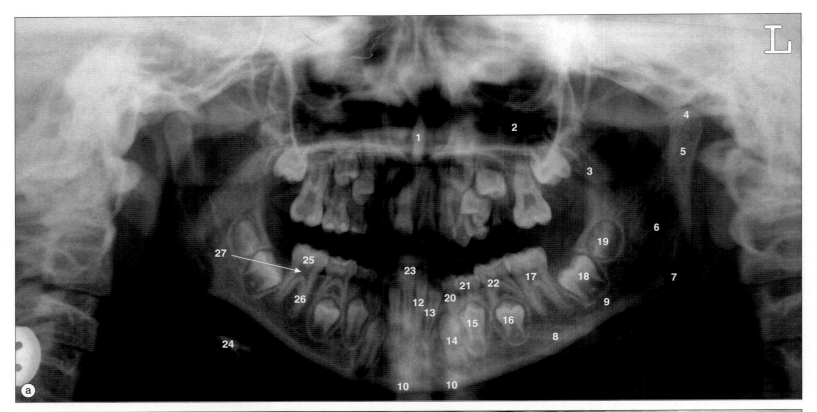

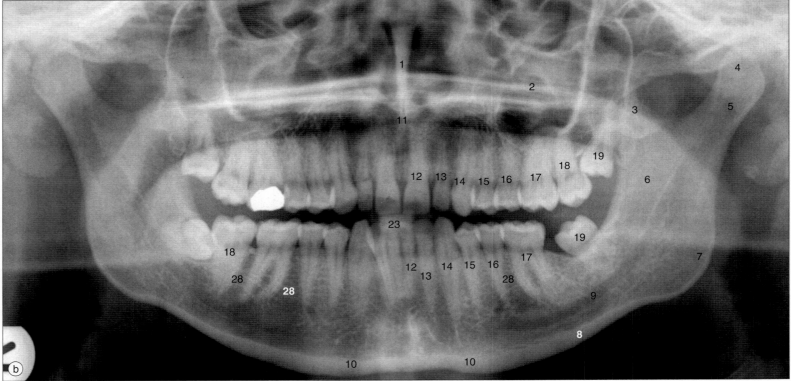

Dental panoramic tomogram (orthopantomogram) of (a) a 6-year-old child, (b) an adult.

1. Nasal septum	8. Mandibular body	15. Anterior premolar	22. Deciduous posterior premolar
2. Maxillary sinus (antrum)	9. Mandibular canal	16. Posterior premolar	23. Bite block
3. Coronoid process of mandible	10. Mental tubercle	17. First molar	24. Hyoid bone
4. Mandibular condylar head	11. Anterior nasal spine	18. Second molar	25. Crown of tooth
5. Mandibular condylar neck	12. Medial incisor	19. Third molar (wisdom tooth)	26. Root of tooth
6. Mandibular ramus	13. Lateral incisor	20. Deciduous canine tooth	27. Pulp chamber of tooth
7. Angle of mandible	14. Canine tooth	21. Deciduous anterior premolar	28. Alveolar bone

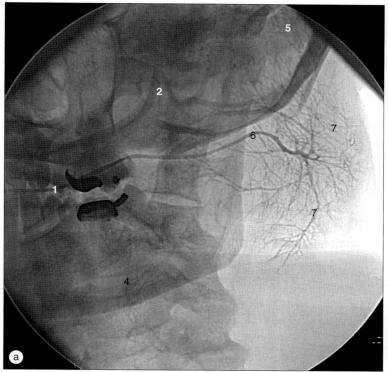

(a) Parotid sialogram.

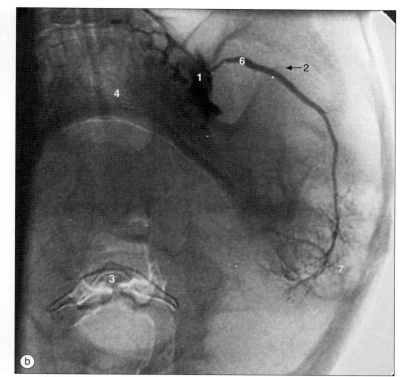

(b) Parotid sialogram, submentovertical projection.

1. Catheter
2. Coronoid process of mandible
3. Hyoid bone
4. Mandible
5. Mastoid process
6. Parotid (Stensen's) duct
7. Secondary ductules

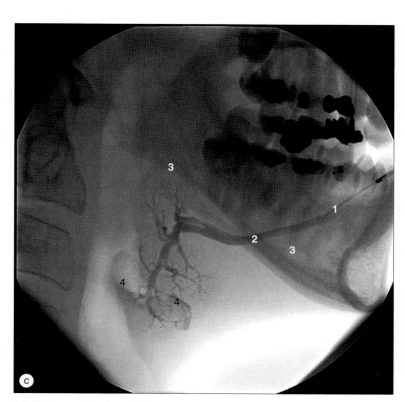

(c) Submandibular sialogram.

1. Catheter
2. Main submandibular (Wharton's) duct
3. Mandible
4. Secondary ductules

Table of Variations

Variant	Frequency	Clinical implications
Thyroid: Zuckerkandl tubercle	66%	May be mistaken for a thyroid nodule, mass or lymph node. It is a projection of normal thyroid tissue from the posterior or lateral lobes of the thyroid gland. It is an important surgical landmark due to its close proximity to the recurrent laryngeal nerve and superior parathyroid gland. Recognition on CT imaging can obviate the need for biopsy and avoid potential recurrent laryngeal nerve injury. However, it should be noted that disease (e.g. thyroid carcinoma) can still occur within this normal variant.
Thyroid: pyramidal lobe	10–30%	Seen as a third thyroid lobe and likely related to a remnant of the thyroglossal duct. It usually arises from the isthmus upwards along the midline or is shifted towards the left of the neck, usually located anterior to the thyroid cartilage.
Common faciolingual arterial trunk	20%	Awareness is needed to avoid inadvertent section of either the lingual or facial arteries in facial flap surgery.
Thyroidea ima artery	1.5–12.5%	The thyroidea ima artery can arise from the brachiocephalic trunk, right CCA, aortic arch or internal thoracic artery. It ascends on the anterior surface of the trachea and supplies both trachea and thyroid. It is often associated with absent inferior thyroid arteries. If unrecognised at surgery, it can be a source of brisk and potentially difficult to control bleeding, as the cut vessel may retract behind the manubrium.
Thyroglossal duct remnants (and ectopic thyroid, including lingual)	7%	Thyroglossal duct (TGD) remnants are one of the most common congenital asymptomatic masses of the neck. The midline TGD cyst is associated with ectopic thyroid in 40%. The presence of duct remnants may lead to abnormal phonation and epithelial carcinomas.
		As a standalone pathology, imaging manifestation of ectopic thyroid is very rare (although microscopically seen in up to 10% along the TGD course). 90% of cases of TGD are solely present at the tongue base, seen as a well-defined posterior glossal mass. This lingual thyroid results from total failure of the normal caudal thyroid migration from the foramen caecum; it exhibits normal histology and functionality. MR signal characteristics include T1 iso to hyperintense to muscle, variable T2 and homogeneous contrast enhancement. A thyroid isotope scan is excellent at not only confirming the diagnosis, but also identifying the presence of any thyroid tissue elsewhere in the neck.
Common carotid bifurcation, high and low levels	Ultrahigh: 3% High: 12–31% Low: 11–15%	Awareness needed for surgical approach to neck and skull base surgery. High level at hyoid bone (C2) and low level below upper border of thyroid cartilage.
Variant relationship of origins of the external and internal carotid arteries	Medial: 37% Anterior: 10% Anterolateral: 1.7–4%	The usual anteromedial position of the ECA to ICA was found in 51.7% of cases. In 1.7% the ECA origin was lateral to that of the ICA. Such variations must be given utmost importance before planning for any neck surgeries to avoid postoperative complications. Characteristic Doppler waveforms between the intracranial and extracranial circulations should obviate confusion on carotid arterial assessment.
Duplication and fenestration of the internal jugular vein	0.4%	These variants can be diagnosed on CTA. Inferiorly, the suprascapular artery may pass between two parts of the vein on the right and omohyoid muscle on the left (also documented to pass through are the C2–3 anterior rami and lateral branch of the spinal accessorius nerve). The variations are important because the IJV is intensively used in clinical procedures.

CCA, *Common carotid artery;* CT, *computed tomography;* CTA, *CT angiography;* ECA, *external carotid artery;* ICA, *internal carotid artery;* IJV, *internal jugular vein;* MR, *magnetic resonance;* MRA, *MR angiography.*

4 | Vertebral column and spinal cord

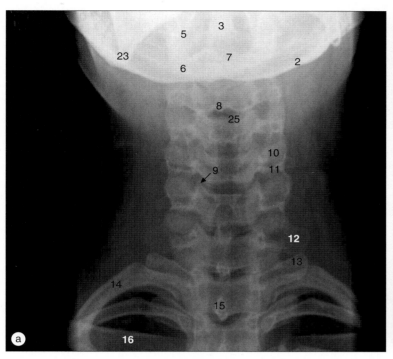
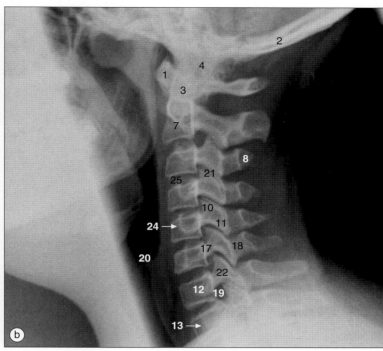

(a) Cervical spine, anteroposterior radiograph, (b) cervical spine, lateral radiograph.

1. Anterior arch of C1 (atlas)
2. Basiocciput
3. Odontoid peg of C2 (axis)
4. Occipital condyle
5. Lateral mass of C1
6. Lateral mass of C2
7. Body of C2
8. Spinous process of C3
9. Uncovertebral joint (Luschka) of C5/6
10. Superior articular process of C5
11. Inferior articular process of C5
12. Transverse process of C7
13. Transverse process of T1
14. First rib
15. Spinous process of T1
16. Clavicle
17. Pedicle of C6
18. Lamina of C6
19. Intervertebral foramen of C7/T1 (for C8 nerve root)
20. Epiglottis
21. Facet (zygapophyseal joint) of C3/4
22. Pars interarticularis of C7
23. Angle of mandible
24. Transverse process of C5
25. Intervertebral disc at C3/4

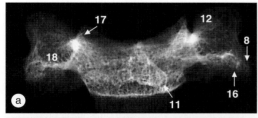
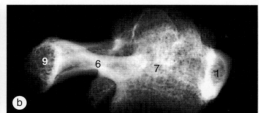
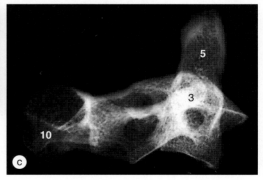
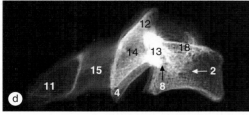

Radiographs of desiccated cervical vertebrae.
(a) AP view C4.
(b) Lateral view C1.
(c) Lateral view C2.
(d) Lateral view C4.

1. Anterior arch of atlas (first cervical vertebra)
2. Anterior tubercle of transverse process of C4
3. Body of axis (second cervical vertebra)
4. Inferior articular process (facet) of C4
5. Odontoid process (dens) of axis (second cervical vertebra)
6. Posterior arch of atlas (first cervical vertebra)
7. Body of atlas (first cervical vertebra)
8. Posterior tubercle of transverse process of C4
9. Posterior tubercle of atlas (first cervical vertebra)
10. Spinous process of axis (second cervical vertebra)
11. Spinous process of C4
12. Superior articular process (facet) of C4
13. Pedicle of C4
14. Pars interarticularis of C4
15. Lamina of C4
16. Intertubercular lamella of C4 transverse process
17. Posterolateral lip (uncus) of C4
18. Body of transverse process of C4

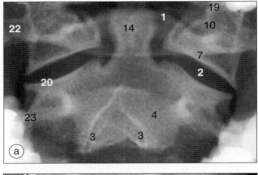

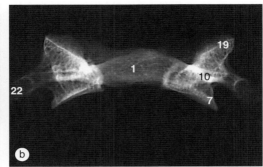

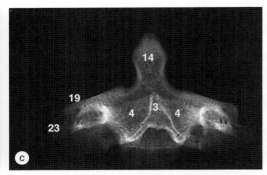

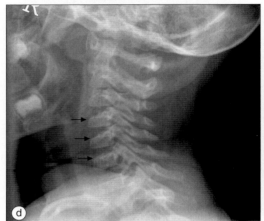

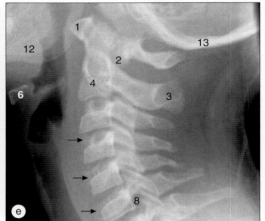

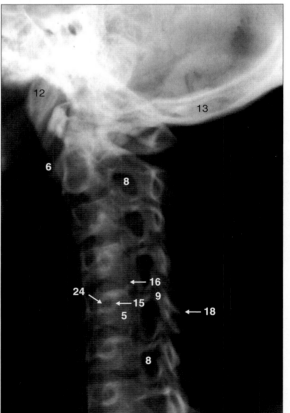

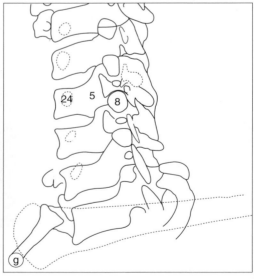

1. Anterior arch of atlas (first cervical vertebra)
2. Atlanto-axial joint
3. Bifid spinous process of axis (second cervical vertebra)
4. Body of axis (second cervical vertebra)
5. Body of fifth cervical vertebra
6. Hyoid bone
7. Inferior articular process (facet) of atlas (first cervical vertebra)
8. Intervertebral foramen
9. Lamina of fifth cervical vertebra
10. Lateral mass of atlas (first cervical vertebra)
11. Left first rib
12. Mandible
13. Occipital bone
14. Odontoid process (dens) of axis (second cervical vertebra)
15. Posterior tubercle of transverse process of fifth cervical vertebra
16. Posterolateral lip (uncus) of fifth cervical vertebra
17. Right first rib
18. Spinous process of fifth cervical vertebra
19. Superior articular process (facet) of atlas (first cervical vertebra)
20. Superior articular process (facet) of axis (second cervical vertebra)
21. Trachea
22. Transverse process of atlas (first cervical vertebra)
23. Transverse process of axis (second cervical vertebra)
24. Transverse process of fifth cervical vertebra

(a) Atlas (first cervical vertebra) and axis (second cervical vertebra), 'open mouth' anteroposterior radiograph.
(b) Dried atlas (first cervical vertebra), anteroposterior radiograph.
(c) Dried axis (second cervical vertebra), anteroposterior radiograph.
(d) Cervical spine lateral radiograph of a 3-year-old. The atlanto-axial joint can normally be up to 5 mm (up to 3 mm in adults).
(e) Cervical spine lateral radiograph of a 9-year-old. Note normal physiological wedging of the vertebral bodies (arrows) due to unossified superior endplate apophyses.
(f) Oblique radiograph of an adult cervical spine.
(g) Line drawing of (f).

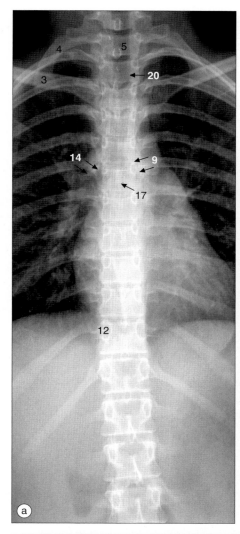

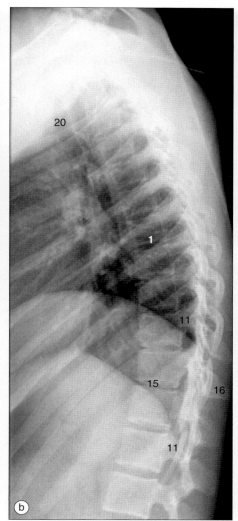

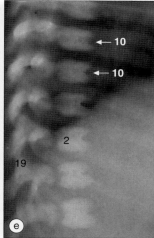

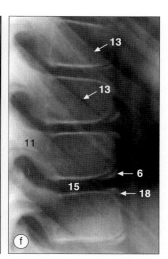

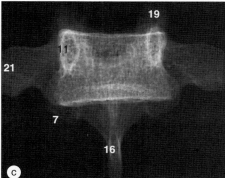

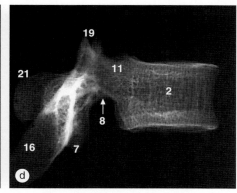

1. Body of sixth thoracic vertebra
2. Body of vertebra
3. Clavicle
4. First rib
5. First thoracic vertebra
6. Inferior annular epiphysial discs for vertebral body
7. Inferior articular process (facet)
8. Inferior vertebral notch
9. Left main bronchus
10. Neonatal cleft
11. Pedicle
12. Pedicle of eleventh thoracic vertebra
13. Ribs
14. Right main bronchus
15. Site of intervertebral disc
16. Spinous process
17. Spinous process of sixth thoracic vertebra
18. Superior annular epiphysial discs for vertebral body
19. Superior articular process (facet)
20. Trachea
21. Transverse process

(a) Thoracic spine, anteroposterior radiograph.
(b) Thoracic spine, lateral radiograph.
(c) Dried thoracic vertebra, anteroposterior radiograph.

(d) Dried sixth thoracic vertebra, lateral radiograph.
Thoracic spine, (e) of a 7-day-old neonate, (f) of a 12-year-old child, lateral radiograph.

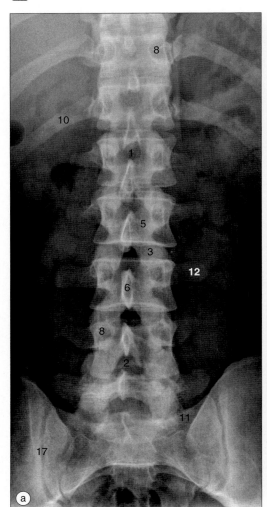

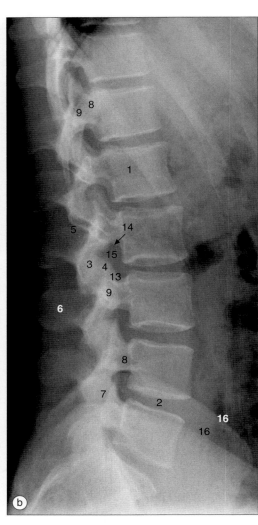

(a) Lumbar spine, anteroposterior radiograph.
(b) Lumbar spine, lateral radiograph.
(c) Dried second lumbar vertebra, anteroposterior radiograph.
(d) Dried second lumbar vertebra, lateral radiograph.
(e) Lumbar spine, oblique radiograph.

1. Body of L1
2. Intervertebral disc at L4/5
3. Inferior articular process (facet) of L2
4. Superior articular process (facet) of L3
5. Lamina of L2
6. Spinous process of L3
7. Facet (zygapophyseal joint) of L4/5
8. Pedicle
9. Pars interarticularis
10. Right twelfth rib
11. Sacral promontory
12. Transverse process of L3
13. Mammillary process
14. Inferior vertebral notch of L2
15. Neural foramen of L2/3 (for L2 root)
16. Iliac crest
17. Sacroiliac joint

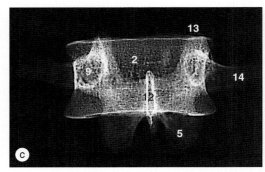

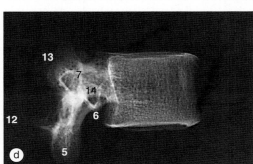

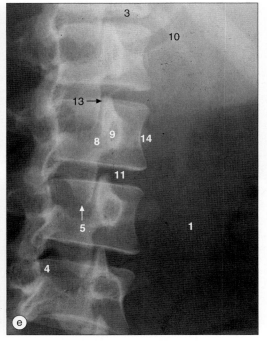

1. Psoas muscle outline
2. Body of second lumbar vertebra
3. Inferior end plate of twelfth thoracic vertebra
4. Body of fourth lumbar vertebra
5. Inferior articular process (facet) of second lumbar vertebra
6. Inferior vertebral notch of second lumbar vertebra
7. Mammillary process of second lumbar vertebra
8. Pars interarticularis
9. Pedicle of second lumbar vertebra
10. Twelfth rib
11. Intervertebral disc space between L2 and L3
12. Spinous process of second lumbar vertebra
13. Superior articular process (facet) of second lumbar vertebra
14. Transverse process of second lumbar vertebra

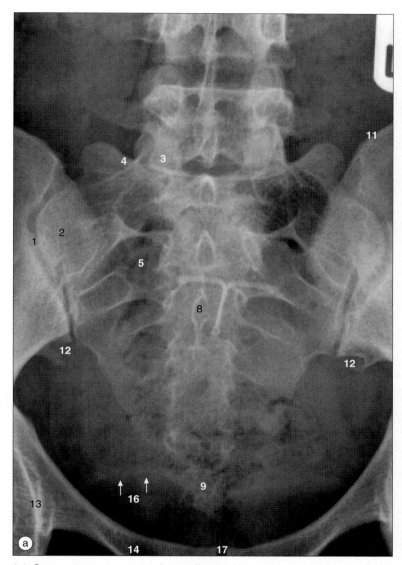

(a) Sacrum, anteroposterior radiograph.

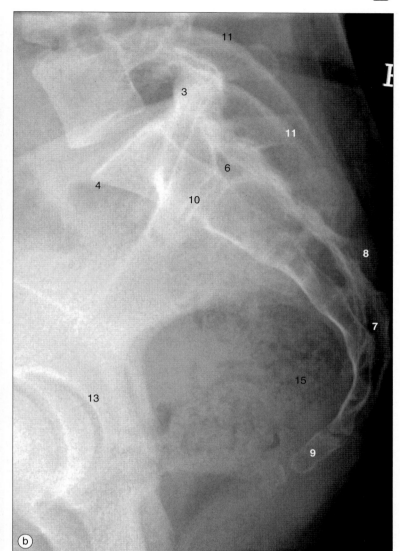

(b) Sacrum and coccyx, lateral radiograph.

1. Sacroiliac joint
2. Ala of sacrum
3. Superior articular process of sacrum
4. Sacral promontory
5. Sacral foramen (S1/2 for right S1 root)
6. Upper part of sacral canal
7. Lower part of sacral canal
8. Spinous tubercle on median sacral crest
9. Coccyx
10. Rudimentary S1/2 disc space
11. Iliac crest
12. Preauricular (paraglenoid) sulcus
13. Acetabular roof
14. Superior pubic ramus
15. Rectum
16. Levator ani (outlined by fat in ischioanal fossa)
17. Symphysis pubis

The preauricular (paraglenoid) sulcus is a characteristic of the female pelvis and is due to bone resorption at the insertion of the anterior sacroiliac ligament. It is prominent in parous women.

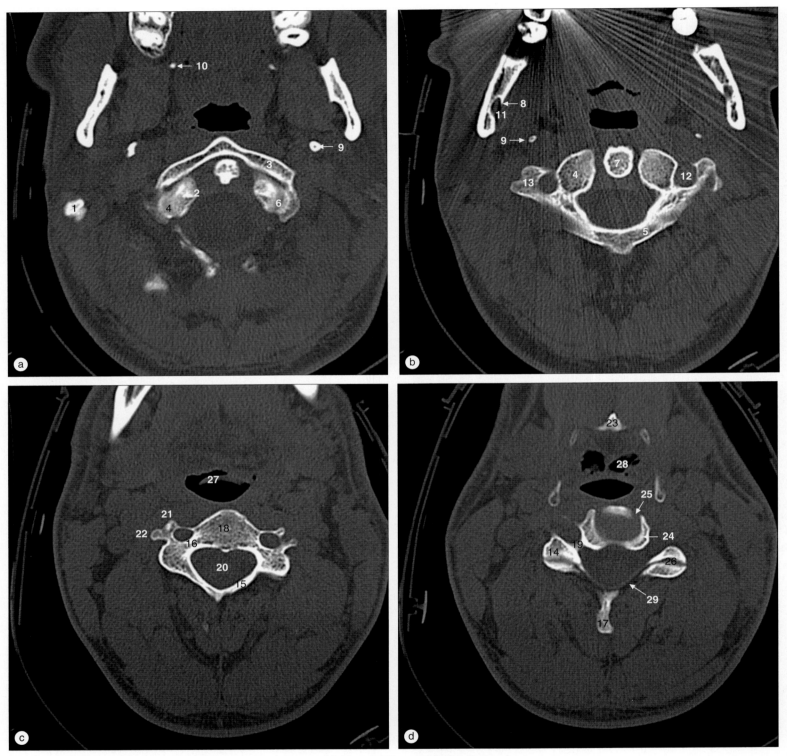

Axial CT images of the upper cervical spine at (**a, b**) C1/2, (**c**) C2 and (**d**) C2/3 level.

1. Mastoid process (tip)
2. Transverse ligament (attachment)
3. Anterior arch of atlas (C1)
4. Lateral mass of atlas
5. Posterior arch of C1
6. Groove for vertebral artery
7. Odontoid process (dens) of axis (C2)
8. Lingula of mandible
9. Styloid process
10. Hamulus of medial pterygoid plate
11. Inferior alveolar foramen of mandibular ramus
12. Foramen transversarium of C1
13. Transverse process of C1
14. Inferior articular process of C2
15. Lamina of C2
16. Pedicle of C2
17. Spinous process of C2
18. Body of C2
19. Intervertebral foramen of C2/3
20. Spinal cord
21. Anterior tubercle of transverse process of C2
22. Posterior tubercle of transverse process of C2
23. Thyroid cartilage
24. Uncus of C3 vertebral body
25. Uncovertebral joint (of Luschka) at C2/3
26. Facet (zygapophyseal) joint at C2/3
27. Epiglottis
28. Vallecula
29. Ligamentum flavum

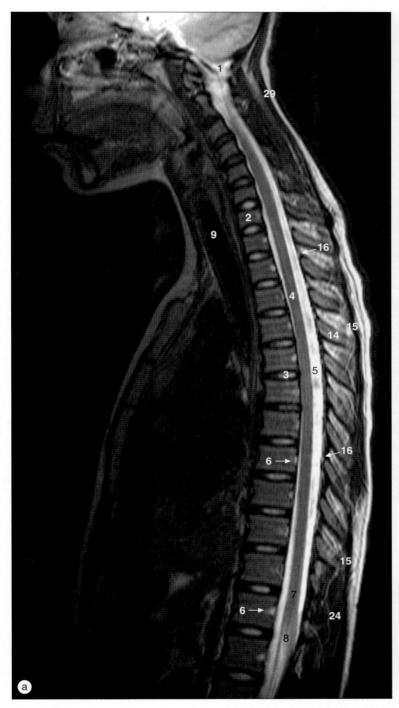

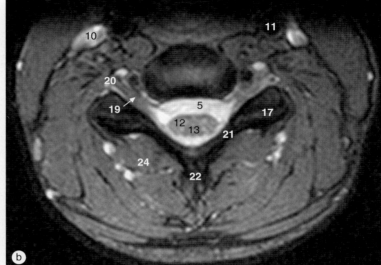

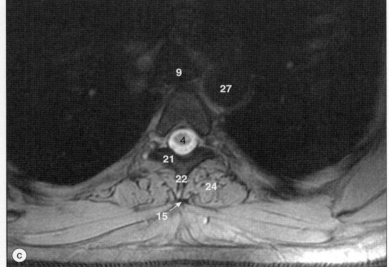

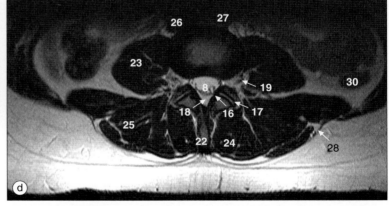

T2w MR images of the spine, (a) sagittal wide field of view and axial sections from the (b) cervical, (c) thoracic and (d) lumbar regions.

1. Foramen magnum
2. Body of C7
3. Nucleus pulposus of T5/6 intervertebral disc
4. Spinal cord
5. Cerebrospinal fluid (CSF) in subarachnoid space (flow void artefact)
6. Basivertebral vein

7. Conus medullaris
8. Cauda equina
9. Trachea
10. Internal jugular vein
11. Common carotid artery
12. Grey matter of spinal cord
13. White matter of spinal cord
14. Spinous process of T4
15. Supraspinous ligament

16. Ligamentum flavum
17. Facet (zygapophyseal) joint
18. Epidural fat
19. Dorsal root ganglion
20. Spinal nerve root
21. Lamina
22. Spinous process
23. Psoas major muscle
24. Erector spinae muscle

25. Multifidus muscle
26. Inferior vena cava
27. Aorta
28. Thoracolumbar fascia
29. Ligamentum nuchae
30. Descending colon

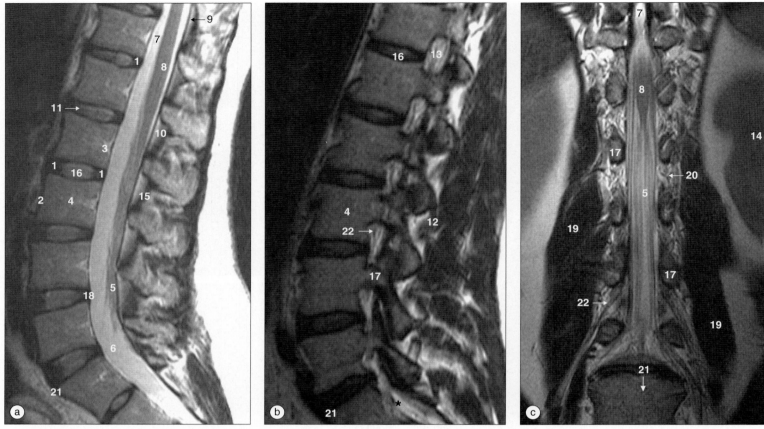

Lumbosacral spine, **(a)** sagittal, **(b)** parasagittal, **(c)** coronal MR images. Note rudimentary S1/2 disc on sagittal sequence.

1. Annulus fibrosus
2. Anterior longitudinal ligament
3. Basivertebral vein
4. Body of third lumbar vertebra
5. Cauda equina
6. Caudal lumbar thecal sac
7. CSF
8. Conus medullaris
9. Dural sac
10. Epidural space (fat filled)
11. Internuclear cleft
12. Interspinous ligament
13. Intervertebral foramen
14. Kidney
15. Ligamentum flavum
16. Nucleus pulposus
17. Pedicle
18. Posterior longitudinal ligament and annulus fibrosus
19. Psoas muscle
20. Radicular vessels
21. Sacral promontory
22. Spinal nerve root in intervertebral foramen

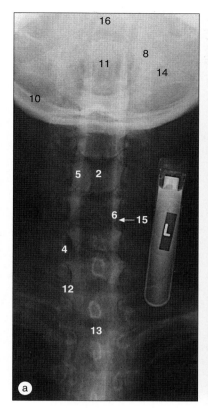

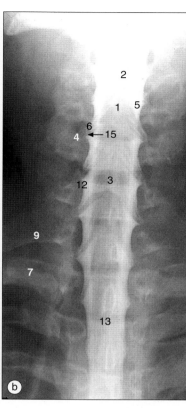

Cervical myelogram, with the neck (a) extended, (b) slightly flexed, anteroposterior radiographs.

Nonionic water-soluble contrast medium is introduced into the lumbar subarachnoid space via a lumbar puncture. The patient is positioned prone, with the neck hyperextended, and strapped onto a tilting table. The contrast medium is then run up into the cervical region to demonstrate the cervical spinal cord and exiting nerve roots. There are eight cervical nerve roots; the roots of the eighth cervical nerve exit through the intervertebral foramina between the seventh cervical vertebra and the first thoracic vertebra. The normal cervical cord enlargement (3) (for the brachial plexus) extends from the third cervical vertebra to the second thoracic vertebra. It is maximal at the fifth cervical vertebra and should not be mistaken for an intramedullary lesion.

1. Anterior spinal artery (impression)
2. Cervical cord
3. Cervical cord enlargement
4. Cervical spinal nerve exiting through intervertebral foramen
5. Contrast medium in cervical subarachnoid space
6. Dorsal root of spinal nerve
7. First rib
8. Lateral mass of atlas (first cervical vertebra)
9. Normal large transverse process of seventh cervical vertebra
10. Occiput
11. Odontoid process (dens)
12. Root of eighth cervical nerve
13. Thoracic cord
14. Transverse foramen
15. Ventral root of spinal nerve
16. Vertebral artery

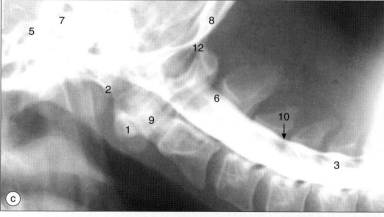

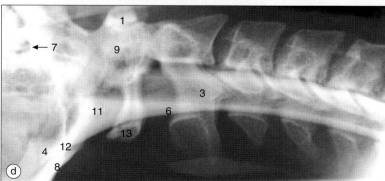

Cervical myelogram, with the patient (c) prone, (d) supine, lateral radiographs.

1. Anterior arch of atlas (first cervical vertebra)
2. Anterior rim of foramen magnum
3. Cervical cord
4. Cisterna magna (cerebellomedullary cistern)
5. Clivus
6. Contrast medium in cervical subarachnoid space
7. External acoustic meatus
8. Occiput
9. Odontoid (process) dens
10. Posterior indentation on theca from ligamentum flavum
11. Posterior inferior cerebellar artery
12. Posterior rim of foramen magnum
13. Posterior tubercle of atlas (first cervical vertebra)

Lumbar radiculogram, (a) lateral, (b) oblique, (c) anteroposterior radiographs. Nonionic water-soluble contrast medium is introduced into the lumbar subarachnoid space via a lumbar puncture. The nerve roots of the cauda equina are well demonstrated and exit through the intervertebral foramina. The nerve roots extending from the conus to the terminal thecal sac pass below the pedicle of the corresponding vertebra. The thecal sac terminates at the level of the first/second sacral vertebrae. The filum terminale may be seen. Tilting the prone patient slightly head down allows the contrast to flow cranially and outlines the conus and lower thoracic cord. The cord is uniform in size from the second to the tenth thoracic vertebra, at which point its second, smaller expansion (for the lumbosacral plexus) extends from the tenth thoracic vertebra to the level of the first lumbar vertebra. The conus medullaris usually terminates at the first/second lumbar vertebrae but may be seen at a level above and below as a normal variant.

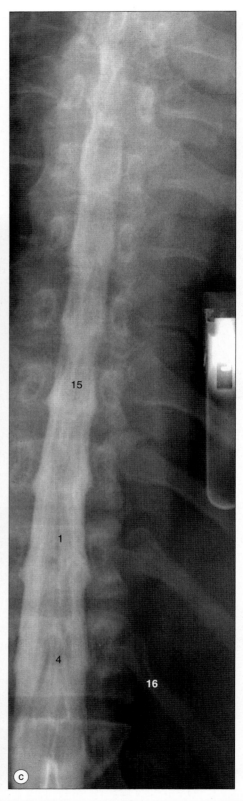

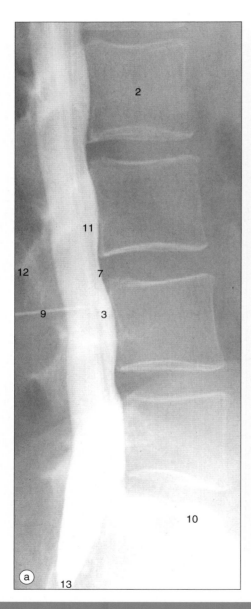

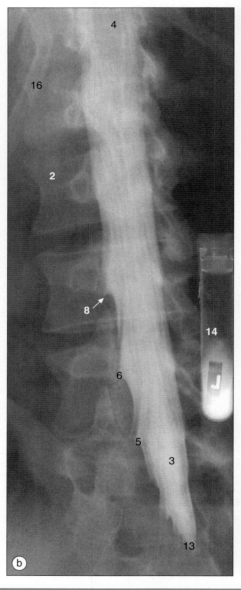

1. Anterior median fissure
2. Body of second lumbar vertebra
3. Contrast medium in subarachnoid space
4. Conus medullaris
5. Fifth lumbar spinal nerve
6. Fourth lumbar spinal nerve
7. Intervertebral disc indentations in anterior thecal margin
8. Lateral extension of subarachnoid space around spinal nerve roots
9. Lumbar puncture needle in space between third and fourth lumbar vertebrae
10. Sacral promontory
11. Spinal nerves within subarachnoid space (cauda equina)
12. Spinous process of third lumbar vertebra
13. Terminal theca at first/second sacral vertebra
14. Test tube containing contrast medium to indicate tilt of patient
15. Thoracic cord
16. Twelfth rib

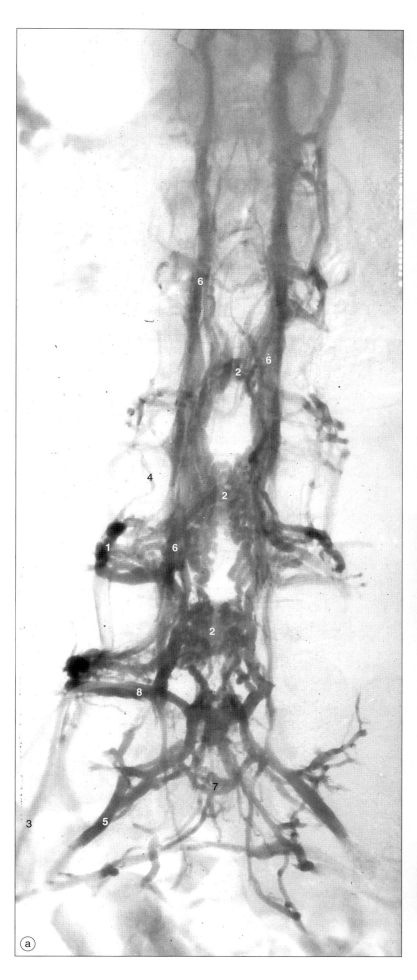

(a) Subtracted lumbar venogram.

Since the advent of CT and MR imaging techniques, lumbar venography is rarely performed. However, the anatomy of the vertebral veins is optimally demonstrated by this technique. Venous drainage of the spinal cord is longitudinally arranged via plexi, which anastomose freely with the internal (6) and external (1 and 4) vertebral venous plexi, which also communicate (4 and 2). Note how the internal veins bend laterally at the level of the disc interspace and medially at the level of pedicles, where they unite via a connecting vein (2).

1. Ascending lumbar veins
2. Basivertebral veins
3. Catheter in common iliac vein
4. Intervertebral veins
5. Lateral sacral veins
6. Longitudinal vertebral venous plexi
7. Sacral venous plexus
8. Tip of catheter in intravertebral vein

(b) Spinal arteriogram.

1. Anterior spinal artery
2. Arteria radicularis magna (Adamkiewicz)
3. Normal transdural stenosis of the arteria radicularis magna
4. Selective catheterisation of left eleventh intercostal artery

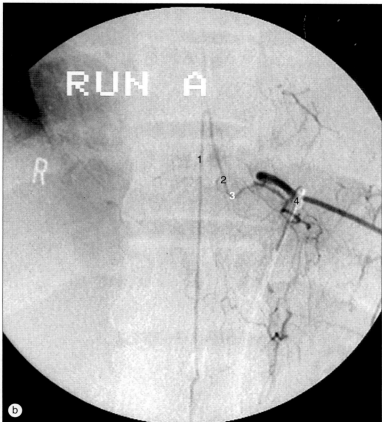

(b)

Bonus e-materials

Slidelines for radiograph features:
Anteroposterior radiograph of the cervical
spine, Lateral radiograph of the cervical spine,
Lateral radiograph of the lumbar spine, Supine
radiograph of the abdomen, Anteroposterior
radiograph of the pelvis (female)

Selected pages from Imaging Atlas 4e

Tutorials: Tutorials 3a, 3b

Single best answer (SBA) self-assessment
questions

Table of Variations

Variant	Frequency	Clinical implications
Lumbosacral transitional vertebrae (LSTV)	15–20%	Nonrecognition of this variant and/or poor description in the report can lead to operations or procedures performed at the wrong level. Lumbarisation of S1 (assimilation of S1 to lumbar spine) is less common than sacralisation, occurring in ~2% of the population. It manifests as the presence of six rib-free lumbar-type vertebrae, which may result in squaring of highest sacral (transitional) vertebra and the presence of facet joints (even rudimentary) and intervertebral disc between S1 and S2. Sacralisation of L5 (assimilation of L5 to the sacrum) is more common than lumbarisation, occurring in ~17% of the population. This is typified by the presence of four rib-free lumbar type vertebrae, which may be associated with wedging of the lowest lumbar (transitional) vertebra and hypoplastic or absent facet joints or intervertebral disc. Nothing replaces accurate and diligent description of which numbering system has been used in all cases where the anatomy is non-standard. The iliolumbar ligament is a relatively constant landmark on which to base numbering, because it arises from the transverse process of L5 in 96% (although not always identified on MRI). An association of low back pain (Bertolotti's syndrome) remains controversial, but there is an increased risk of disc degeneration at the level above the LSTV.
Limbus vertebra	5–20%	Limbus vertebra is a well-corticated osseous density, usually of the anterosuperior vertebral body corner, that occurs secondary to herniation of the nucleus pulposus through the vertebral body endplate beneath the ring apophysis. These are closely related to Schmorl nodes and should not be confused with limbus fractures. Limbus vertebrae should be well corticated and occupy the expected location of a normal vertebral body corner; the anterosuperior corner of a single vertebral body in the mid lumbar spine is the most common presentation.
Conjoined lumbosacral nerve roots (CNR)	6–8%	CNR is the most common nerve root developmental anomaly of the cauda equina (twice as common as two roots in the same foramen, the next most common anomaly). CNR are two adjacent nerve roots which share a common dural envelope at some time during their coursing from the thecal sac. Multimodality imaging incidence is reported in 6% of MRI and 8% of cadaveric studies. CNR should be considered in the differential diagnosis of herniated intervertebral discs. CNR occur in over 5% of cases which were classified preoperatively as 'disc herniation'. Postarachnoiditic adhesions of the cauda may appear similar. Inadvertent nerve root injury/battered nerve syndrome can result if the second nerve in the field is not appreciated. Diagnosis can be made with high-quality MRI with coronal views (still challenging despite improvements in technology) or intraoperatively. CNR itself does not usually cause symptoms alone. The clinical picture that should raise awareness is a prodrome of claudication with or without radiculopathy. Decompression of the bony canal of the nerve root exit zone is performed with outcomes comparable to those of disc herniations, provided surgical management addresses the pathology of lateral recess stenosis.
Arcuate foramen	8%	The arcuate foramen (or foramen arcuale atlantis, posterior ponticle, ponticulus posticus or Kimerle foramen) is a common normal variant of the atlas, easily appreciated on a lateral plain film of the cranio-cervical junction. It is an osseous/calcific bridge from the posterior aspects of the lateral mass of the atlas to the posterior arch, forming an arch. It is thought to develop by calcification/ossification of the oblique atlanto-occipital ligaments. The atlantic portion (V3) of the vertebral arteries passes through this foramen. Incidence range is 1–15% and is more common in females. It has a variable morphology and may be complete or incomplete, unilateral or bilateral and is associated with tethering and dissection of the vertebral artery from repetitive cervical flexion-extension. It is linked to upper cervical syndrome, vertigo, Barre-Lieou syndrome and common migraines.
Atlanto-occipital assimilation (AOA)	0.25–1%	AOA is typically asymptomatic, but symptoms from neurovascular compression can occur. Fusion of C1 to the occiput can be either **complete** (C1 not identifiable) or **incomplete** (C1 partially identifiable). AOA is associated with fusion of C2-C3 (in 50%), basilar invagination, cleft palate, cervical ribs and urinary tract anomalies.

MRI, *Magnetic resonance imaging.*

5 | Upper limb

(a) Shoulder, anteroposterior radiograph.

1. Acromion of scapula
2. Anatomical neck of humerus
3. Clavicle
4. Coracoid process of scapula
5. Glenoid fossa of scapula
6. Greater tubercle (tuberosity) of humerus
7. Head of humerus
8. Lesser tubercle (tuberosity) of humerus
9. Scapula
10. Surgical neck of humerus

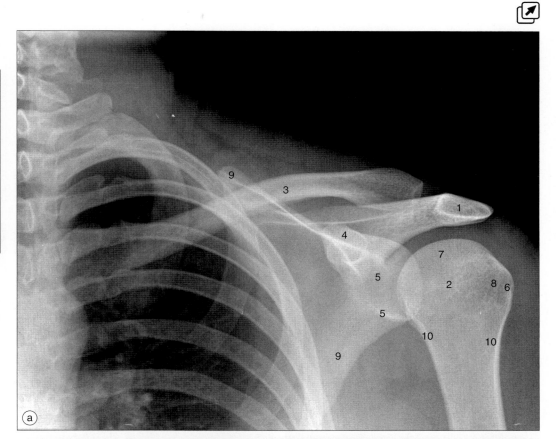

(b) Shoulder, axial (supero-inferior) radiograph.

1. Acromion of scapula
2. Clavicle
3. Coracoid process of scapula
4. Glenoid fossa of scapula
5. Greater tubercle (tuberosity) of humerus
6. Head of humerus
7. Intertubercular groove of humerus
8. Lesser tubercle (tuberosity) of humerus
9. Spine of scapula

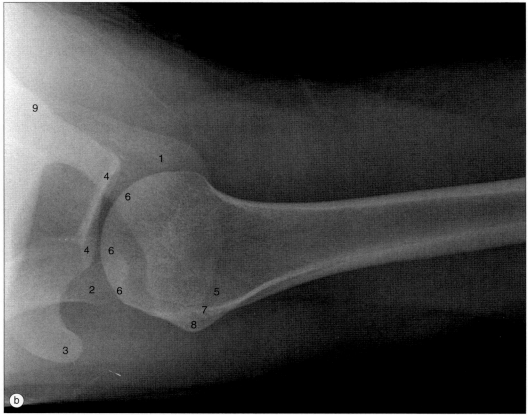

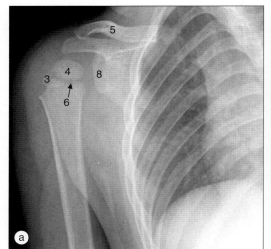

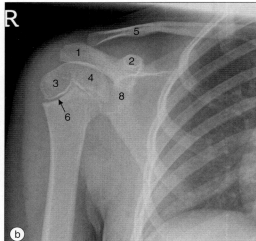

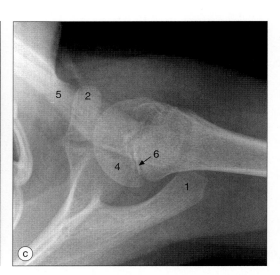

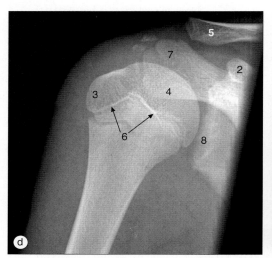

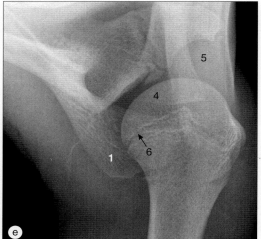

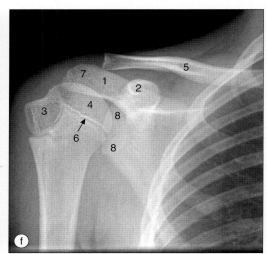

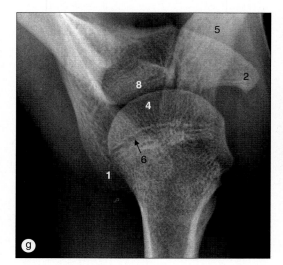

Shoulder, (a) anteroposterior radiograph of a 1-year-old child, (b) anteroposterior radiograph and (c) axial radiographs of a 6-year-old child, (d) anteroposterior and (e) axial radiographs of a 12-year-old child, (f) anteroposterior and (g) axial radiographs of a 14-year-old child.

1. Acromion of scapula
2. Centre for coracoid process
3. Centre for greater tubercle (tuberosity) of humerus
4. Centre for head of humerus
5. Clavicle
6. Epiphysial line
7. Centre for acromion (multicentric)
8. Glenoid fossa of scapula

Clavicle (m)	Appears	Fused
Lateral end	5 wiu	20 + yrs
Medial end	15 yrs	20 + yrs
Scapula (c)		
Body	8 wiu	15 yrs
Coracoid	<1 yr	20 yrs
Coracoid base	Puberty	15–20 yrs
Acromion	Puberty	15–20 yrs

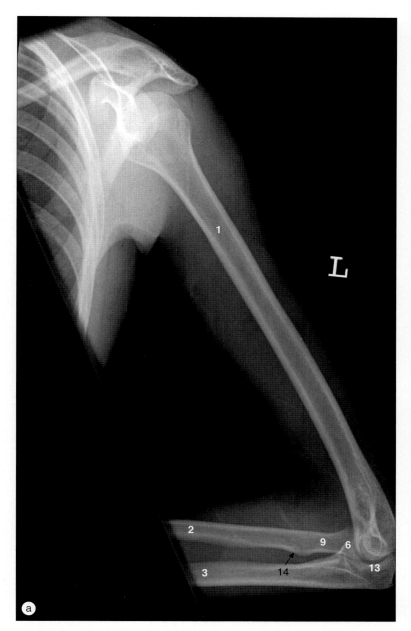

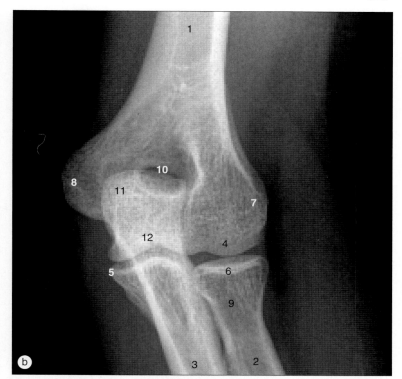

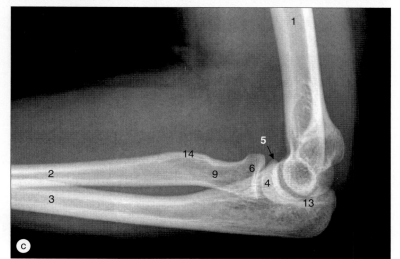

(a) Humerus, lateral radiograph, (b) elbow, anteroposterior radiograph, (c) elbow, lateral radiograph.

1. Humerus
2. Radius
3. Ulna
4. Capitulum of humerus
5. Coronoid process of ulna
6. Head of radius
7. Lateral epicondyle of humerus
8. Medial epicondyle of humerus
9. Neck of radius
10. Olecranon fossa of humerus
11. Olecranon of ulna
12. Trochlea of humerus
13. Trochlear notch of ulna
14. Tuberosity of radius

Humerus (c)	Appears	Fused
Shaft	8 wiu	15–20 yrs
Head	1–6 mths	15–20 yrs
Greater tubercle	6 mths–1 yr	15–20 yrs
Lesser tubercle	3–5 yrs	18–20 yrs
Capitulum	4 mths–1 yr	13–16 yrs
Medial trochlea	10 yrs	13–16 yrs
Medial epicondyle	3–6 yrs	13–16 yrs
Lateral epicondyle	9–12 yrs	13–16 yrs

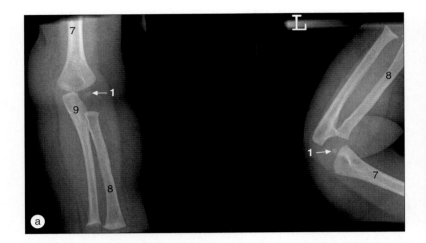

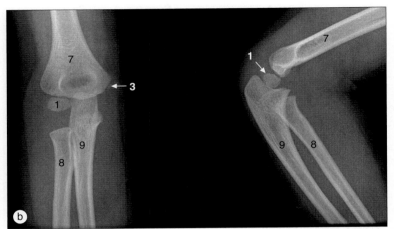

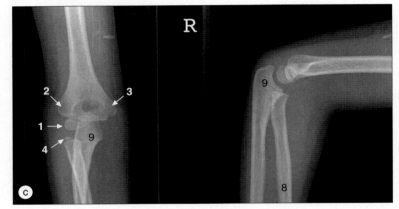

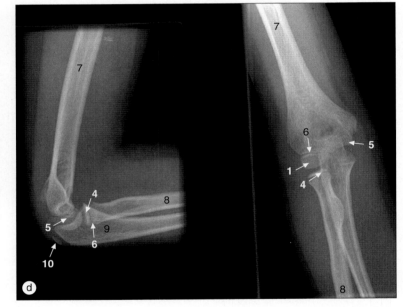

Elbow radiographs, (a) 7-month-old child, (b) 3-year-old child, (c) 6-year-old child, (d) 9-year-old child.

Radius (c)	Appears	Fused
Shaft	8 wiu	
Proximal	4–6 yrs	13–16 yrs
Distal	1 yr	16–18 yrs
Ulna (c)		
Shaft	8 wiu	
Proximal	8–10 yrs	13–15 yrs
Distal	5–7 yrs	16–18 yrs

1. Centre for capitulum
2. Centre for lateral epicondyle
3. Centre for medial epicondyle
4. Centre for radial head
5. Centre for trochlea
6. Epiphysial line
7. Humerus
8. Radius
9. Ulna
10. Centre for olecranon

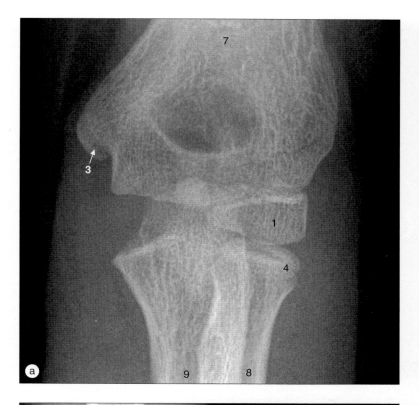

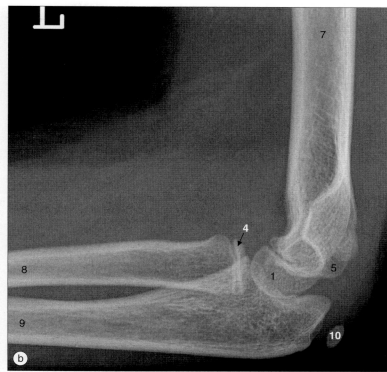

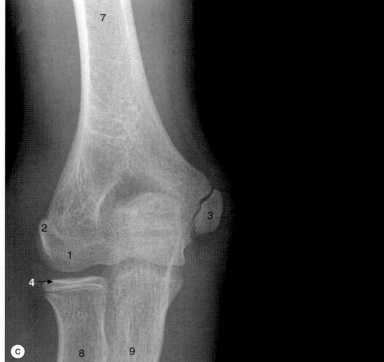

Elbow radiographs, (a) and (b) 11-year-old child, (c) and (d) 14-year-old child.

1. Centre for capitulum
2. Centre for lateral epicondyle
3. Centre for medial epicondyle
4. Centre for radial head
5. Centre for trochlea
6. Epiphyseal line
7. Humerus
8. Radius
9. Ulna
10. Centre for olecranon

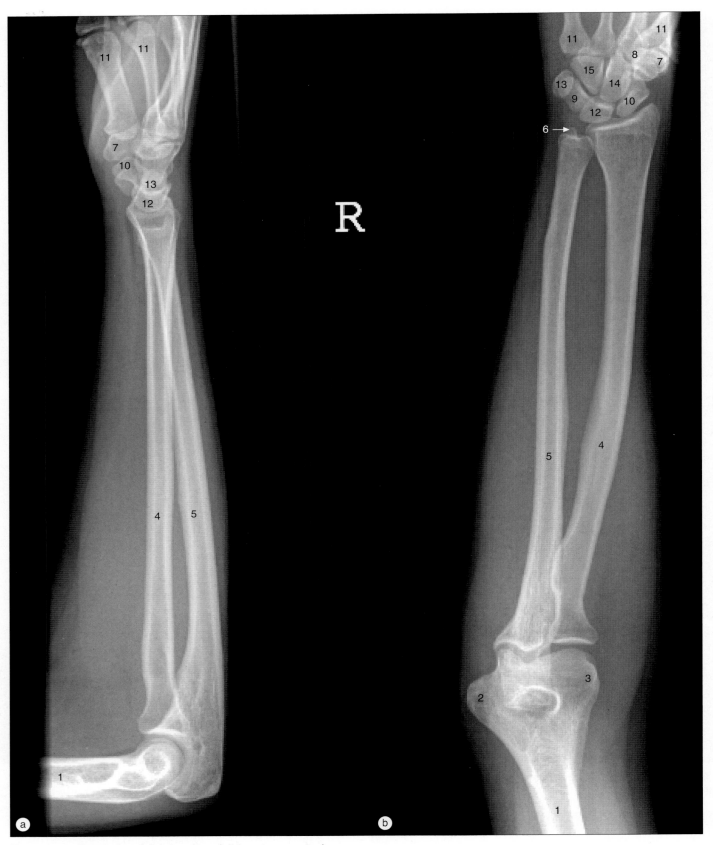

Forearm radiographs, (a) lateral and (b) anteroposterior.

1. Humerus
2. Medial epicondyle of humerus
3. Lateral epicondyle of humerus
4. Radius
5. Ulna
6. Styloid of ulna
7. Trapezium
8. Trapezoid
9. Triquetral
10. Scaphoid
11. Metacarpals
12. Lunate
13. Pisiform
14. Capitate
15. Hamate

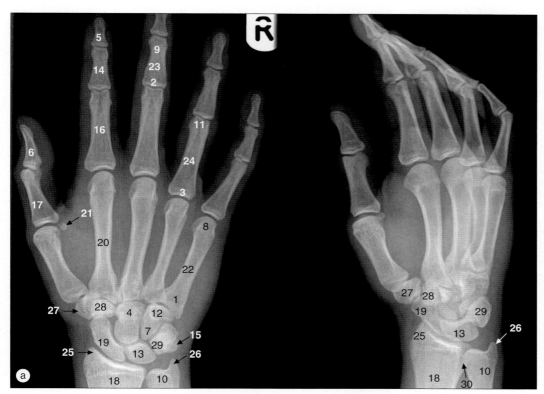

(a) Bones of the hand, dorsopalmar and oblique radiographs.

1. Base of fifth metacarpal	**12.** Hook of hamate	**23.** Shaft of middle phalanx of middle finger
2. Base of middle phalanx of middle finger	**13.** Lunate	**24.** Shaft of proximal phalanx of ring finger
3. Base of proximal phalanx of ring finger	**14.** Middle phalanx of index finger	**25.** Styloid process of radius
4. Capitate	**15.** Pisiform	**26.** Styloid process of ulna
5. Distal phalanx of index finger	**16.** Proximal phalanx of index finger	**27.** Trapezium
6. Distal phalanx of thumb	**17.** Proximal phalanx of thumb	**28.** Trapezoid
7. Hamate	**18.** Radius	**29.** Triquetral
8. Head of fifth metacarpal	**19.** Scaphoid	**30.** Ulnar notch of radius
9. Head of middle phalanx of middle finger	**20.** Second metacarpal	**31.** Base of metacarpal
10. Head of ulna	**21.** Sesamoid bone	
11. Head of proximal phalanx of ring finger	**22.** Shaft of fifth metacarpal	

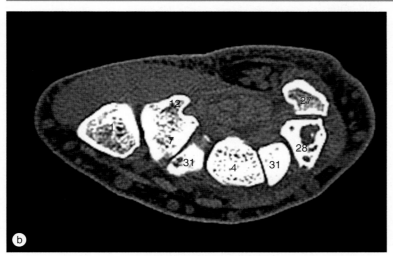

(b) Axial CT image through carpal tunnel.

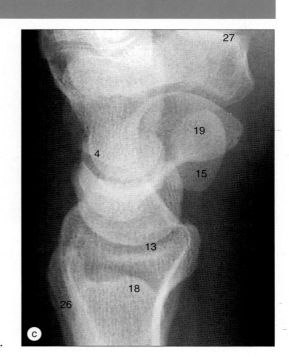

(c) Bones of the wrist, lateral radiograph.

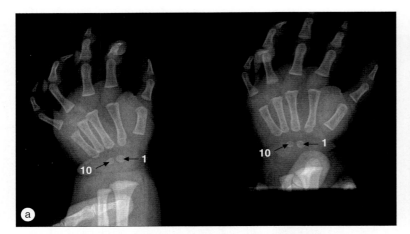

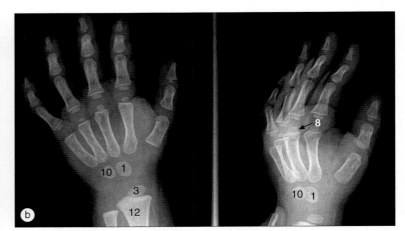

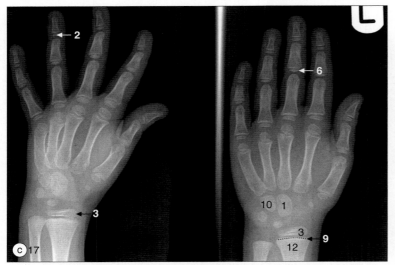

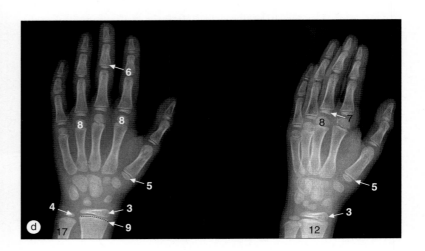

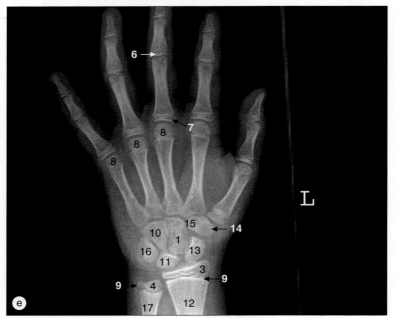

Bones of the hand (dorsopalmar radiographs), (a) of a
10-month-old child, (b) of a 2-year-old child, (c) of a 6-year-old
child, (d) of a 9-year-old child, to illustrate centres of
ossification, (e) of an 11-year-old child.

Carpus (c)	Appears	Fused
Capitate	1–3 mths	
Hamate	2–4 mths	
Triquetral	2–3 yrs	
Lunate	2–4 yrs	
Scaphoid	4–6 yrs	
Trapezium	4–6 yrs	
Trapezoid	4–6 yrs	
Pisiform (sesamoid)	8–12 yrs	
Metacarpals (c)		
Shaft	9 wiu	
Head	1–2 yrs	14–19 yrs
Phalanges (c)		
Shaft	8–12 wiu	
Base	1–3 yrs	14–18 yrs

1. Capitate
2. Centre for distal phalanx of ring finger
3. Centre for distal radius
4. Centre for distal ulna
5. Centre for first metacarpal
6. Centre for middle phalanx of middle finger
7. Centre for proximal phalanx of middle finger
8. Centre for second metacarpal (applies
   to second to fifth metacarpals)
9. Epiphysial line
10. Hamate
11. Lunate
12. Radius
13. Scaphoid
14. Trapezium
15. Trapezoid
16. Triquetral
17. Ulna

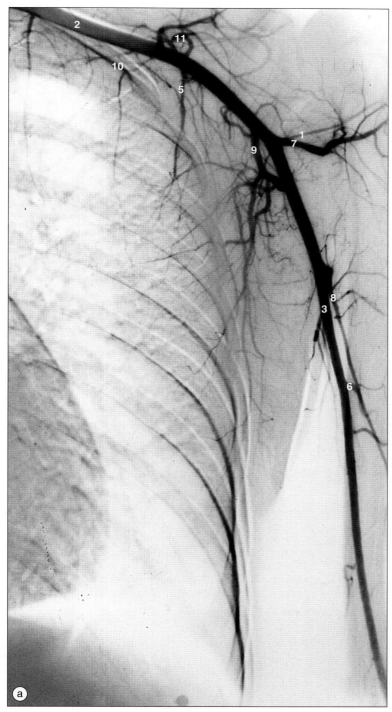

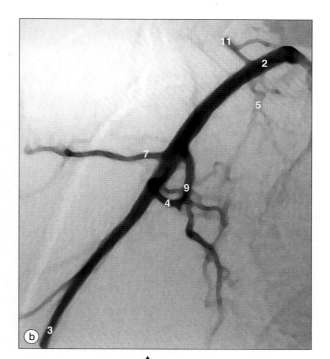

1. Anterior circumflex
   humeral artery
2. Axillary artery
3. Brachial artery
4. Circumflex scapular artery
5. Lateral thoracic artery
6. Muscular branches of
   brachial artery
7. Posterior circumflex
   humeral artery
8. Profunda brachii artery
9. Subscapular artery
10. Superior thoracic artery
11. Thoraco-acromial artery

Axillary arteriograms, (a) subtracted, (b) digitally subtracted,
(c) and (d) brachial arteriograms.

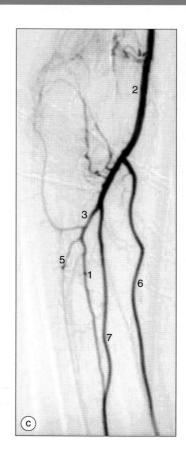

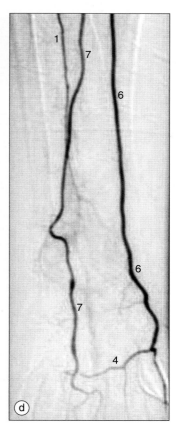

1. Anterior interosseous artery
2. Brachial artery
3. Common interosseous artery
4. Deep palmar arch
5. Posterior interosseous artery
6. Radial artery
7. Ulnar artery

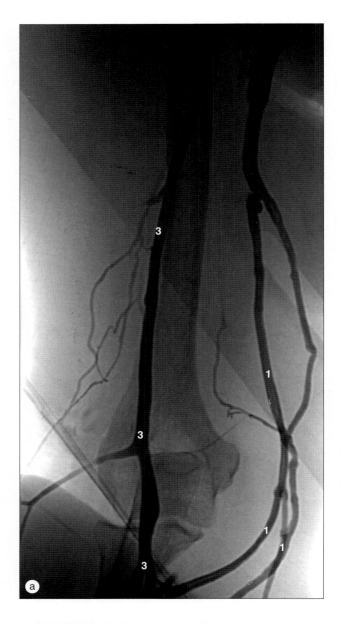

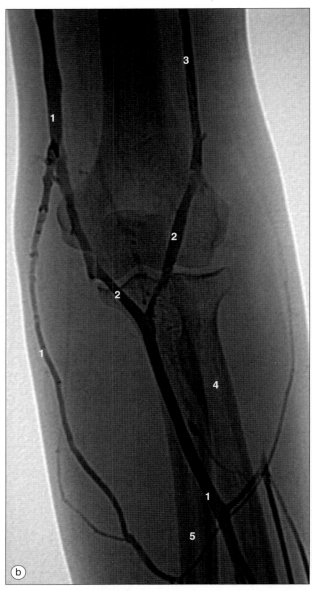

(a) and (b) Upper limb venograms, (c) superior vena cavogram.

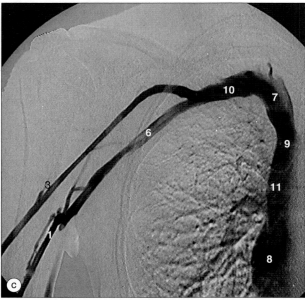

1. Basilic vein
2. Median cubital vein
3. Cephalic vein
4. Radius
5. Ulna
6. Axillary vein
7. Brachiocephalic vein
8. Right atrium
9. Site of entry of left brachiocephalic vein
10. Subclavian vein
11. Superior vena cava

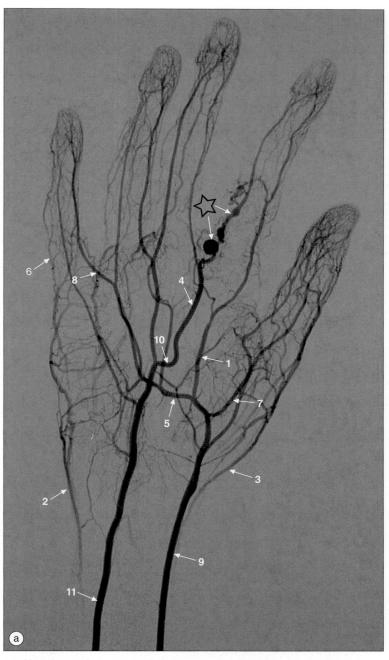

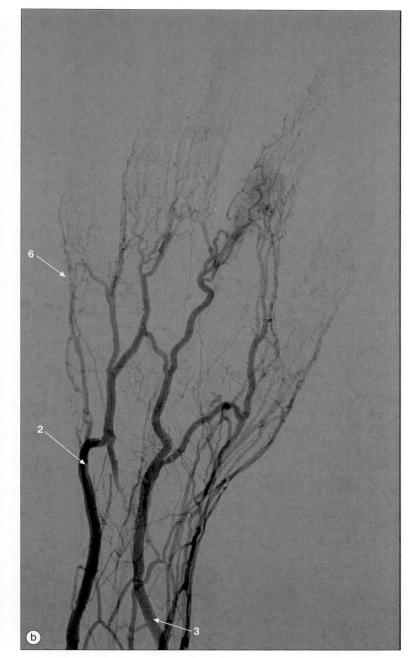

(a) Hand arteriogram and (b) venogram (digital subtraction).
Note venous component of arteriovenous malformation
(unlabelled) in figure (b).
With permission from Standring, S, Gray's Anatomy: The
Anatomical Basis of Clinical Practice, 41st ed, 2015, London,
Elsevier. Figure 065043f & Figure 065043k. *aneurysm index
finger.

1. Arteria radialis indicis
2. Basilic vein
3. Cephalic vein
4. Common palmar digital artery
5. Deep palmar arch
6. Digital vein
7. Princeps pollicis artery

8. Proper palmar digital artery (little finger)
9. Radial artery
10. Superficial palmar arch (incomplete)
11. Ulnar artery
☆. Arteriovenous malformation of digital artery of index finger.

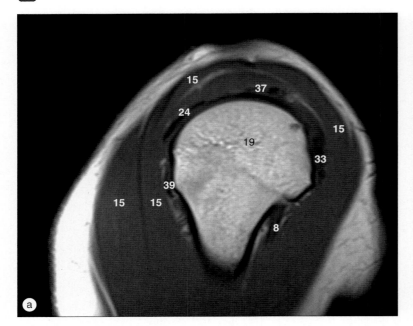

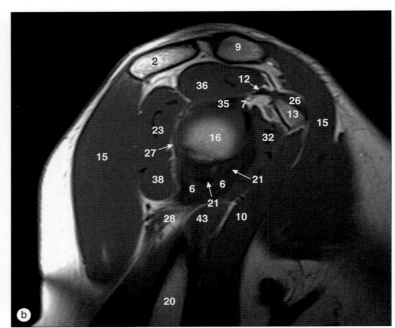

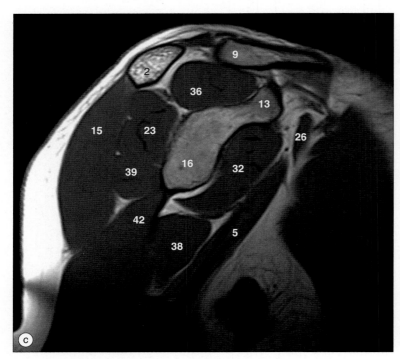

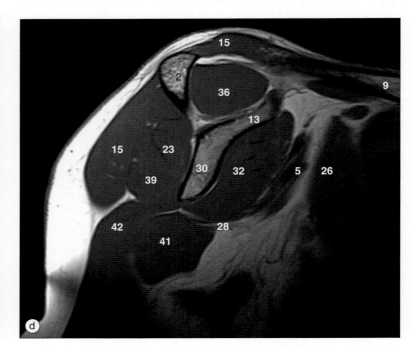

Shoulder, sagittal MR images, from medial to lateral.

1. Acromioclavicular joint	**6.** Axillary recess of glenohumeral joint	**12.** Coracohumeral ligament
2. Acromion	**7.** Biceps brachii muscle, short head	**13.** Coracoid process
3. Anterior capsule of shoulder joint	**8.** Biceps brachii tendon, long head	**14.** Deltoid tendon
4. Anterior labrum	**9.** Clavicle	**15.** Deltoid muscle
5. Axillary vessels (and surrounding brachial plexus cords)	**10.** Coracobrachialis muscle	**16.** Glenoid of scapula
	11. Coracoclavicular ligament	**17.** Glenoid fossa

Numbers 1–43 are common to pages 76–77.

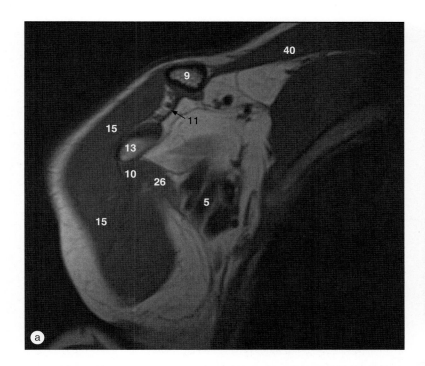

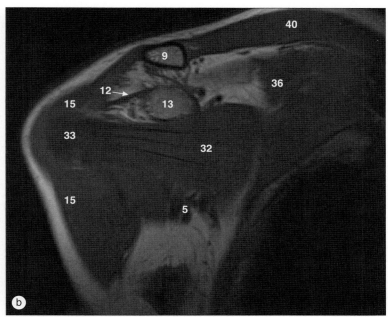

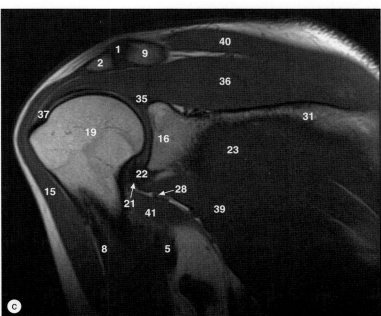

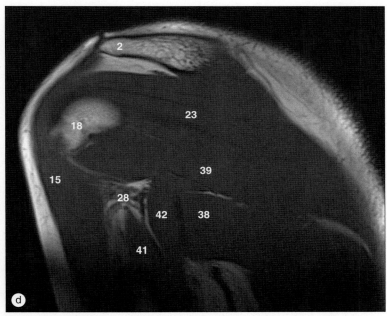

Shoulder, coronal MR images, from anterior to posterior.

18. Greater tuberosity of humerus	**27.** Posterior part of capsule of shoulder joint	**35.** Superior glenoid labrum
19. Head of humerus	**28.** Posterior circumflex humeral vessels	**36.** Supraspinatus muscle
20. Humerus	(and axillary nerve)	**37.** Supraspinatus tendon
21. Inferior glenohumeral ligament	**29.** Posterior glenoid labrum	**38.** Teres major muscle
22. Inferior glenoid labrum	**30.** Scapula	**39.** Teres minor muscle
23. Infraspinatus muscle	**31.** Spine of scapula	**40.** Trapezius muscle
24. Infraspinatus tendon	**32.** Subscapularis muscle	**41.** Triceps brachii muscle, medial head
25. Middle glenohumeral ligament	**33.** Subscapularis tendon	**42.** Triceps brachii muscle, lateral head
26. Pectoralis minor muscle	**34.** Superior glenohumeral ligament	**43.** Triceps brachii muscle, long head

Numbers 1–43 are common to pages 76–77.

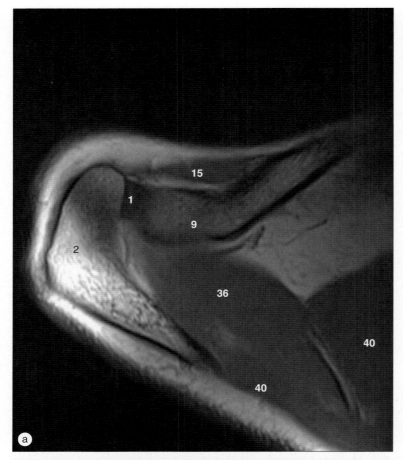

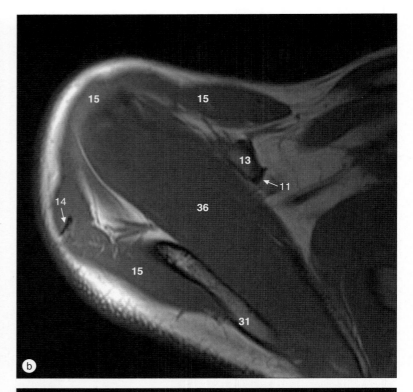

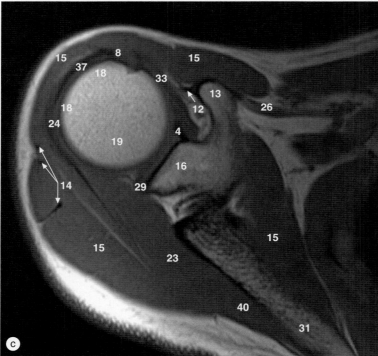

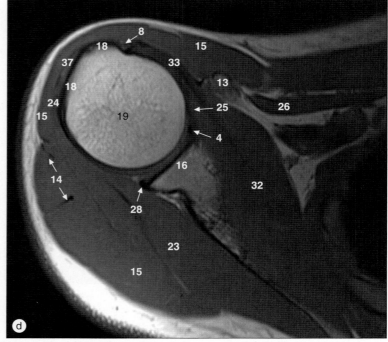

Shoulder, axial MR images, from superior to inferior.

1. Acromioclavicular joint	6. Axillary recess of glenohumeral joint	12. Coracohumeral ligament
2. Acromion	7. Biceps brachii muscle, short head	13. Coracoid process
3. Anterior capsule of shoulder joint	8. Biceps brachii tendon, long head	14. Deltoid tendon
4. Anterior labrum	9. Clavicle	15. Deltoid muscle
5. Axillary vessels (and surrounding brachial plexus cords)	10. Coracobrachialis muscle	16. Glenoid of scapula
	11. Coracoclavicular ligament	17. Glenoid fossa

Numbers 1–43 are common to pages 78–79.

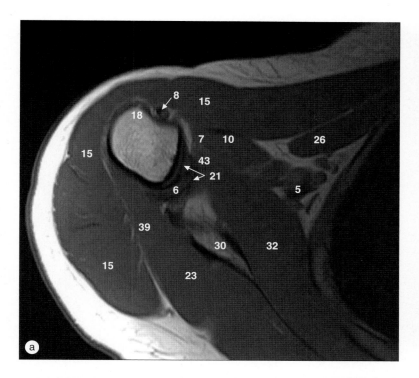

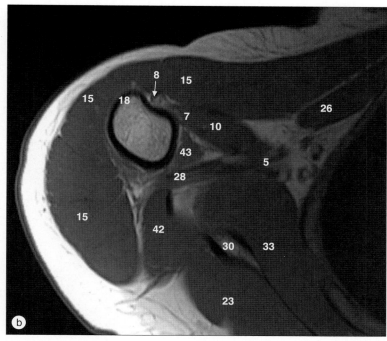

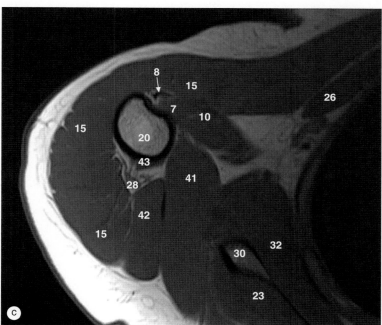

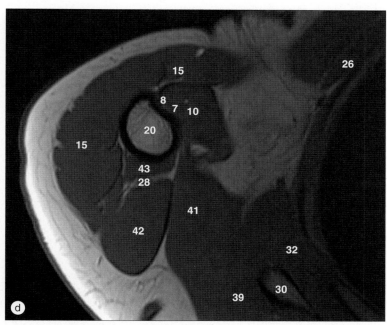

Shoulder, axial MR images, from superior to inferior.

18. Greater tuberosity of humerus
19. Head of humerus
20. Humerus
21. Inferior glenohumeral ligament
22. Inferior glenoid labrum
23. Infraspinatus muscle
24. Infraspinatus tendon
25. Middle glenohumeral ligament
26. Pectoralis minor muscle

27. Posterior part of capsule of shoulder joint
28. Posterior circumflex humeral vessels (and axillary nerve)
29. Posterior glenoid labrum
30. Scapula
31. Spine of scapula
32. Subscapularis muscle
33. Subscapularis tendon
34. Superior glenohumeral ligament

35. Superior glenoid labrum
36. Supraspinatus muscle
37. Supraspinatus tendon
38. Teres major muscle
39. Teres minor muscle
40. Trapezius muscle
41. Triceps brachii muscle, medial head
42. Triceps brachii muscle, lateral head
43. Triceps brachii muscle, long head

Numbers 1–43 are common to pages 78–79.

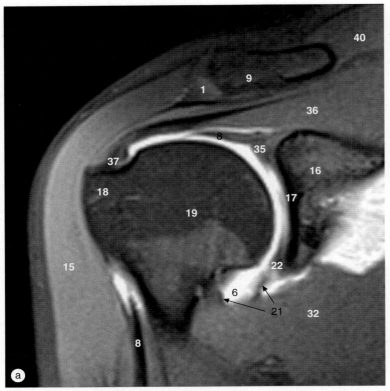

(a) Shoulder, coronal T1-weighted fat-saturated MR arthrogram.

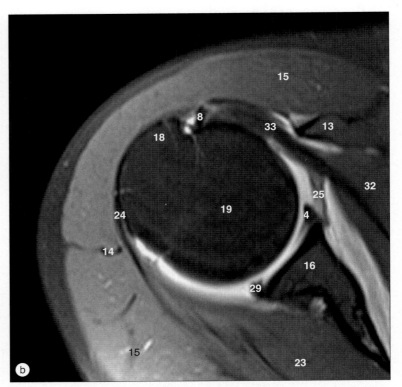

(b) Shoulder, axial T1-weighted fat-saturated MR arthrogram.

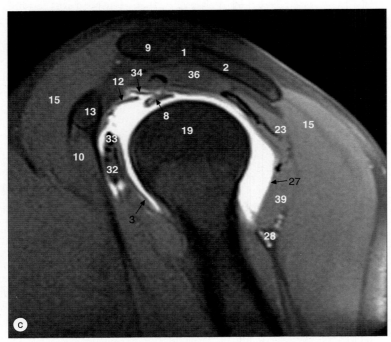

(c) Shoulder, sagittal T1-weighted fat-saturated MR arthrogram.

For label key see pages 76–77 and pages 78–79.

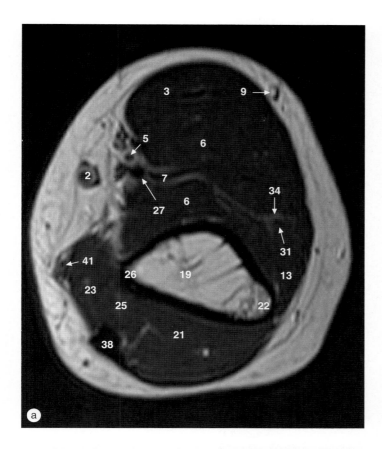

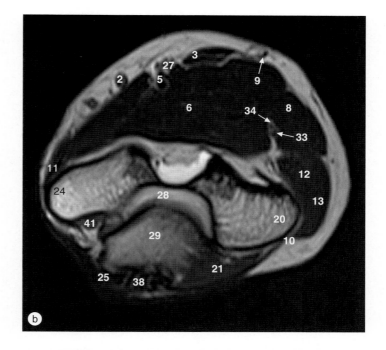

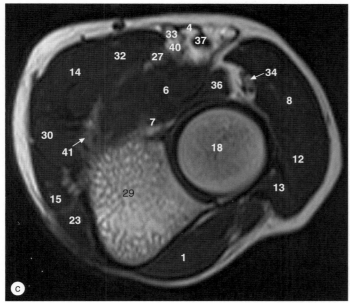

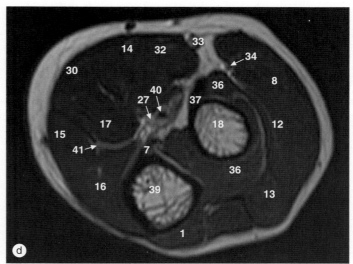

Elbow, axial MR images, from superior to inferior.

1. Anconeus muscle	13. Extensor carpi radialis longus muscle	22. Lateral supracondylar ridge	35. Radius
2. Basilic vein	14. Flexor carpi radialis muscle	23. Long head of triceps muscle	36. Supinator muscle
3. Biceps brachii muscle	15. Flexor carpi ulnaris muscle	24. Medial epicondyle	37. Tendon of biceps brachii muscle
4. Bicipital aponeurosis	16. Flexor digitorum profundus muscle	25. Medial head of triceps muscle	38. Tendon of triceps brachii muscle
5. Brachial artery	17. Flexor digitorum superficialis muscle	26. Medial supracondylar ridge	39. Ulna
6. Brachialis muscle	18. Head of radius	27. Median nerve	40. Ulnar artery
7. Brachialis tendon	19. Humerus	28. Olecranon fossa of humerus	41. Ulnar nerve
8. Brachioradialis muscle	20. Lateral epicondyle	29. Olecranon process of ulna	
9. Cephalic vein	21. Lateral head of triceps brachii muscle	30. Palmaris longus muscle	
10. Common extensor origin		31. Profunda brachii artery	
11. Common flexor origin		32. Pronator teres muscle	
12. Extensor carpi radialis brevis muscle		33. Radial artery	
		34. Radial nerve	

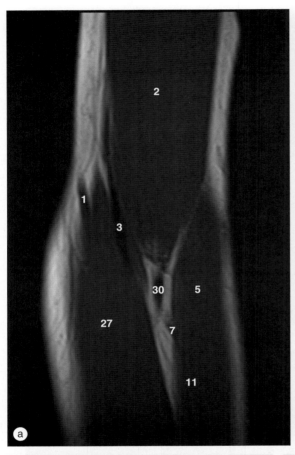

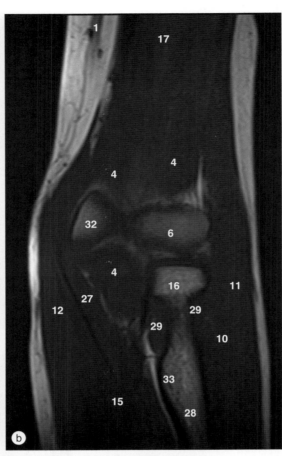

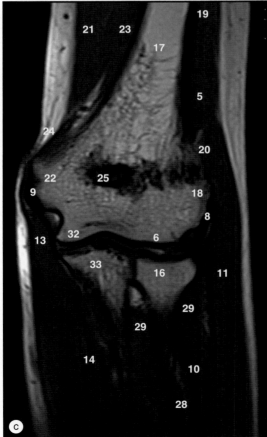

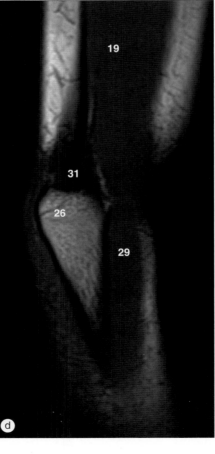

1. Basilic vein
2. Biceps brachii muscle
3. Brachial artery
4. Brachialis muscle
5. Brachioradialis muscle
6. Capitulum of humerus
7. Cephalic vein
8. Common extensor origin
9. Common flexor origin
10. Extensor carpi radialis brevis muscle
11. Extensor carpi radialis longus muscle
12. Flexor carpi radialis muscle
13. Flexor carpi ulnaris muscle
14. Flexor digitorum profundus muscle
15. Flexor digitorum superficialis muscle
16. Head of radius
17. Humerus
18. Lateral epicondyle
19. Lateral head of triceps muscle
20. Lateral supracondylar ridge
21. Long head of triceps muscle
22. Medial epicondyle
23. Medial head of triceps muscle
24. Medial supracondylar ridge
25. Olecranon fossa of humerus
26. Olecranon process of ulnar
27. Pronator teres muscle
28. Radius
29. Supinator muscle
30. Tendon of biceps brachii muscle
31. Tendon of triceps muscle
32. Trochlea of humerus
33. Tuberosity of radius
34. Ulnar

Elbow, coronal MR images, from anterior to posterior.

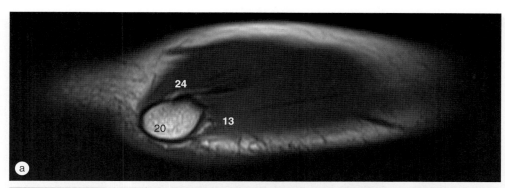

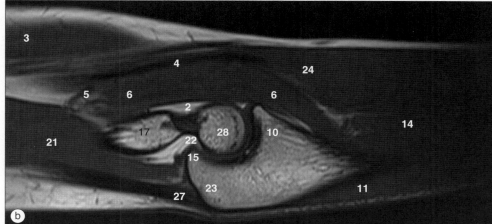

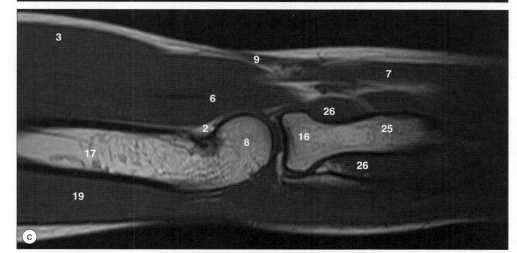

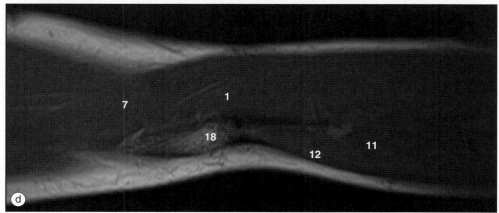

1. Abductor pollicis longus
2. Anterior fat pad
3. Biceps brachii muscle
4. Biceps brachii tendon
5. Brachial artery
6. Brachialis muscle
7. Brachioradialis muscle
8. Capitulum of humerus
9. Cephalic vein
10. Coronoid process
11. Extensor carpi radialis brevis
12. Extensor carpi radialis longus
13. Flexor carpi ulnaris
14. Flexor digitorum profundus muscle
15. Flexor digitorum superficialis muscle
16. Head of radius
17. Humerus
18. Lateral epicondyle
19. Lateral head of triceps muscle
20. Medial epicondyle
21. Medial head of triceps muscle
22. Olecranon fossa of humerus
23. Olecranon process of ulna
24. Pronator teres muscle
25. Radius
26. Supinator muscle
27. Tendon of triceps muscle
28. Trochlea of humerus

Elbow, sagittal MR images, from medial to lateral.

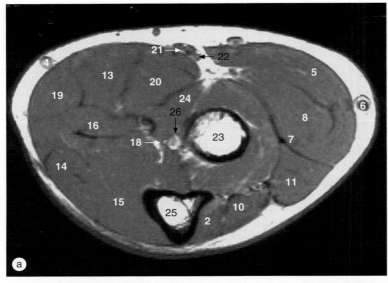

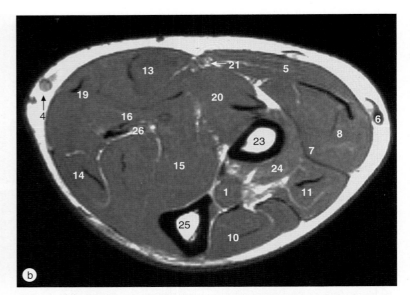

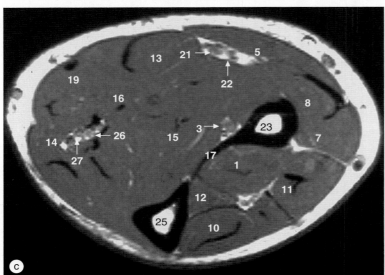

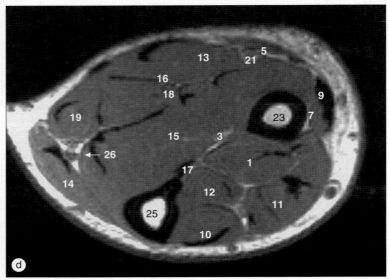

(a)–(d) Forearm, axial MR images, from superior to inferior.

1. Abductor pollicis longus muscle	10. Extensor carpi ulnaris muscle	19. Palmaris longus muscle
2. Anconeus muscle	11. Extensor digitorum muscle	20. Pronator teres muscle
3. Anterior interosseous artery	12. Extensor pollicis longus muscle	21. Radial artery
4. Basilic vein	13. Flexor carpi radialis muscle	22. Radial nerve
5. Brachioradialis muscle	14. Flexor carpi ulnaris muscle	23. Radius
6. Cephalic vein	15. Flexor digitorum profundus muscle	24. Supinator muscle
7. Extensor carpi radialis brevis muscle	16. Flexor digitorum superficialis muscle	25. Ulna
8. Extensor carpi radialis longus muscle	17. Interosseous membrane	26. Ulnar artery
9. Extensor carpi radialis longus tendon	18. Median nerve	27. Ulnar nerve

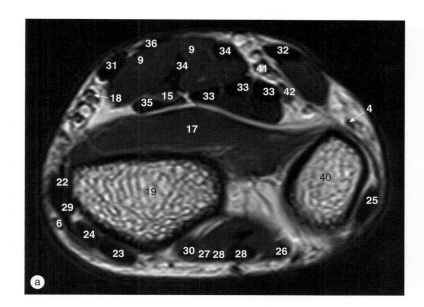

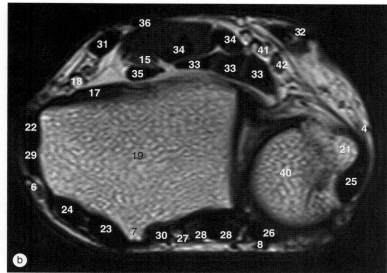

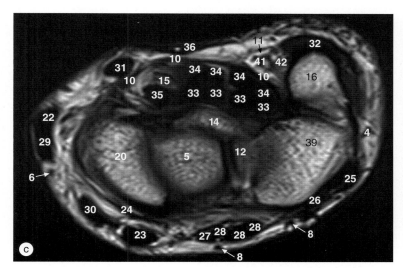

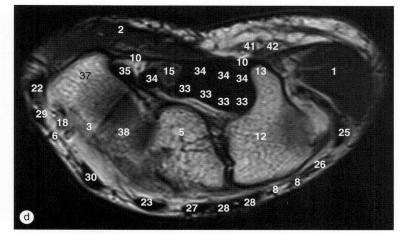

Wrist, axial MR images, from superior to inferior.

1. Abductor digiti minimi muscle	17. Pronator quadratus muscle	30. Tendon of extensor pollicis longus muscle
2. Abductor pollicis brevis muscle	18. Radial artery	31. Tendon of flexor carpi radialis muscle
3. Base of first metacarpal	19. Radius	32. Tendon of flexor carpi ulnaris muscle
4. Basilic vein	20. Scaphoid	33. Tendon of flexor digitorum profundus muscle
5. Capitate	21. Styloid process of ulna	
6. Cephalic vein	22. Tendon of abductor pollicis longus muscle	34. Tendon of flexor digitorum superficialis muscle
7. Dorsal tubercle of radius	23. Tendon of extensor carpi radialis brevis muscle	35. Tendon of flexor pollicis longus muscle
8. Dorsal venous arch		36. Tendon of palmaris longus muscle
9. Flexor digitorum superficialis muscle	24. Tendon of extensor carpi radialis longus muscle	37. Trapezium
10. Flexor retinaculum	25. Tendon of extensor carpi ulnaris muscle	38. Trapezoid
11. Guyon's canal	26. Tendon of extensor digiti minimi muscle	39. Triquetral
12. Hamate	27. Tendon of extensor indicis muscle	40. Ulna
13. Hook of hamate	28. Tendon of extensor digitorum muscle	41. Ulnar artery
14. Lunate	29. Tendon of extensor pollicis brevis muscle	42. Ulnar nerve
15. Median nerve		
16. Pisiform		

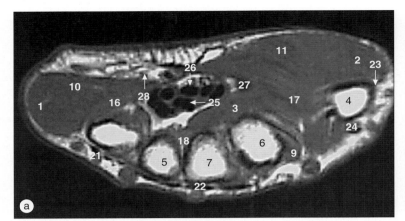

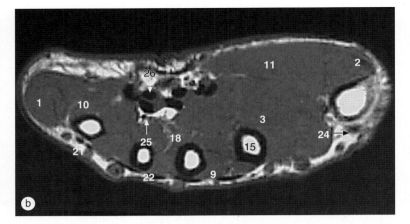

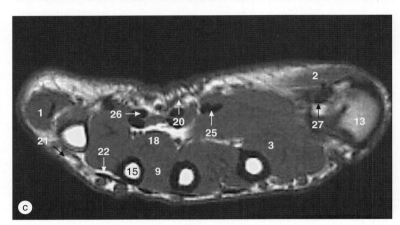

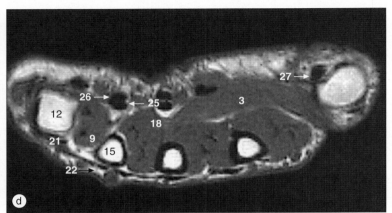

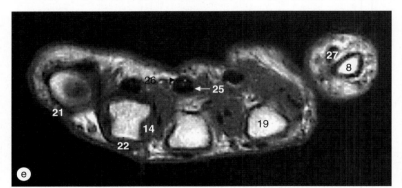

(a)–(e) Hand, axial MR images, from superior to inferior.

1. Abductor digiti minimi muscle
2. Abductor pollicis brevis muscle
3. Adductor pollicis muscle
4. Base of first metacarpal
5. Base of fourth metacarpal
6. Base of second metacarpal
7. Base of third metacarpal
8. Distal phalanx of thumb
9. Dorsal interossei muscles
10. Flexor digiti minimi muscle
11. Flexor pollicis brevis muscle
12. Head of fifth metacarpal
13. Head of first metacarpal
14. Lumbrical muscle
15. Metacarpal shaft
16. Opponens digiti minimi muscle
17. Opponens pollicis muscle
18. Palmar interossei muscles
19. Proximal phalanx of index finger
20. Superficial palmar arch
21. Tendon of extensor digiti minimi muscle
22. Tendon of extensor digitorum muscle
23. Tendon of extensor pollicis brevis muscle
24. Tendon of extensor pollicis longus muscle
25. Tendon of flexor digitorum profundus muscle
26. Tendon of flexor digitorum superficialis muscle
27. Tendon of flexor pollicis longus muscle
28. Ulnar artery

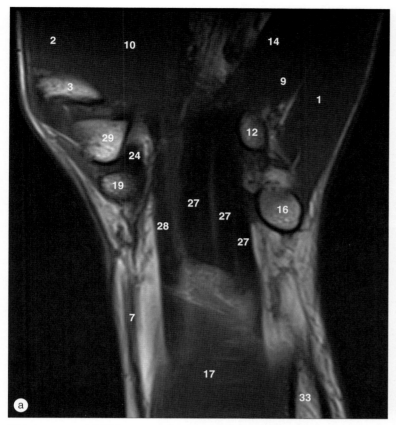

Wrist, coronal MR images, from anterior to posterior.

1. Abductor digiti minimi muscle	**14.** Opponens digiti minimi muscle	**26.** Tendon of flexor digitorum profundus muscle
2. Abductor pollicis brevis muscle	**15.** Palmar interossei muscle	**27.** Tendon of flexor digitorum superficialis muscle
3. Base of first metacarpal	**16.** Pisiform	
4. Base of third metacarpal	**17.** Pronator quadratus muscle	**28.** Tendon of flexor pollicis longus muscle
5. Base of fifth metacarpal	**18.** Radius (physeal scar)	**29.** Trapezium
6. Capitate	**19.** Scaphoid	**30.** Trapezoid
7. Cephalic vein	**20.** Scapholunate ligament	**31.** Triangular fibrocartilage
8. Distal radioulnar joint	**21.** Tendon of abductor pollicis longus muscle	**32.** Triquetral
9. Flexor digiti minimi muscle	**22.** Tendon of extensor carpi ulnaris muscle	**33.** Ulna
10. Flexor pollicis brevis	**23.** Tendon of extensor digitorum muscle	**34.** Ulnar styloid
11. Hamate	**24.** Tendon of flexor carpi radialis muscle	
12. Hook of hamate	**25.** Tendon of flexor carpi ulnaris muscle	
13. Lunate		

Numbers 1–34 are common to pages 87–88.

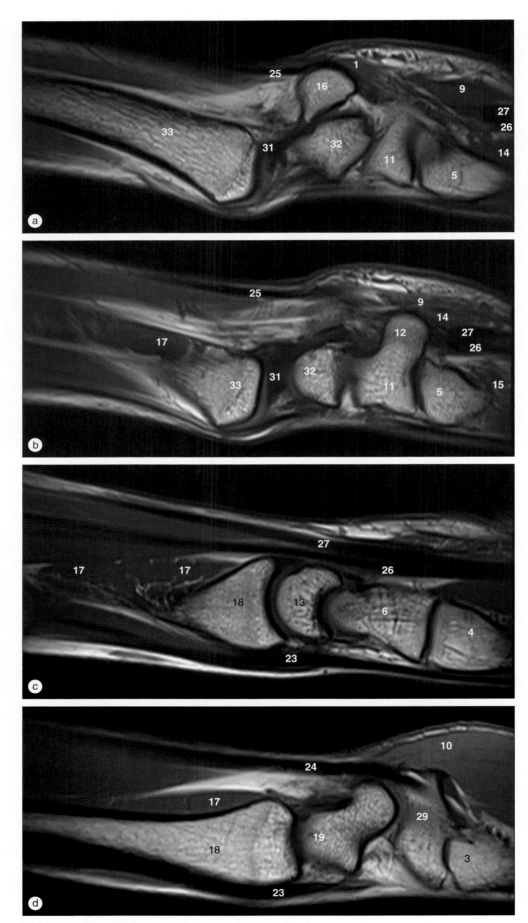

Wrist, sagittal MR images, from medial to lateral.

For label key see page 87.

Bonus e-materials

Slidelines for radiograph features:
Anteroposterior radiograph of the left shoulder,
Axial radiograph of the left shoulder,
Anteroposterior radiograph of the right elbow,
Lateral radiograph of the right elbow,
Dorsopalmar radiograph of the right wrist,
Lateral radiograph of the right wrist

Multi-tier labelling in slideshow/test yourself:
T1-weighted sagittal oblique MRI through the
shoulder

Selected pages from Imaging Atlas 4e

Tutorials: Tutorial 4

Ultrasound videos: Video 5.1 Dynamic
ultrasound of the extensor compartment of
the forearm (transverse), Video 5.2 Dynamic
ultrasound of the finger extensors at the
dorsal aspect of the wrist (transverse), Video
5.3 Dynamic ultrasound of flexor digitorum
tendons in the hand (longitudinal), Video 5.4
Dynamic ultrasound of flexor pollicis longus
(transverse)

Single best answer (SBA) self-assessment
questions

Table of Variations

Variant	Frequency	Clinical implications
Accessory head of flexor pollicis longus (Gantzer's muscle)	45–74%	May cause anterior interosseous nerve syndrome.
Accessory abductor digiti minimi	24%	Anterior to ulnar nerve in Guyon's canal, may cause ulnar nerve compression.
Radial artery origin from mid brachial artery	10–25%	Awareness in harvesting for CABG, forearm flaps, fistula for renal dialysis.
Accessory extensor carpi radialis brevis	12–24%	Mimics forearm soft tissue mass and causes false diagnosis of split tendon to ECR in second extensor compartment.
Sublabral foramen glenohumeral joint	14% (7–40%)	Mistaken for labral tear on MR arthrography. May vary from few millimeters to whole of the anterosuperior quadrant, age-related; 19–24 yrs 7% and 61–96 yrs 40%. Associated with increased incidence of cordlike middle glenohumeral ligament.
Anconeus epitrochlearis	11%	Parallels cubital tunnel retinaculum at elbow; association with cubital tunnel syndrome.
Palmaris longus (muscular variant)	7%	May cause pseudomass in forearm or median or ulnar nerve compression; commonly overlooked on MRI.
Accessory flexor digitorum superficialis	3%	May cause pseudomass in palm; associated with carpal tunnel syndrome (originates from FDS beneath flexor retinaculum).
Extensor digitorum brevis manus	1.6%	Pseudomass on dorsum of hand; often clinically misdiagnosed as ganglion, synovitis or carpal boss (originates in dorsal wrist capsule deep to extensor retinaculum). Can mimic giant cell tumour of tendon sheath on MRI (low T1 and T2 signal), but ultrasound reveals dynamic contraction. Usually painless, firms on finger extension – used surgically to repair ruptured tendons. Occasionally associated with extensor tendon tenosynovitis.
Radial artery axillary origin	1%	Awareness in harvesting for CABG, forearm flaps, fistula for renal dialysis.
Superficial ulnar artery at elbow/forearm	1–2%	Usually associated with high origin; mistaken for basilic vein and ligated in flap elevation; located underneath deep fascia.
Buford complex within glenohumeral joint	1.2–6.5%	Absent anterosuperior labrum and cordlike middle glenohumeral ligament replaces the functionality of the deficient labrum; mistaken for labral/ SLAP tear.

CABG, *Coronary artery bypass graft*; ECR, *extensor carpi radialis*; FDS, *flexor digitorum superficialis*; MR, *magnetic resonance*; MRI, *MR imaging*; SLAP, *superior labral anterior posterior*.

6 Breast and axilla

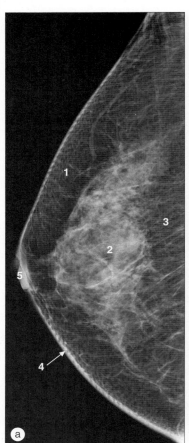

Craniocaudal (CC) view.

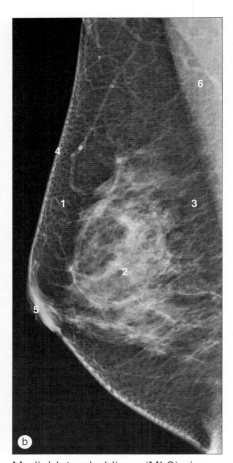

Medial lateral oblique (MLO) view.

1. Premammary zone
2. Mammary zone
3. Retromammary zone
4. Skin
5. Nipple
6. Pectoralis muscle

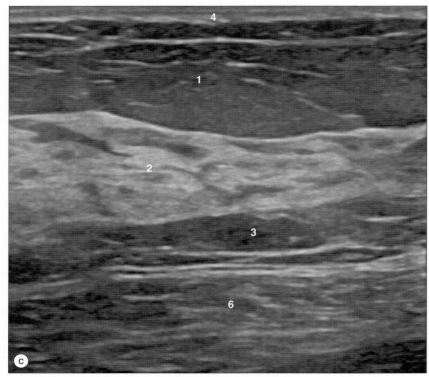

Ultrasound view.

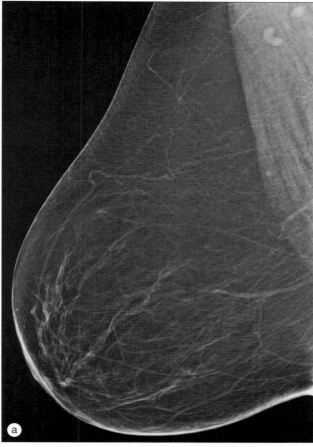

Fatty breast tissue.

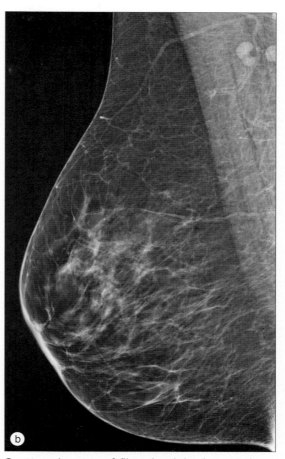

Scattered areas of fibroglandular breast tissue.

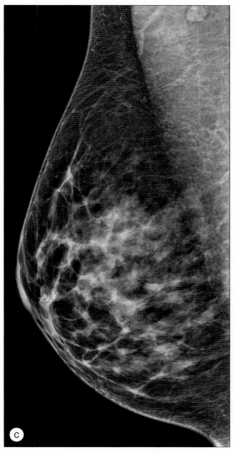

Heterogeneously dense breast tissue.

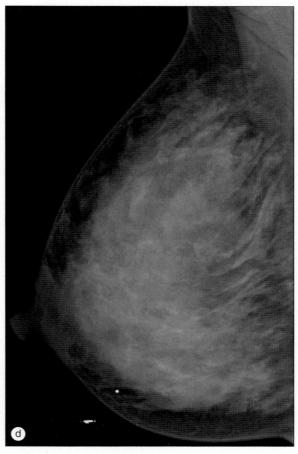

Extremely dense breast tissue.

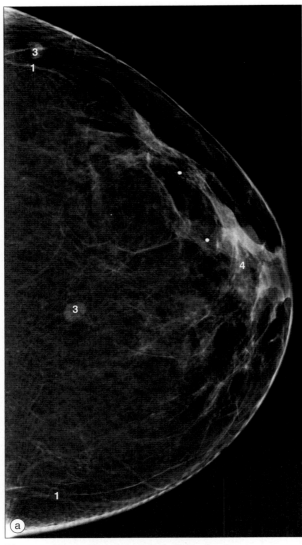

Mammogram (Craniocaudal (CC) view).

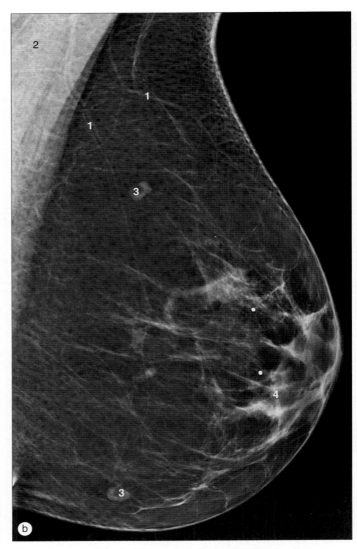

Mammogram (Medial lateral oblique (MLO) view).

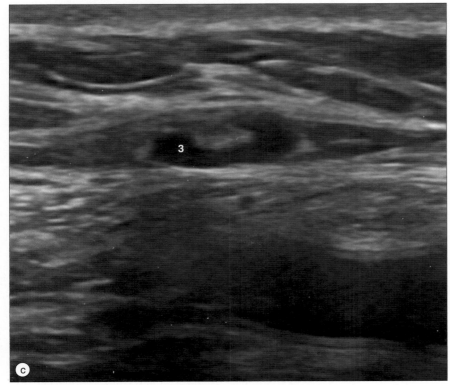

Ultrasound of breast.

1. Blood vessel
2. Pectoralis muscle
3. Lymph node
4. Fibroglandular tissue

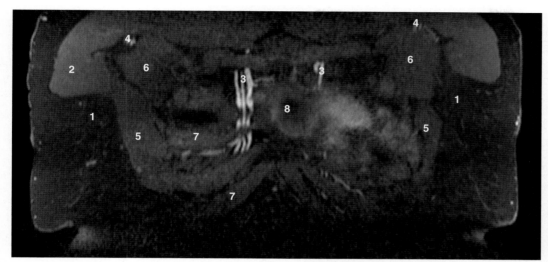

Coronal T1-weighted fat-saturated MR image post contrast of the chest wall.

1. Axillary tail breast tissue
2. Deltoid muscle
3. Internal thoracic artery and veins
4. Lateral thoracic artery and veins
5. Pectoralis major muscle
6. Pectoralis minor muscle
7. Ribs
8. Sternum, body

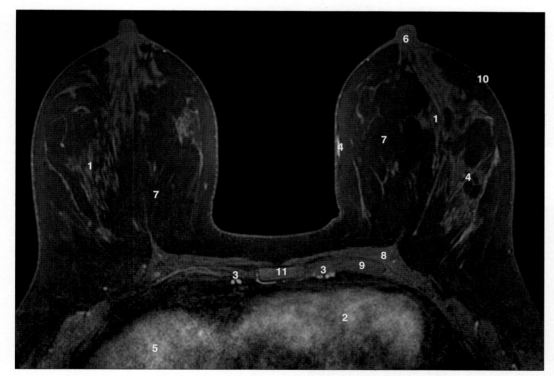

Axial T1-weighted fat-saturated MR image post contrast at the mid portion of the breast.

1. Fibroglandular tissue, scattered density
2. Heart
3. Internal thoracic artery and veins
4. Intramammary vessels
5. Liver
6. Nipple–areolar complex
7. Non-enhancing mammary fat
8. Pectoralis major muscle
9. Rib
10. Skin
11. Sternum, body

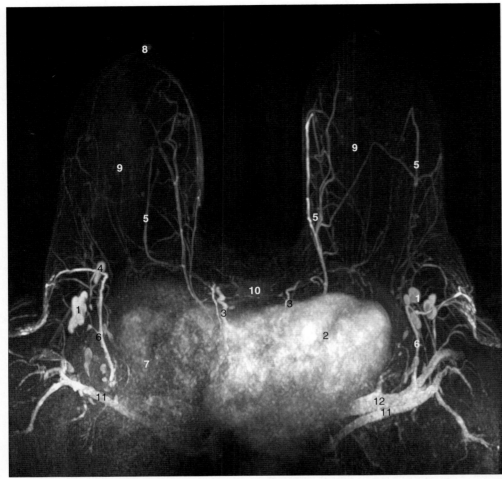

Maximal intensity projection (MIP) axial projection.

1. Axillary lymph nodes, normal (level 1)
2. Heart
3. Internal thoracic artery and veins
4. Intramammary lymph node (axillary tail)
5. Intramammary vessels
6. Lateral thoracic artery
7. Liver
8. Nipple–areolar complex
9. Non-enhancing mammary fibroglandular tissue
10. Sternum, body
11. Subclavian artery
12. Subclavian vein

Sagittal T1-weighted fat-saturated MR image post contrast.

1. Axillary lymph nodes, normal (level 1)
2. Intramammary lymph node (axillary tail)
3. Lateral thoracic artery
4. Liver
5. Non-enhancing mammary fibroglandular tissue
6. Pectoralis major muscle
7. Pectoralis minor muscle

Bonus e-materials

Selected pages from Imaging Atlas 4e

Tutorials: Tutorial 5g

Single best answer (SBA) self-assessment
questions

Table of Variations

Variant	Frequency	Clinical implications
Congenital inversion of the nipple	3%	Present at birth. Not to be confused with later developing inversion, which can be a sign of malignancy. Can result in functional problems during lactation. May be a source of chronic mastitis.
Polymastia (accessory breast tissue)	1–2%	Breast tissue can occur any place along the milk line from the axilla to the groin. The majority of breast development is on the anterior chest wall.
Polythelia (accessory nipples)	0.22–5.6%	Most common congenital anomaly of the breast.
Poland's syndrome	1–3/100,00 births	Unilateral hypoplasia of breast, hemithorax and pectoral muscle.
Asymmetric breast tissue	3%	Differing amounts of breast tissue in each breast. The important point is comparison to prior breast imaging examinations, as a new asymmetry can be a sign of cancer. Stability across mammograms is the best sign of a benign finding.
Sternalis muscle	8%	The presence of a sternalis muscle is considered a normal variant, however it can mimic a mass on mammographic imaging. It is a muscle that is orientated vertically from the infraclavicular region to near the caudal aspect of the sternum. It is located medial on the chest wall in the parasternal location (medial edge of pectoralis major muscle) and may be unilateral or bilateral. If present, it is best seen on the craniocaudal mammographic image. Ultrasound can be useful to evaluate a possible sternalis muscle seen on mammography.

7 Thorax: non cardiac

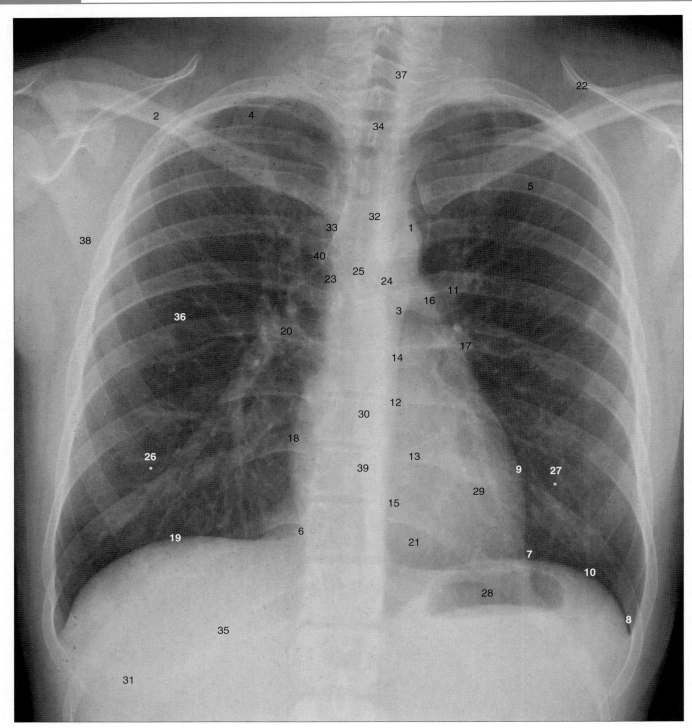

Chest radiograph, postero-anterior projection.

1. Arch of aorta (aortic knuckle or knob)
2. Clavicle
3. Descending aorta
4. First rib, anterior
5. Fifth rib, posterior
6. Position of inferior vena cava
7. Left cardiophrenic angle
8. Left costophrenic angle
9. Left ventricular border
10. Left dome of diaphragm
11. Left pulmonary artery
12. Position of aortic valve
13. Position of mitral valve
14. Position of pulmonary valve
15. Position of tricuspid valve
16. Pulmonary trunk
17. Region of tip of auricle of left atrium
18. Right atrial border
19. Right dome of diaphragm
20. Right pulmonary artery
21. Right ventricle
22. Spine of scapula
23. Right main bronchus
24. Left main bronchus
25. Carina
26. BB marker on right nipple
27. BB marker on left nipple
28. Gas in fundus of stomach
29. Position of left ventricle
30. Position of left atrium
31. Position of liver
32. Manubrium
33. Superior vena cava
34. Trachea
35. Twelfth rib, posterior
36. Right horizontal fissure
37. First thoracic vertebrae
38. Blade of scapula
39. Azygoesophageal recess
40. Position of azygos arch

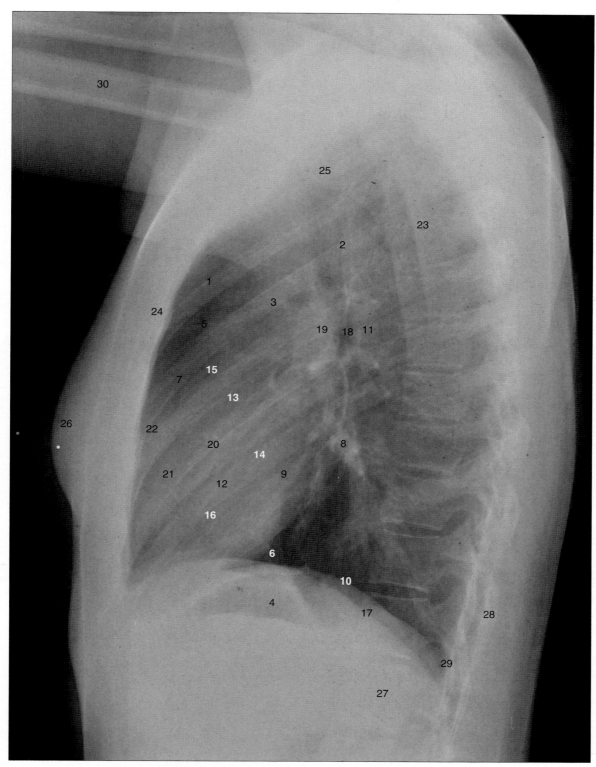

Chest radiograph, right lateral projection.

1. Anterior mediastinal space	**8.** Left atrial border of heart	**18.** Right main bronchus	**27.** First lumbar vertebral body
2. Arch of aorta (aortic knuckle or knob)	**9.** Left atrium	**19.** Right main pulmonary artery	**28.** Eleventh rib
3. Ascending aorta	**10.** Left dome of diaphragm	**20.** Right oblique fissure	**29.** Posterior costophrenic angle
4. Gas in fundus of stomach	**11.** Left main pulmonary artery	**21.** Right ventricle	**30.** Humerus
5. Horizontal fissure	**12.** Left oblique fissure	**22.** Right ventricular border of heart	
6. Inferior vena cava	**13.** Position of aortic valve	**23.** Scapula	
7. Infundibulum of right ventricle (below) with pulmonary trunk (above)	**14.** Position of mitral valve	**24.** Sternum	
	15. Position of pulmonary valve	**25.** Trachea	
	16. Position of tricuspid valve	**26.** Left breast shadow	
	17. Right dome of diaphragm		

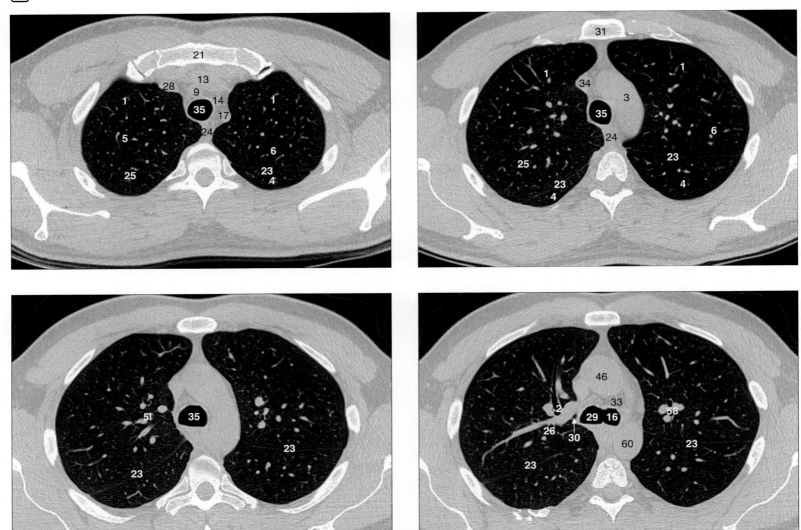

Lungs, axial, high resolution CT images, from superior to inferior.

1. Anterior segment of superior lobe
2. Anterior segmental bronchus
3. Aortic arch
4. Apical segment of inferior lobe
5. Apical segment of right superior lobe
6. Apicoposterior segment of left superior lobe
7. Right pulmonary artery
8. Left pulmonary artery
9. Brachiocephalic trunk
10. Bronchus intermedius
11. Horizontal fissure

12. Lateral segment of middle lobe
13. Left brachiocephalic vein
14. Left common carotid artery
15. Left inferior lobe bronchus
16. Left main bronchus
17. Left subclavian artery
18. Left superior lobe bronchus
19. Right superior pulmonary vein
20. Lingular segmental bronchus
21. Manubrium of sternum
22. Medial segment of middle lobe
23. Oblique fissure

24. Oesophagus
25. Posterior segment of superior lobe
26. Posterior segmental bronchus
27. Pulmonary artery
28. Right brachiocephalic vein
29. Right main bronchus
30. Right upper lobe bronchus
31. Sternum
32. Superior lingular segment
33. Superior pericardial recess

Numbers 1–62 are common to pages 98–101.

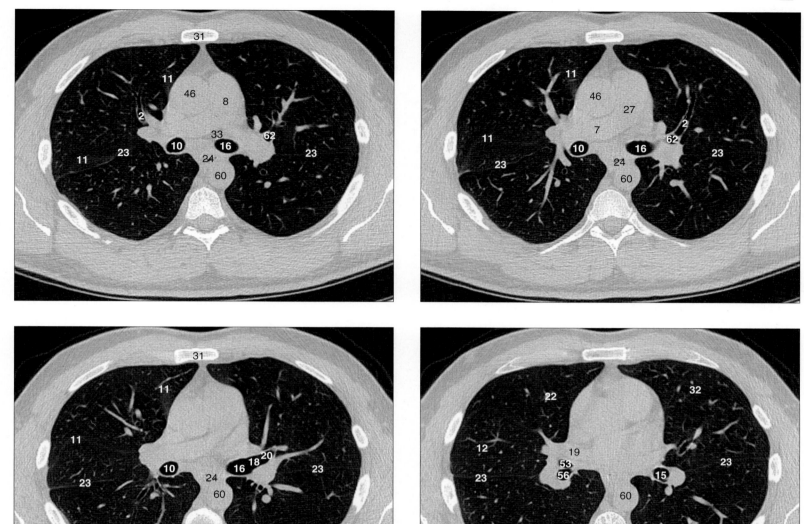

Lungs, axial, high resolution CT images, from superior to inferior.

34. Superior vena cava	**45.** Lateral basal segmental bronchus	**54.** Posterior basal segment of inferior lobe
35. Trachea	**46.** Ascending aorta	**55.** Posterior basal segmental bronchus
36. Anterior basal segment inferior lobe	**47.** Lateral segmental bronchus of middle lobe	**56.** Right inferior lobe bronchus
37. Anterior basal segmental bronchus	**48.** Liver	**57.** Right inferior pulmonary vein
38. Apical segment of inferior lobe bronchus	**49.** Medial basal segment of inferior lobe	**58.** Apicoposterior bronchi
39. Heart	**50.** Medial basal segmental bronchus	**59.** Pericardium
40. Hemiazygos vein	**51.** Apical segmental bronchus	**60.** Descending aorta
41. Inferior lingular segment	**52.** Medial segmental bronchus of middle lobe	**61.** Superior lingular segmental bronchus
42. Inferior lingular segmental bronchus		**62.** Apicoposterior bronchus
43. Azygos vein	**53.** Middle lobe bronchus	
44. Lateral basal segment of inferior lobe		

Numbers 1–62 are common to pages 98–101.

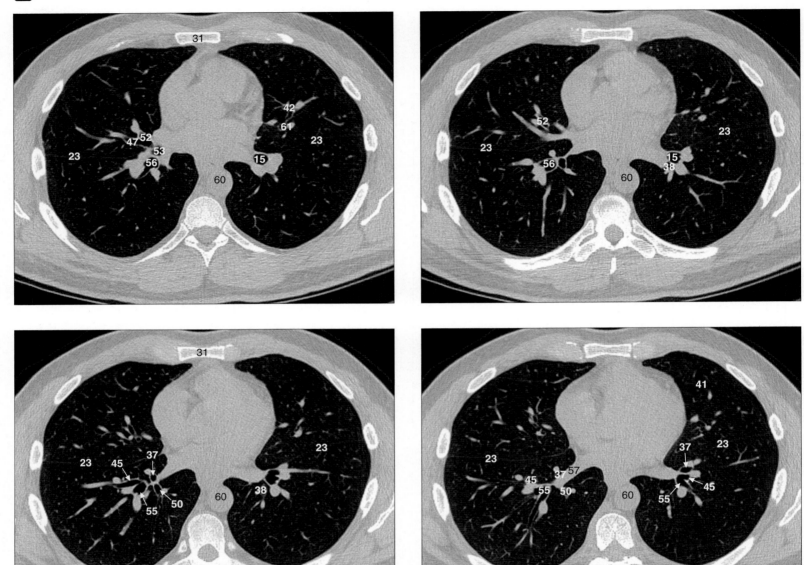

Lungs, high resolution CT images, from superior to inferior.

1. Anterior segment superior lobe
2. Anterior segmental bronchus
3. Aortic arch
4. Apical segment inferior lobe
5. Apical segment right superior lobe
6. Apicoposterior segment left superior lobe
7. Right pulmonary artery
8. Left pulmonary artery
9. Brachiocephalic trunk
10. Bronchus intermedius
11. Horizontal fissure
12. Lateral segment middle lobe
13. Left brachiocephalic vein
14. Left common carotid artery
15. Left inferior lobe bronchus
16. Left main bronchus
17. Left subclavian artery
18. Left superior lobe bronchus
19. Right superior pulmonary vein
20. Lingular segmental bronchus
21. Manubrium of sternum
22. Medial segment middle lobe
23. Oblique fissure
24. Oesophagus
25. Posterior segment superior lobe
26. Posterior segmental bronchus
27. Pulmonary artery
28. Right brachiocephalic vein
29. Right main bronchus
30. Right upper lobe bronchus
31. Sternum
32. Superior lingular segment
33. Superior pericardial recess

Numbers 1–62 are common to pages 98–101.

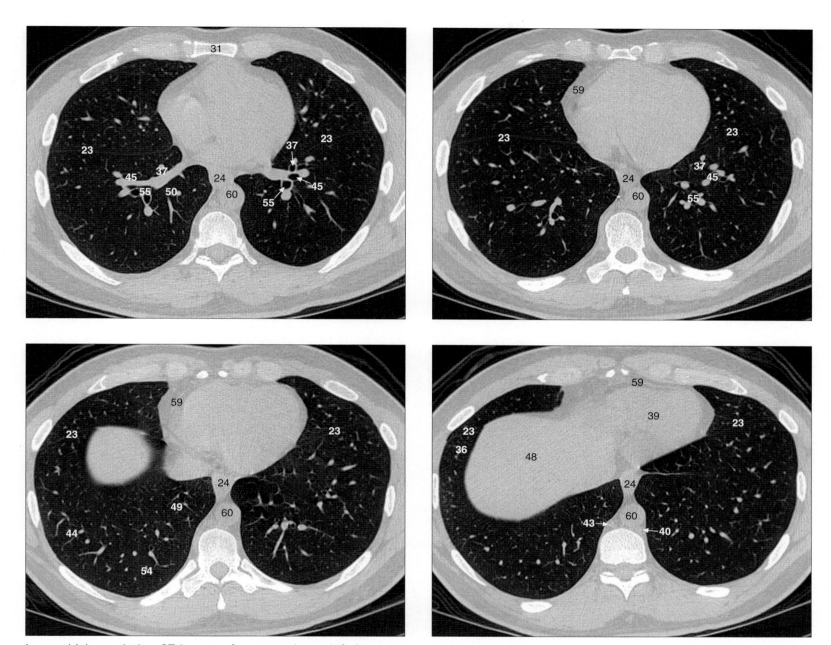

Lungs, high resolution CT images, from superior to inferior.

34. Superior vena cava
35. Trachea
36. Anterior basal segment inferior lobe
37. Anterior basal segmental bronchus
38. Apical segment inferior lobe bronchus
39. Heart
40. Hemiazygos vein
41. Inferior lingular segment
42. Inferior lingular segmental bronchus
43. Azygos vein
44. Lateral basal segment inferior lobe

45. Lateral basal segmental bronchus
46. Ascending aorta
47. Lateral segmental bronchus of middle lobe
48. Liver
49. Medial basal segment inferior lobe
50. Medial basal segmental bronchus
51. Apical segmental bronchus
52. Medial segmental bronchus of middle lobe
53. Middle lobe bronchus

54. Posterior basal segment inferior lobe
55. Posterior basal segmental bronchus
56. Right inferior lobe bronchus
57. Right inferior pulmonary vein
58. Apicoposterior bronchi
59. Pericardium
60. Descending aorta
61. Superior lingular segmental bronchus
62. Apicoposterior bronchus

Numbers 1–62 are common to pages 98–101.

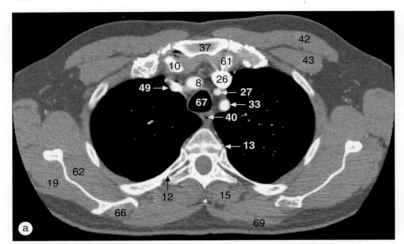

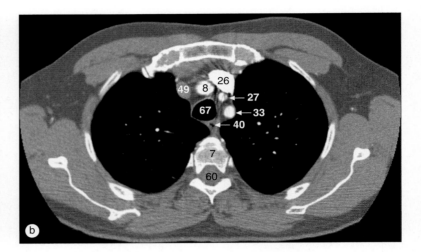

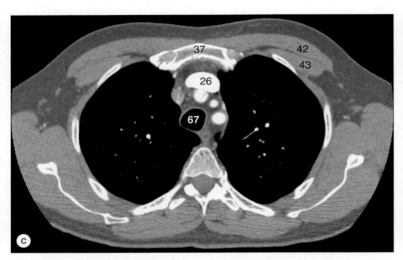

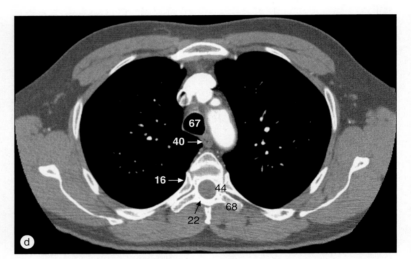

(a)–(t) Contrasted enhanced axial CT images of the chest, mediastinum, from superior to inferior.

1. Anterior interventricular branch of left coronary artery	**12.** Costotransverse joint	**24.** Left atrial appendage (auricle)
	13. Costovertebral joint	**25.** Left atrium
2. Aortic valve	**14.** Descending aorta	**26.** Left brachiocephalic vein
3. Arch of aorta (aortic knuckle or knob)	**15.** Erector spinae muscle	**27.** Left common carotid artery
4. Ascending aorta	**16.** Head of rib	**28.** Left hemidiaphragm
5. Azygos vein	**17.** Hemiazygos vein	**29.** Left inferior lobe bronchus
6. Sternum, body	**18.** Inferior vena cava	**30.** Left inferior pulmonary vein
7. Body of vertebra	**19.** Infraspinatus muscle	**31.** Left main bronchus
8. Brachiocephalic trunk	**20.** Interatrial septum	**32.** Left pulmonary artery
9. Carina (bifurcation of trachea)	**21.** Internal thoracic artery and vein	**33.** Left subclavian artery
10. Clavicle	**22.** Lamina	**34.** Left superior lobe bronchus
11. Coronary sinus	**23.** Latissimus dorsi muscle	**35.** Left superior pulmonary vein

Numbers 1–71 are common to pages 102–105.

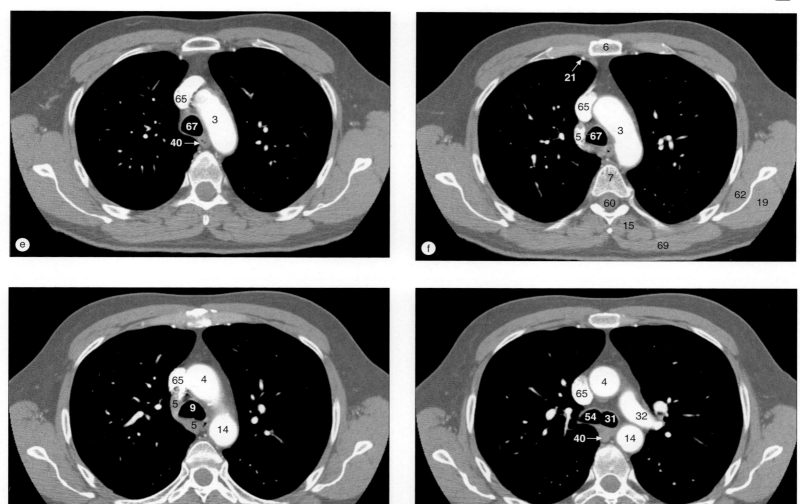

(a)–(t) Contrasted enhanced axial CT images of the chest, mediastinum, from superior to inferior.

36. Left ventricular cavity	**49.** Right brachiocephalic vein	**62.** Subscapularis muscle
37. Manubrium of sternum	**50.** Right hemidiaphragm	**63.** Superior lobe branch of right pulmonary artery
38. Mitral valve	**51.** Right inferior lobe bronchus	
39. Muscular interventricular septum	**52.** Right inferior pulmonary vein	**64.** Superior pericardial recess
40. Oesophagus	**53.** Right lobe of liver	**65.** Superior vena cava
41. Papillary muscles	**54.** Right main bronchus	**66.** Supraspinatus muscle
42. Pectoralis major muscle	**55.** Right pulmonary artery	**67.** Trachea
43. Pectoralis minor muscle	**56.** Right superior lobe bronchus	**68.** Transverse process
44. Pedicle	**57.** Right superior pulmonary vein	**69.** Trapezius muscle
45. Pericardium	**58.** Right ventricular cavity	**70.** Tricuspid valve
46. Pulmonary trunk	**59.** Serratus anterior muscle	**71.** Xiphisternum
47. Right atrial appendage (auricle)	**60.** Spinal canal	
48. Right atrium	**61.** Sternoclavicular joint	

Numbers 1–71 are common to pages 102–105.

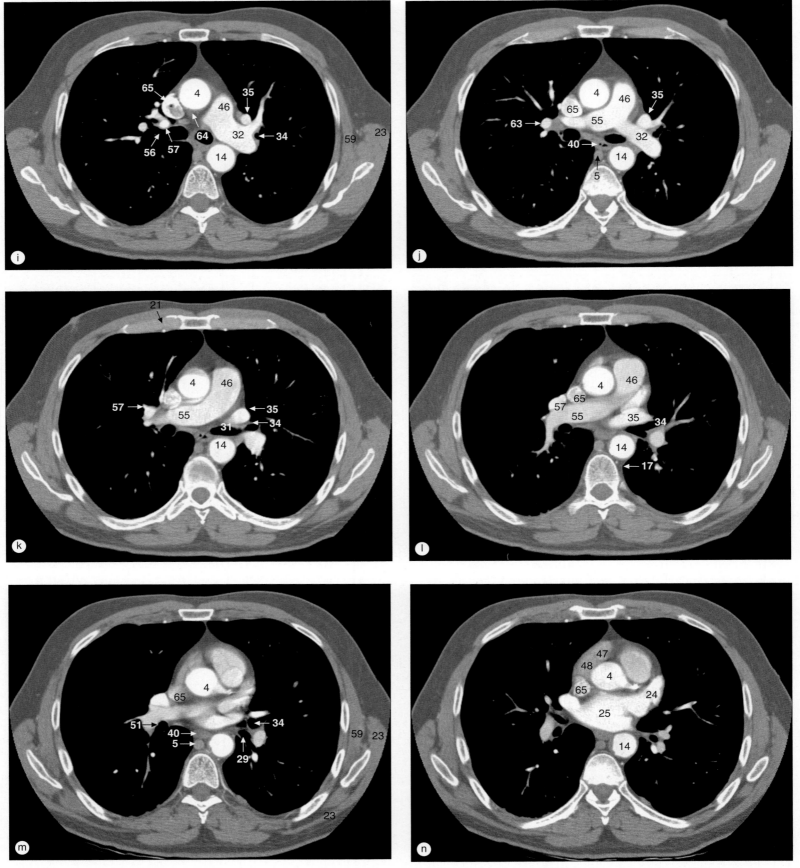

(a)–(t) Contrasted enhanced axial CT images of the chest, mediastinum, from superior to inferior. See pages 102–103 for key.

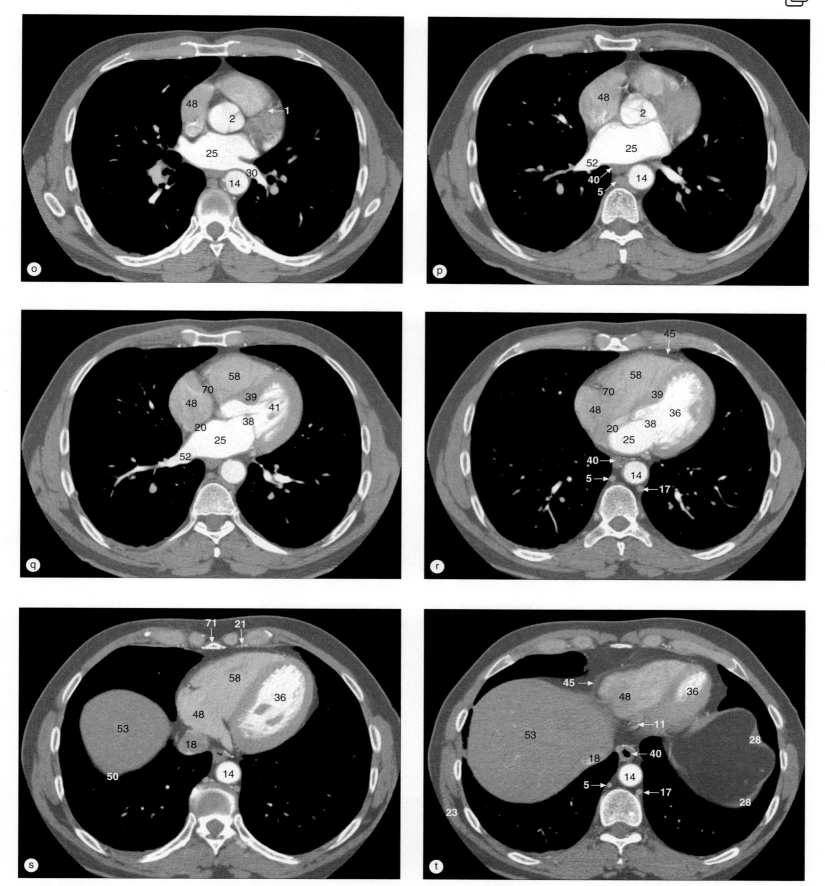

(a)–(t) Contrasted enhanced axial CT images of the chest, mediastinum, from superior to inferior. See pages 102–103 for key.

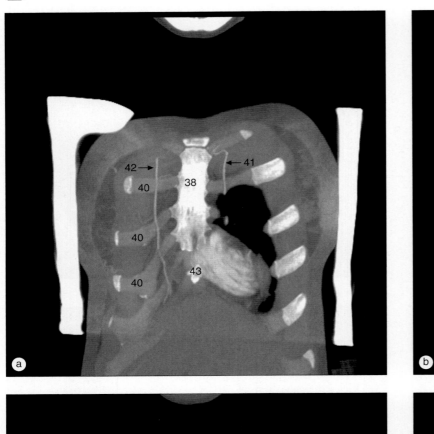

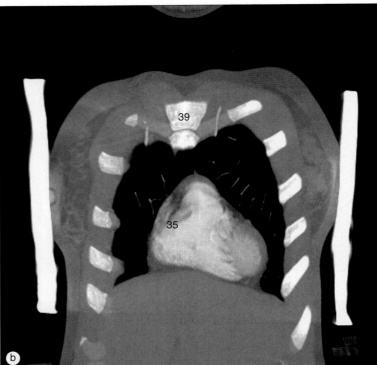

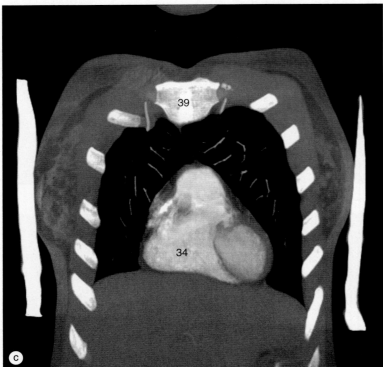

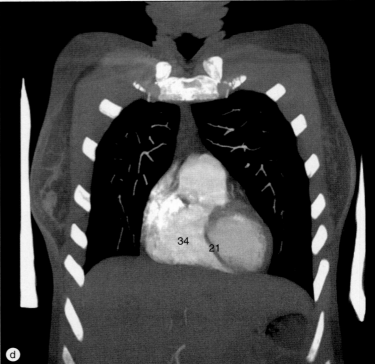

(a)–(p) Contrast enhanced coronal CT images of the chest, from anterior to posterior.

1. Aortic valve	**9.** Interatrial septum	**17.** Left superior pulmonary vein
2. Arch of aorta (aortic knuckle or knob)	**10.** Left atrial appendage (auricle)	**18.** Left ventricular cavity
3. Ascending aorta	**11.** Left atrium	**19.** Left ventricular wall
4. Brachiocephalic trunk	**12.** Left brachiocephalic vein	**20.** Membranous interventricular septum
5. Carina (bifurcation of trachea)	**13.** Left common carotid artery	**21.** Muscular interventricular septum
6. Clavicle	**14.** Left main bronchus	**22.** Papillary muscles
7. Descending aorta	**15.** Left pulmonary artery	**23.** Pericardium
8. Inferior vena cava	**16.** Left subclavian artery	**24.** Pulmonary trunk

Numbers 1–51 are common to pages 106–109.

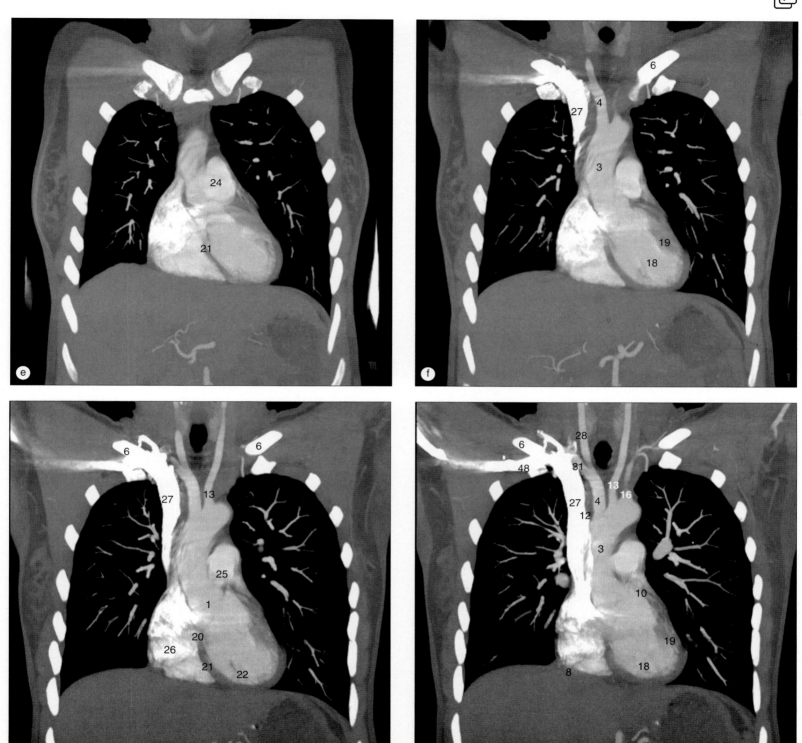

(a)–(p) Contrast enhanced coronal CT images of the chest, from anterior to posterior.

25. Pulmonary valve	**34.** Right ventricular cavity	**43.** Xiphisternum
26. Right atrium	**35.** Right ventricular wall	**44.** Tricuspid valve
27. Right brachiocephalic vein	**36.** Superior vena cava	**45.** Mitral valve
28. Right common carotid artery	**37.** Trachea	**46.** Left axillary artery
29. Right main bronchus	**38.** Sternum	**47.** Left subclavian artery
30. Right pulmonary artery	**39.** Manubrium	**48.** Right subclavian vein
31. Right subclavian artery	**40.** Anterior costal cartilage	**49.** Left inferior pulmonary vein
32. Right superior lobe pulmonary artery	**41.** Left internal thoracic (mammary) artery	**50.** Abdominal aorta
33. Right superior pulmonary vein	**42.** Right internal thoracic (mammary) artery	**51.** Right inferior pulmonary vein

Numbers 1–51 are common to pages 106–109.

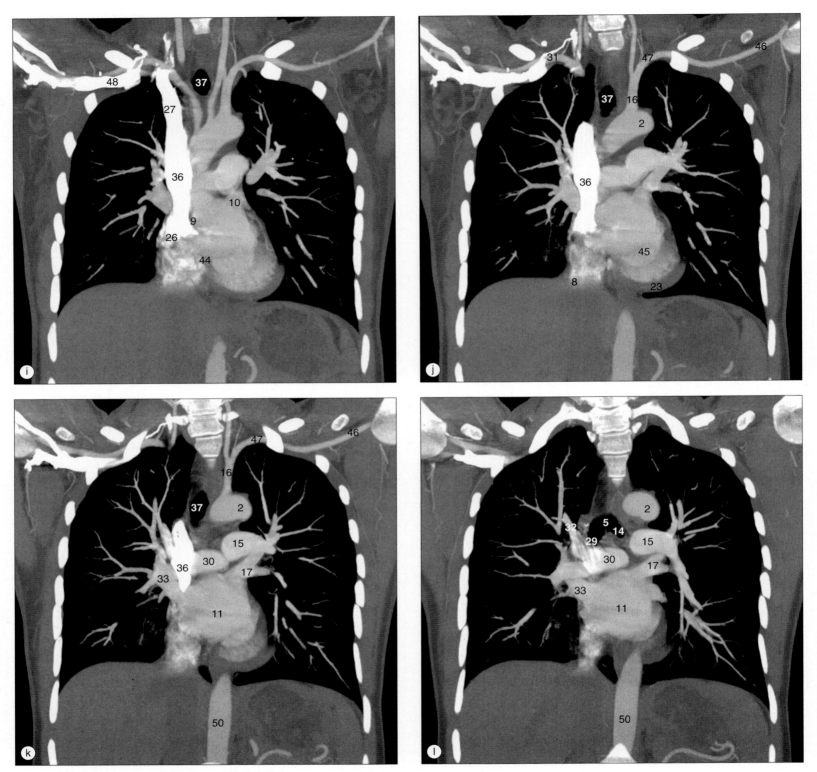

(a)–(p) Contrast enhanced coronal CT images of the chest, from anterior to posterior.

1. Aortic valve	9. Interatrial septum	17. Left superior pulmonary vein
2. Arch of aorta (aortic knuckle or knob)	10. Left atrial appendage (auricle)	18. Left ventricular cavity
3. Ascending aorta	11. Left atrium	19. Left ventricular wall
4. Brachiocephalic trunk	12. Left brachiocephalic vein	20. Membranous interventricular septum
5. Carina (bifurcation of trachea)	13. Left common carotid artery	21. Muscular interventricular septum
6. Clavicle	14. Left main bronchus	22. Papillary muscles
7. Descending aorta	15. Left pulmonary artery	23. Pericardium
8. Inferior vena cava	16. Left subclavian artery	24. Pulmonary trunk

Numbers 1–51 are common to pages 106–109.

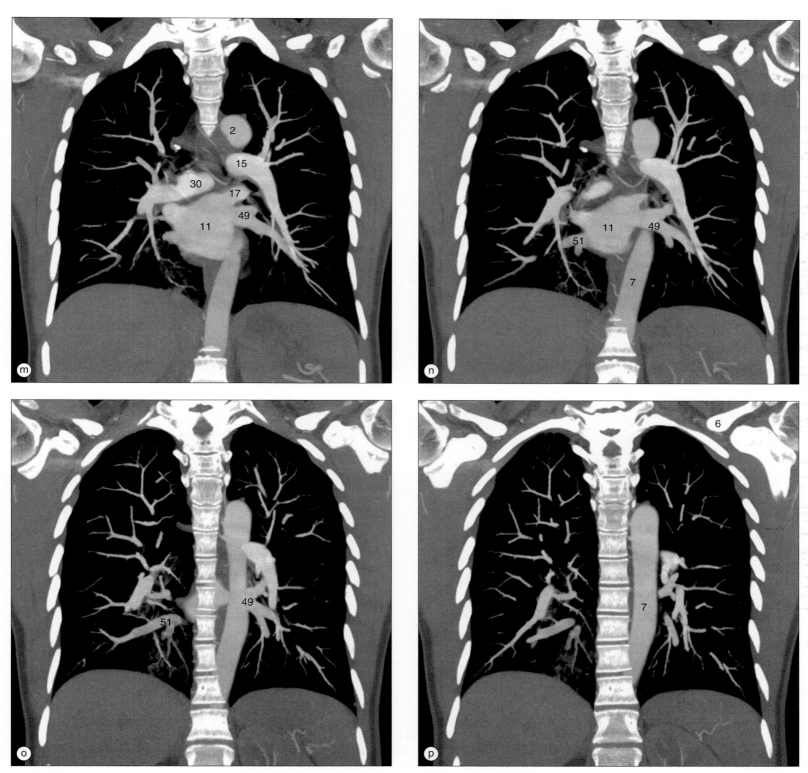

(a)–(p) Contrast enhanced coronal CT images of the chest, from anterior to posterior.

25. Pulmonary valve	34. Right ventricular cavity	43. Xiphisternum
26. Right atrium	35. Right ventricular wall	44. Tricuspid valve
27. Right brachiocephalic vein	36. Superior vena cava	45. Mitral valve
28. Right common carotid artery	37. Trachea	46. Left axillary artery
29. Right main bronchus	38. Sternum	47. Left subclavian artery
30. Right pulmonary artery	39. Manubrium	48. Right subclavian vein
31. Right subclavian artery	40. Anterior costal cartilage	49. Left inferior pulmonary vein
32. Right superior lobe pulmonary artery	41. Left internal thoracic (mammary) artery	50. Abdominal aorta
33. Right superior pulmonary vein	42. Right internal thoracic (mammary) artery	51. Right inferior pulmonary vein

Numbers 1–51 are common to pages 106–109.

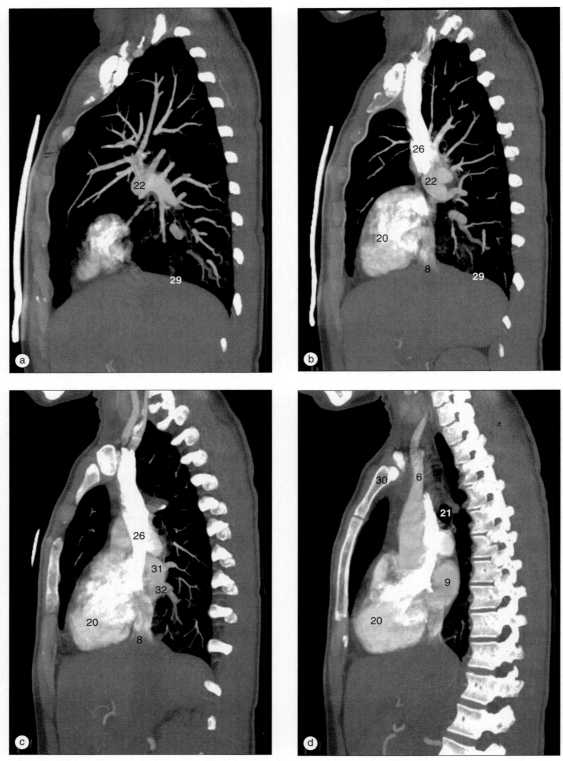

(a)–(p) Contrast enhanced sagittal CT images of the chest, right to left.

1. Aortic valve	8. Inferior vena cava	15. Mitral valve
2. Arch of aorta (aortic knuckle or knob)	9. Left atrium	16. Muscular interventricular septum
3. Ascending aorta	10. Left common carotid artery	17. Pericardium
4. Body of sternum	11. Left main bronchus	18. Pulmonary trunk
5. Body of vertebra	12. Left pulmonary artery	19. Pulmonary valve
6. Brachiocephalic trunk	13. Left subclavian artery	20. Right atrium
7. Descending aorta	14. Left ventricular cavity	21. Right main bronchus

Numbers 1–38 are common to pages 110–113.

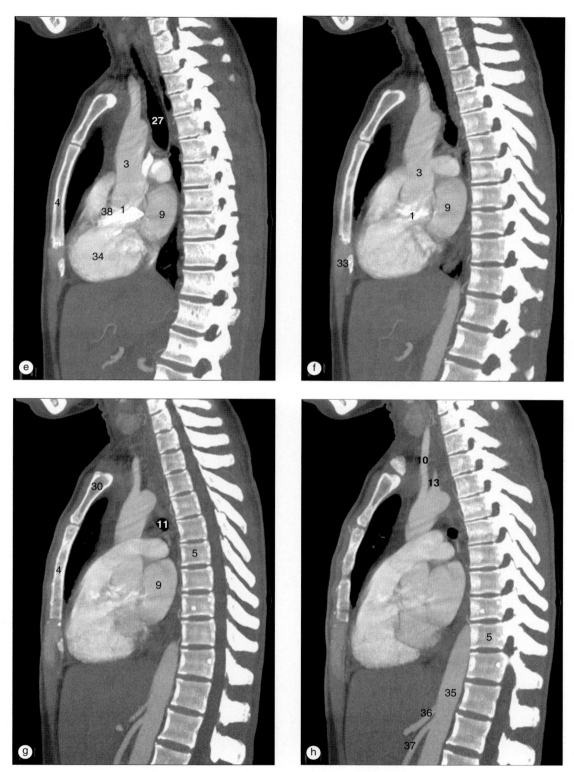

(a)–(p) Contrast enhanced sagittal CT images of the chest, right to left.

22. Right pulmonary artery	**28.** Left dome of diaphragm	**34.** Tricuspid valve
23. Right ventricular cavity	**29.** Right dome of diaphragm	**35.** Abdominal aorta
24. Right ventricular outflow tract	**30.** Manubrium	**36.** Coeliac axis
25. Right ventricular wall	**31.** Right superior pulmonary vein	**37.** Superior mesenteric artery
26. Superior vena cava	**32.** Right inferior pulmonary vein	**38.** Right coronary artery
27. Trachea	**33.** Xiphisternum	

Numbers 1–38 are common to pages 110–113.

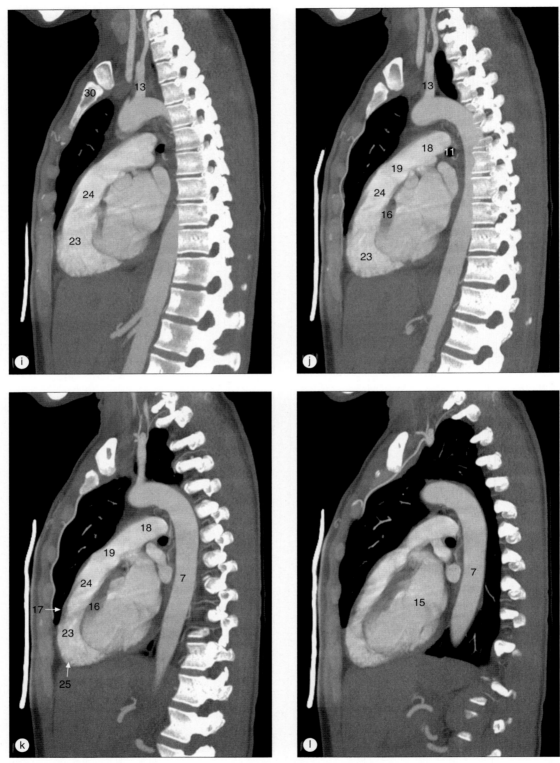

(a)–(p) Contrast enhanced sagittal CT images of the chest, right to left.

1. Aortic valve	**8.** Inferior vena cava	**15.** Mitral valve
2. Arch of aorta (aortic knuckle or knob)	**9.** Left atrium	**16.** Muscular interventricular septum
3. Ascending aorta	**10.** Left common carotid artery	**17.** Pericardium
4. Body of sternum	**11.** Left main bronchus	**18.** Pulmonary trunk
5. Body of vertebra	**12.** Left pulmonary artery	**19.** Pulmonary valve
6. Brachiocephalic trunk	**13.** Left subclavian artery	**20.** Right atrium
7. Descending aorta	**14.** Left ventricular cavity	**21.** Right main bronchus

Numbers 1–38 are common to pages 110–113.

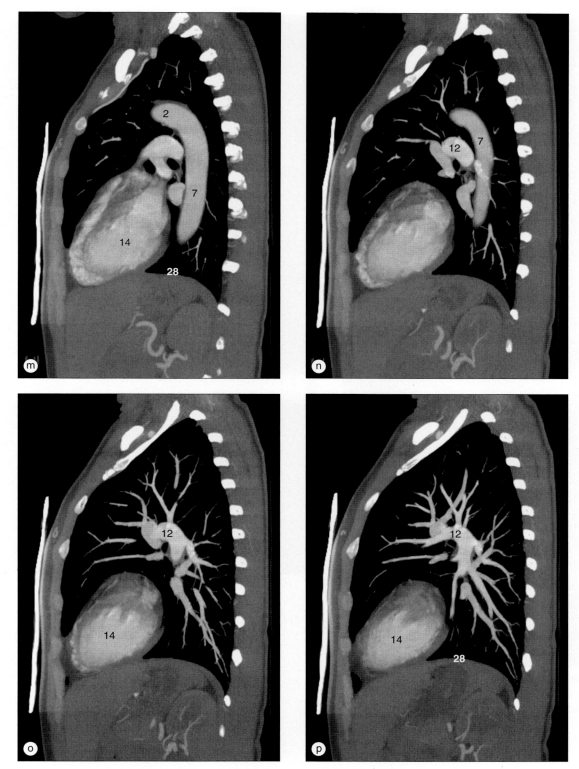

(a)–(p) Contrast enhanced sagittal CT images of the chest, right to left.

22. Right pulmonary artery
23. Right ventricular cavity
24. Right ventricular outflow tract
25. Right ventricular wall
26. Superior vena cava
27. Trachea
28. Left dome of diaphragm
29. Right dome of diaphragm
30. Manubrium
31. Right superior pulmonary vein
32. Right inferior pulmonary vein
33. Xiphisternum
34. Tricuspid valve
35. Abdominal aorta
36. Coeliac axis
37. Superior mesenteric artery
38. Right coronary artery

Numbers 1–38 are common to pages 110–113.

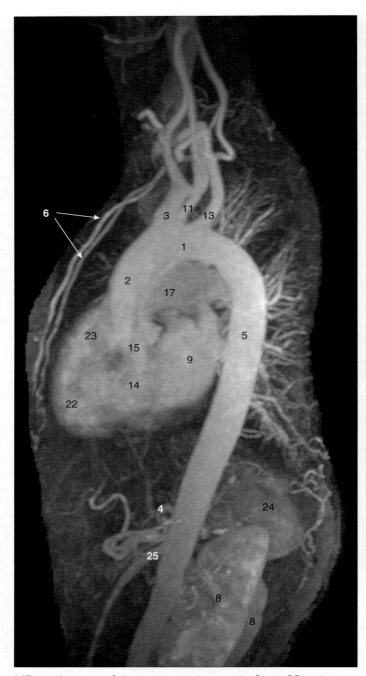

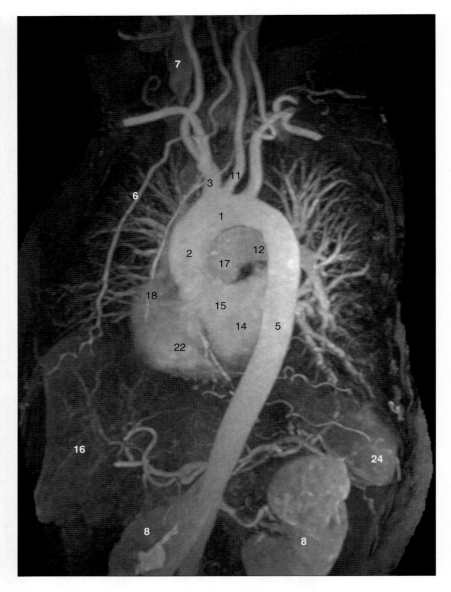

MR angiogram of the aorta and vessels from 3D volume set. Images presented as a series from lateral rotating counterclockwise to anterior projection.

1. Aortic arch	**6.** Internal thoracic artery	**11.** Left common carotid artery
2. Ascending aorta	**7.** Jugular vein	**12.** Left pulmonary artery
3. Brachiocephalic trunk	**8.** Kidney	**13.** Left subclavian artery
4. Celiac artery	**9.** Left atrium	**14.** Left ventricle
5. Descending aorta	**10.** Left brachiocephalic vein	**15.** Left ventricle outflow tract

Numbers 1–26 are common to pages 114–115.

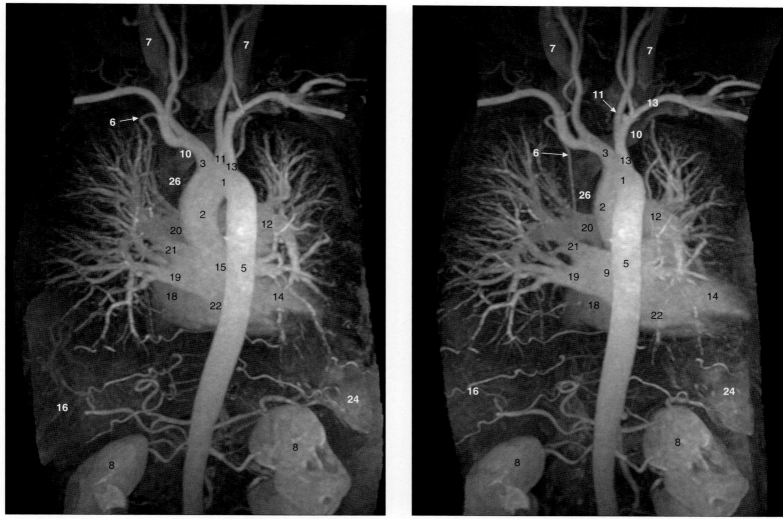

MR angiogram of the aorta and vessels from 3D volume set. Images presented as a series from lateral rotating counterclockwise to anterior projection.

16. Liver	**20.** Right pulmonary artery	**24.** Spleen
17. Main pulmonary artery	**21.** Right superior pulmonary vein	**25.** Superior mesenteric artery
18. Right atrium	**22.** Right ventricle	**26.** Superior vena cava
19. Right inferior pulmonary vein	**23.** Right ventricular outflow tract	

Numbers 1–26 are common to pages 114–115.

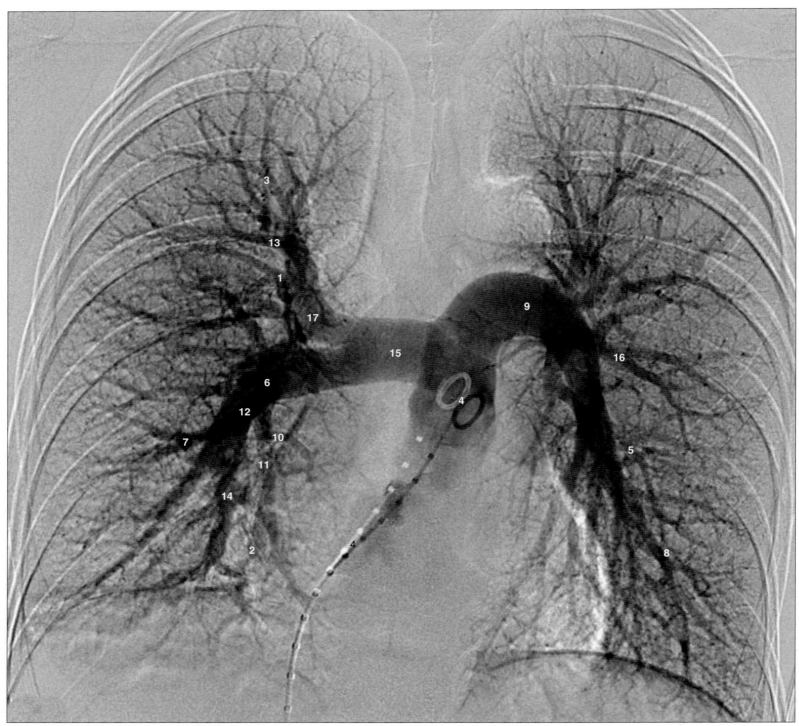

Pulmonary arteriogram, arterial phase.

1. Anterior artery (superior lobe)
2. Anterior basal artery
3. Apical artery (superior lobe)
4. Catheter in main pulmonary artery via a femoral vein, inferior vena cava, right atrium and right ventricle
5. Inferior lingular artery
6. Inferior lobe pulmonary artery
7. Lateral artery (middle lobe)
8. Lateral basal artery
9. Left pulmonary artery
10. Medial artery (middle lobe)
11. Medial basal artery
12. Middle lobe pulmonary artery
13. Posterior artery (superior lobe)
14. Posterior basal artery
15. Right pulmonary artery
16. Superior lingular artery
17. Superior lobe pulmonary artery

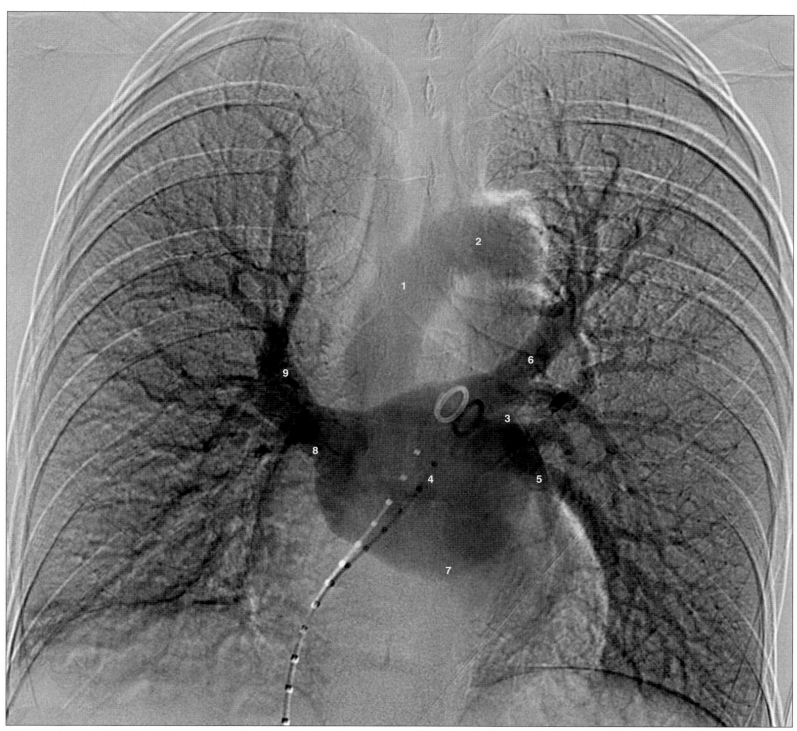

Pulmonary arteriogram, venous phase.

1. Aorta
2. Aortic arch
3. Left atrial appendage (auricle)
4. Left atrium
5. Left inferior pulmonary vein
6. Left superior pulmonary vein
7. Mitral valve
8. Right inferior pulmonary vein
9. Right superior pulmonary vein

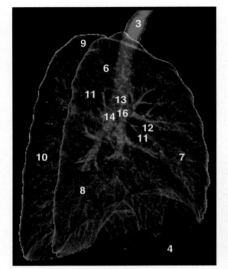

3D lungs and airways RPO.

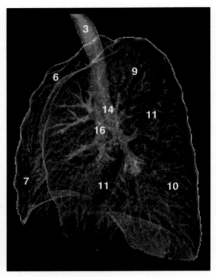

3D lungs and airways LAO.

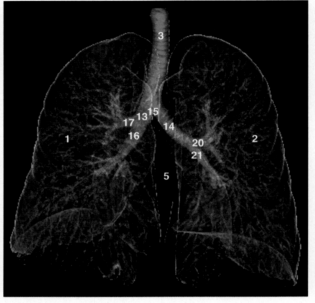

3D lungs and airways AP.

AP = anteroposterior
LAO = left anterior oblique
RAO = right anterior oblique
RPO = right posterior oblique

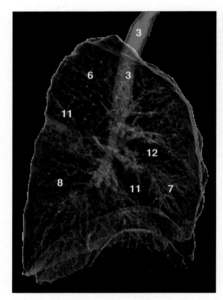

3D lungs and airways Right Lateral.

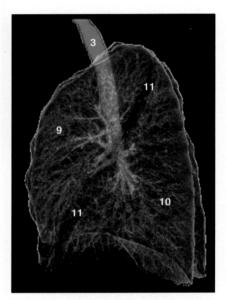

3D lungs and airways Left Lateral.

3D images of the lungs and airways reconstructed from CT scan of the chest. These views of the lungs are similar to those obtained during nuclear medicine V/Q scans.

1. Right lung	15. Carina	29. Right anterior basilar bronchus (RB8)
2. Left lung	16. Bronchus intermedius	30. Right lateral basilar bronchus (RB9)
3. Trachea	17. Right upper lobe bronchus	31. Right posterior basilar bronchus (RB10)
4. Gas in stomach	18. Right middle lobe bronchus	32. Left apical-posterior bronchus (LB1+2)
5. Mediastinum location	19. Right lower lobe bronchus	32a. Left posterior bronchus (LB2)
6. Right upper lobe	20. Left upper lobe bronchus	32b. Left apical bronchus (LB1)
7. Right middle lobe	21. Left lower lobe bronchus	33. Left anterior bronchus (LB3)
8. Right lower lobe	22. Right apical bronchus (RB1)	34. Left superior lingular bronchus (LB4)
9. Left upper lobe	23. Right posterior bronchus (RB2)	35. Left inferior lingular bronchus (LB5)
10. Left lower lobe	24. Right anterior bronchus (RB3)	36. Left superior bronchus (LB6)
11. Oblique (major) fissure	25. Right lateral bronchus (RB4)	37. Left anteromedial basilar bronchus (LB7+8)
12. Horizontal (minor) fissure	26. Right medial bronchus (RB5)	
13. Right main bronchus	27. Right superior bronchus (RB6)	38. Left lateral basilar bronchus (LB9)
14. Left main bronchus	28. Right medial basilar bronchus (RB7)	39. Left posterior basilar bronchus (LB10)

Numbers 1–39 are common to pages 118–119.

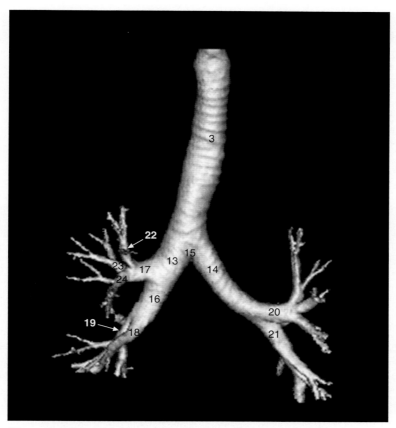

AP tracheobronchial tree, 3D CT reconstruction image.

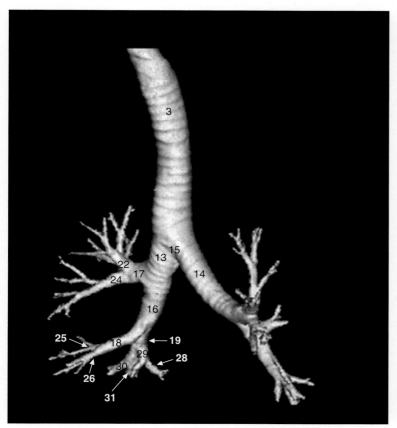

LAO tracheobronchial tree, 3D CT reconstruction image.

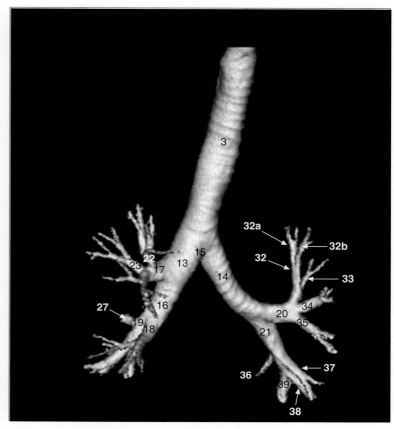

RAO tracheobronchial tree, 3D CT reconstruction image.

For labels see page 118.

Bonus e-materials

Slidelines for radiograph features:
Posteroanterior radiograph of the chest
(female)

Cross-sectional image stack Slideshows: Axial
CT of the chest with intravenous contrast
medium taken in the portal venous phase
(arms raised above head)

Selected pages from Imaging Atlas 4e

Tutorials: Tutorials 5a, 5b, 5d, 5e, 5f

Single best answer (SBA) self-assessment
questions

Table of Variations

Variant	Frequency	Clinical implications
Azygous lobe	1%	Right posterior cardinal vein (precursor of azygous vein) fails to migrate over the apex of the lung and thus penetrates and carries along with it the pleural and traps a portion of the right upper lobe. No clinical sequelae.
Bronchial atresia	1.2 cases per 100,000 males and 0.6 cases per 100,000 females with a male to female ratio of 2:1	Obliteration of the proximal lumen of a segmental bronchus. Emphysematous due to air trapping and may appear similar to pneumothorax or bullous changes. Bronchial atresia is usually benign and asymptomatic. It is often discovered incidentally, with mean age of diagnosis of 17 years. Most do not need surgical intervention.
Congenital diaphragmatic hernia (CDH) (Bochdalek)	0.04% (85–90% of CDH are Bochdalek)	Posterolateral diaphragmatic defect caused by maldevelopment or defective fusion of the cephalic fold of the pleuroperitoneal membranes. Left is more common than right, but can occur on both sides. If the hernia occurs on the right, then liver can herniate into the chest.
Congenital diaphragmatic hernia (Morgagni)	0.04% (1–2% of CDH are Morgagni)	Caused by maldevelopment of septum transversum. More common in the anterior and central location and more common on the right side.

8 | Thorax: cardiac

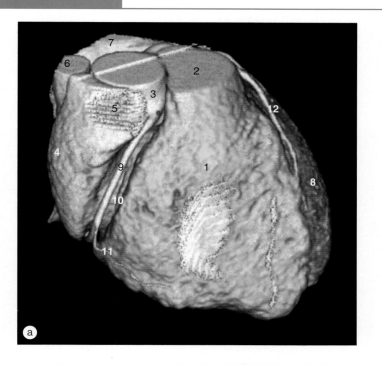

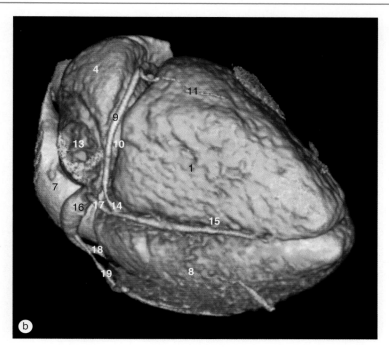

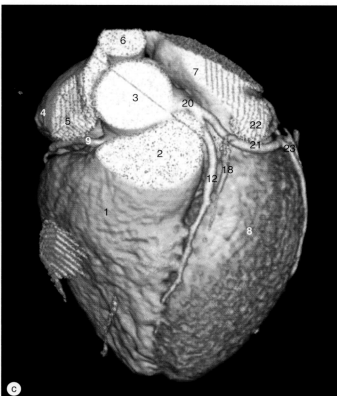

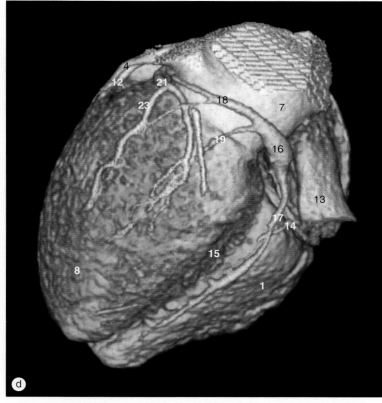

Heart 3D CT reconstruction images. (a) Anterior view. (b) Right inferolateral. (c) Left superolateral. (d) Posteroinferior view.

1. Right ventricle
2. Pulmonary outflow tract
3. Aortic root
4. Right atrium
5. Right atrial appendage (auricle)
6. Superior vena cava
7. Left atrium
8. Left ventricle
9. Right coronary artery
10. Right atrioventricular sulcus
11. Acute marginal branch of right coronary artery
12. Left anterior descending coronary artery
13. Inferior vena cava
14. Posterior interventricular artery
15. Posterior interventricular sulcus
16. Coronary sinus
17. Middle cardiac vein
18. Great cardiac vein
19. Posterior cardiac vein
20. Left main coronary artery
21. Circumflex artery
22. Left atrial appendage
23. Obtuse marginal branch of the curcumflex artery

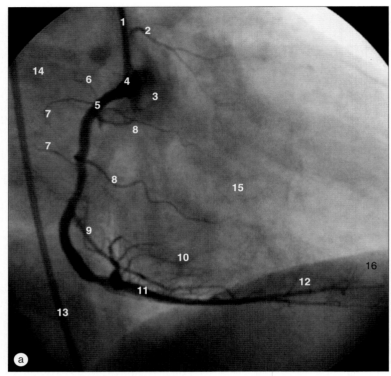

Right coronary arteriogram.

1. Catheter in the ascending aorta
2. Right conal artery
3. Right aortic sinus
4. Ostium of right coronary artery
5. Right coronary artery
6. Artery to the sinoatrial node
7. Right atrial branches
8. Right ventricular branches
9. Acute marginal artery
10. Artery to the atrioventricular node
11. Posterior interventricular artery
12. Septal perforators (from posterior interventricular artery)
13. Catheter in the descending thoracic aorta
14. Area of the right atrium
15. Area of the right ventricle
16. Ventricular apex

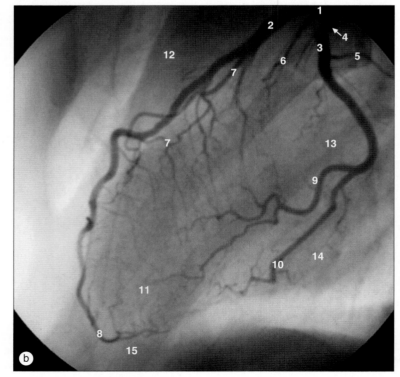

Left coronary arteriogram.

1. Left main stem coronary artery
2. Left anterior interventricular artery (left anterior descending)
3. Circumflex artery
4. Left aortic sinus
5. Artery to the sinoatrial node
6. Diagonal artery
7. Septal perforators from left anterior interventricular artery
8. Left anterior interventricular artery curving around apex of heart
9. Obtuse marginal branch of circumflex artery
10. Posterior interventricular artery (posterior descending artery)
11. Anastomosis between anterior and posterior interventricular arteries
12. Area of right anterior ventricular wall
13. Area of left lateral ventricular wall
14. Inferior wall of left ventricle
15. Apex of the left ventricle

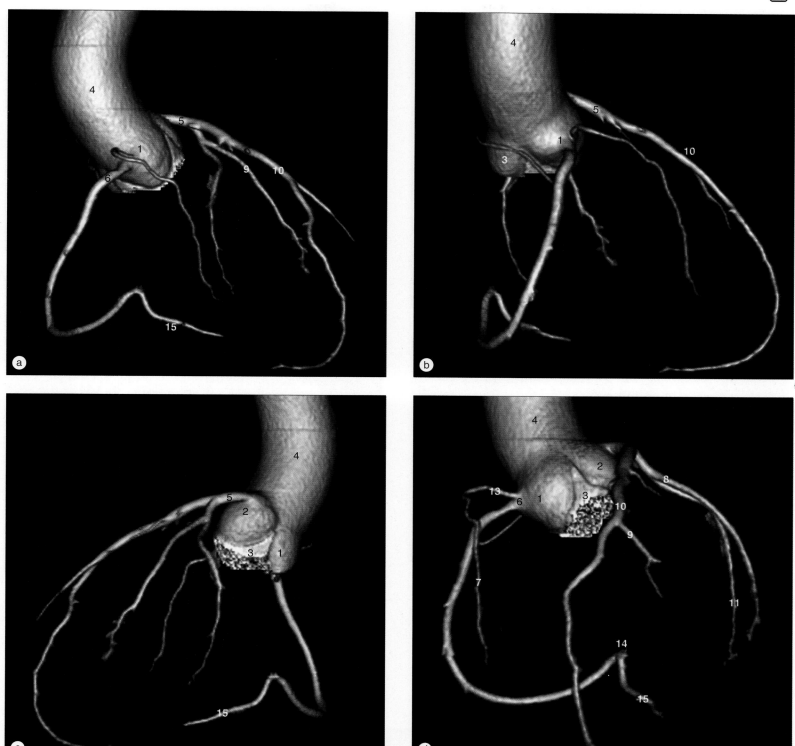

(a)–(d) Coronary angiograms, 3D CT images.

1. Right aortic sinus
2. Left aortic sinus
3. Interleaflet triangle
4. Ascending aorta
5. Left main coronary artery
6. Right main coronary artery
7. Right ventricular branch of right coronary artery
8. Circumflex artery
9. Diagonal artery
10. Left anterior descending artery
11. Obtuse marginal artery
12. Marginal artery
13. Right conal artery
14. Atrioventricular nodal artery
15. Posterior interventricular branch, right coronary artery

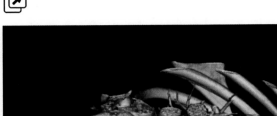

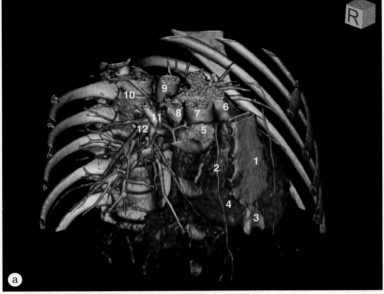

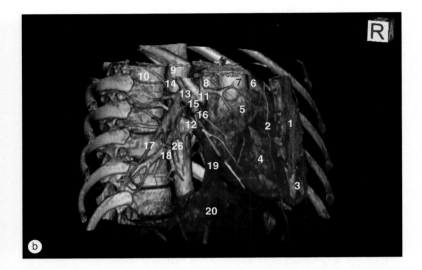

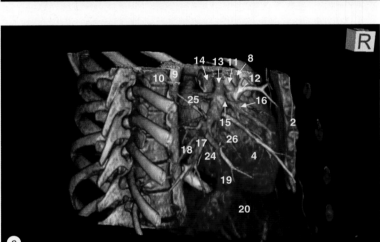

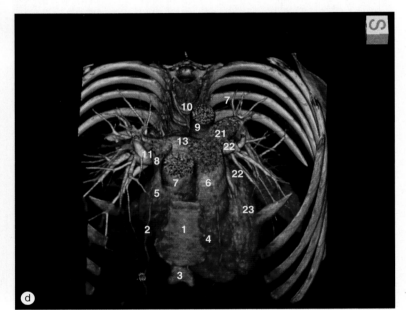

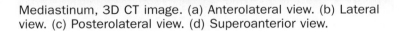

Mediastinum, 3D CT image. (a) Anterolateral view. (b) Lateral view. (c) Posterolateral view. (d) Superoanterior view.

1. Body of sternum
2. Internal thoracic artery
3. Bifid xiphoid process
4. Right ventricle
5. Right atrium
6. Pulmonary trunk
7. Ascending aorta
8. Superior vena cava
9. Descending thoracic aorta
10. Thoracic vertebral body
11. Upper right pulmonary vein
12. Lower right pulmonary vein
13. Right pulmonary artery
14. Superior lobe pulmonary vein
15. Middle lobe pulmonary artery
16. Medial artery (middle lobe)
17. Lateral artery (middle lobe)
18. Posterior basal artery
19. Inferior vena cava
20. Diaphragm
21. Left pulmonary artery
22. Upper left pulmonary vein
23. Left atrium
24. Left ventricle
25. Left atrium
26. Anterior basal artery (lower lobe)

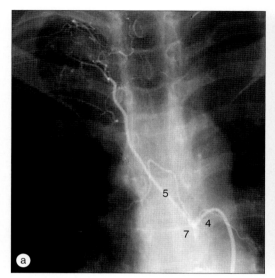
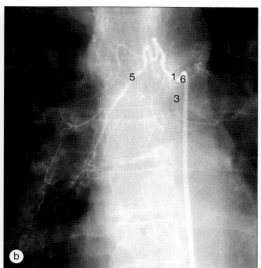
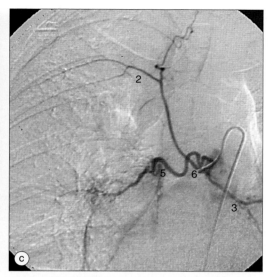

(a)–(c) Right bronchial arteriograms.
There is a great variability in the anatomy of the bronchial arteries, but the majority originate from the descending thoracic aorta, above the level of the left main stem bronchus between the upper border of the fifth thoracic vertebra and the lower border of the sixth thoracic vertebra. The number of bronchial arteries on each side may vary between one and four. Usually, there is one vessel to the right lung and two to the left. Accessory bronchial arteries may arise from the brachiocephalic artery and subclavian arteries or from other branches such as the internal thoracic, pericardiophrenic and oesophageal arteries. In many cases the right bronchial artery arises from an intercostobronchial trunk, but in this example the trunk is very short and divides almost immediately into a right bronchial artery, which is directed towards the hilum, and the first right aortic intercostal artery. Reflux filling of the left bronchial artery is seen.
A second larger bronchial artery which has been catheterised **(b)** has a common trunk arising from the front of the aorta, giving rise to a right and left bronchial artery.

1. Common bronchial trunk
2. Intercostal artery
3. Left bronchial branches
4. Reflux filling of left bronchial artery
5. Right bronchial artery
6. Tip of catheter in common bronchial arterial trunk
7. Tip of catheter in intercostobronchial trunk

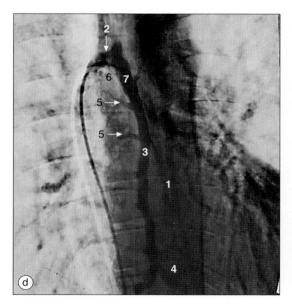

(d) Azygos venogram.
In the thorax the vertebral veins drain into intercostal veins, whilst in the lumbar region the lumbar veins drain into the ascending lumbar veins. The right ascending lumbar vein becomes the azygos vein on entering the thorax, and the left ascending lumbar vein becomes the hemi-azygos vein. At the level of the fourth thoracic vertebra, the azygos vein turns anteriorly (the arch of the azygos) to enter the superior vena cava. The hemi-azygos vein crosses to join the azygos vein at the level of the eighth or ninth thoracic vertebral body. The accessory hemi-azygos vein is continuous with the hemi-azygos vein inferiorly and the left superior intercostal vein superiorly.

1. Accessory hemi-azygos vein
2. Azygos arch
3. Azygos vein
4. Hemi-azygos vein
5. Posterior intercostal veins
6. Subtraction artefact caused by cardiac and catheter movement
7. Tip of catheter introduced via femoral vein into superior vena cava and azygos vein

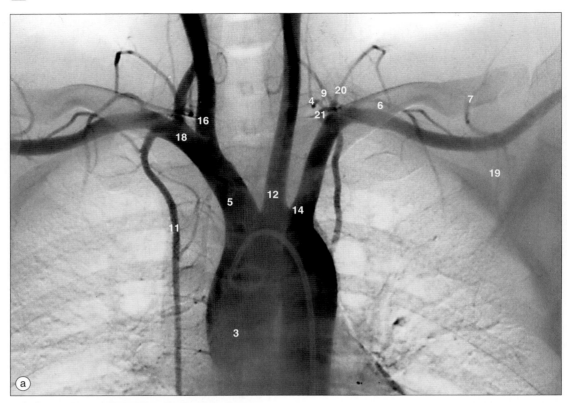

(a) Subtracted arch aortogram, anteroposterior image.
The vertebral artery (22) has a separate origin off the arch, projected over the left common carotid artery in this view. This is a normal variant.

(b) Subtracted arch aortogram, left anterior oblique image.
The origins of the supra-aortic branches are best shown by left anterior oblique projection, so that the origins of the vessels are not superimposed. There are many congenital variations in the way in which the major vessels arise from the aortic arch, but the most common is shown here.

(c) Left ventricular angiogram.

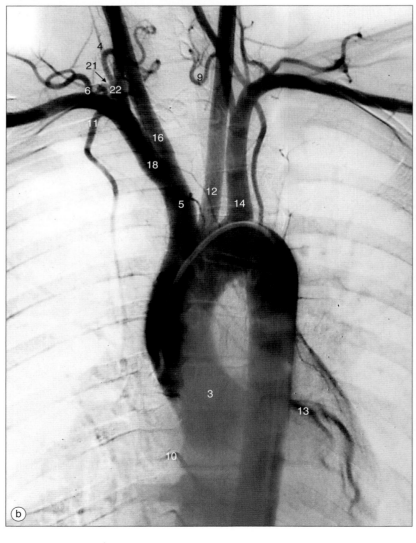

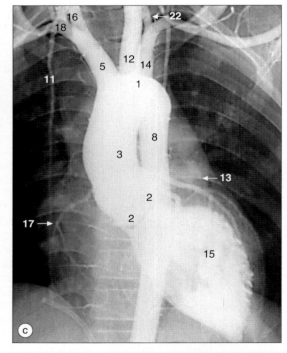

1. Aortic arch	**12.** Left common carotid artery
2. Aortic valve	**13.** Left coronary artery
3. Ascending aorta	**14.** Left subclavian artery
4. Ascending cervical artery	**15.** Left ventricle
5. Brachiocephalic trunk	**16.** Right common carotid
6. Costocervical trunk	artery
7. Deltoid branch of thoraco-	**17.** Right coronary artery
acromial artery	**18.** Right subclavian artery
8. Descending aorta	**19.** Superior thoracic artery
9. Inferior thyroid artery	**20.** Suprascapular artery
10. Intercostal artery	**21.** Thyrocervical trunk
11. Internal thoracic artery	**22.** Vertebral artery

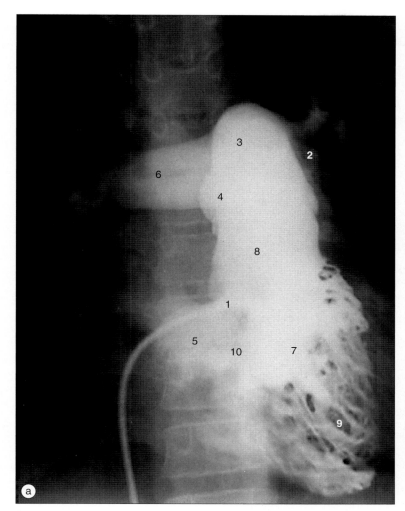

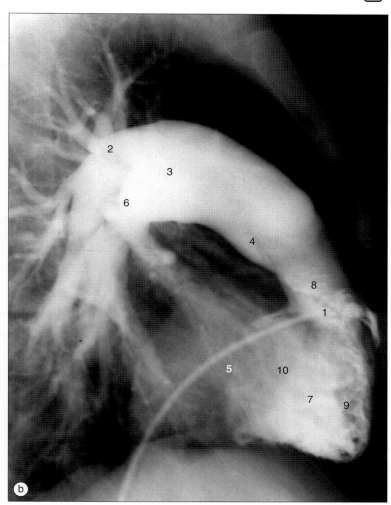

Right ventricular angiograms, (a) anteroposterior projection, (b) lateral projection.

1. Catheter in right ventricle via inferior vena cava and right atrium
2. Left main pulmonary artery
3. Pulmonary artery
4. Pulmonary valve
5. Right atrium
6. Right main pulmonary artery
7. Right ventricle
8. Right ventricular outflow tract
9. Trabeculae of right ventricle
10. Tricuspid valve

Bonus e-materials

Slidelines for radiograph features: Posteroanterior radiograph of the chest (female)

Cross-sectional image stack slideshows: Axial CT of the chest with intravenous contrast medium taken in the portal venous phase (arms raised above head)

Multi-tier labelling in slideshow/test yourself: T2-weighted steady state MRI, four chamber view of the heart

Selected pages from Imaging Atlas 4e

Tutorials: Tutorial 5c

Single best answer (SBA) self-assessment questions

Table of Variations

Variant	Frequency	Clinical implications
Aberrant right subclavian artery	0.5–2%	Tracheoesophageal symptoms and dysphagia (dysphagia lusoria).
Aortic nipple	10%	Pneumomediastinum, or obstructed SVC.
Left common carotid artery has its origin from the brachiocephalic artery proper	<10%	Typically asymptomatic.
Double aortic arch classified as type 1 (both arches patent)	0.5–1%	Oesophageal or tracheal obstruction.
Right brachiocephalic vein drains into left SVC	0.3–0.5%	Implications for planning surgical vascular procedures and IVC filter placement.
Left-sided IVC	<0.5%	Implications for planning surgical vascular procedures and IVC filter placement.

IVC, *Inferior vena cava;* SVC, *superior vena cava.*

9 | Abdomen and pelvis: cross-sectional

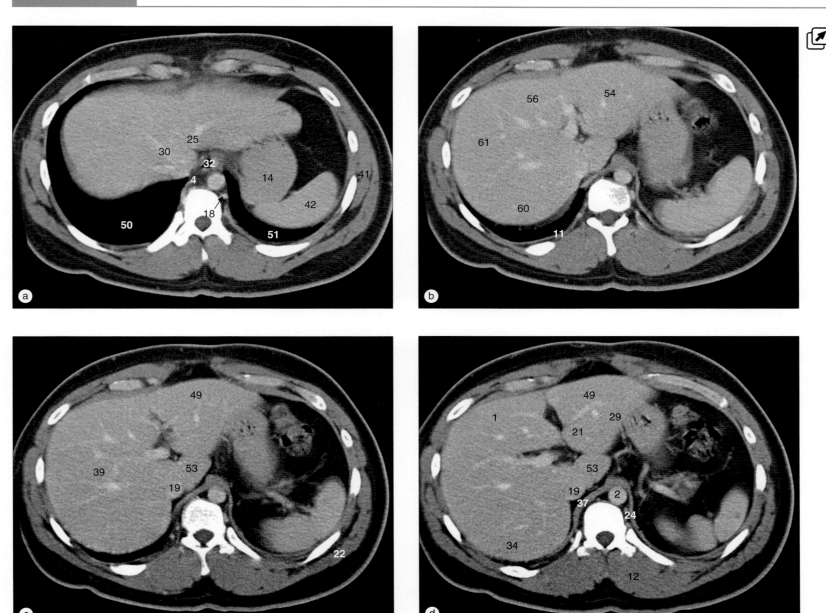

(a)–(h) Abdomen and pelvis in a male, sequential axial CT images, from superior to inferior.
Note: Pages 129–140 show sequential images of the abdomen and pelvis of the same male patient.

1. Anterior segment of right lobe of liver
2. Aorta
3. Descending colon
4. Azygos vein
5. Body of pancreas
6. Body of stomach
7. Body of vertebra
8. Coeliac trunk
9. Common hepatic artery
10. Descending (second) part of duodenum
11. Diaphragm
12. Erector spinae muscles
13. Fissure for falciform ligament
14. Fundus of stomach
15. Gall bladder
16. Greater curvature of stomach
17. Head of pancreas
18. Hemi-azygos vein
19. Inferior vena cava
20. Jejunum
21. Lateral segment of left lobe of liver
22. Latissimus dorsi muscle
23. Left colic (splenic) flexure
24. Left crus of diaphragm
25. Left hepatic vein
26. Left kidney
27. Left suprarenal gland
28. Lesser curvature of stomach
29. Medial segment of left lobe of liver
30. Middle hepatic vein
31. Neck of pancreas
32. Oesophagus
33. Portal vein
34. Posterior segment of right lobe of liver
35. Renal cortex
36. Renal fascia
37. Right crus of diaphragm
38. Right kidney
39. Right lobe of liver

Numbers 1–61 are common to pages 129–130.

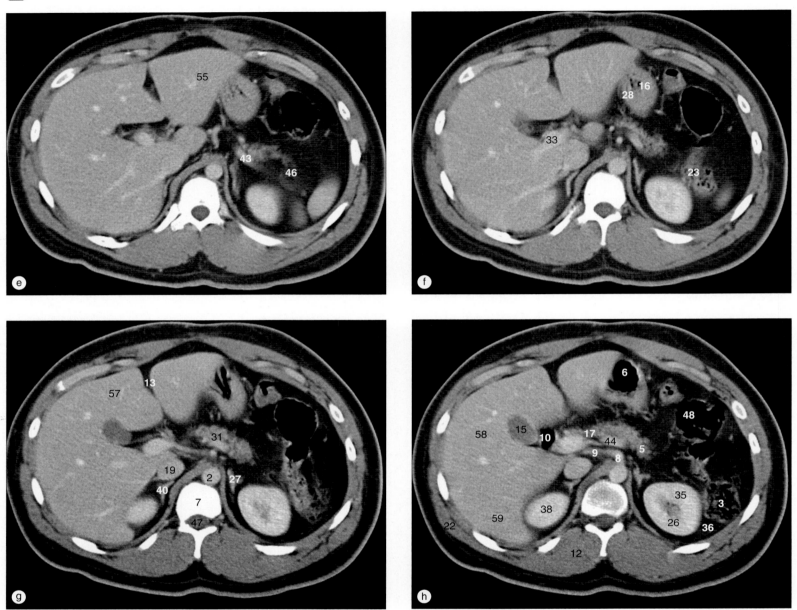

(a)–(h) Abdomen and pelvis in a male, sequential axial CT images, from superior to inferior.

40. Right suprarenal gland
41. Serratus anterior muscle
42. Spleen
43. Splenic artery
44. Splenic vein
45. Superior (first) part of duodenum
46. Tail of pancreas
47. Thecal sac
48. Transverse colon
49. Left lobe of liver

50. Right inferior lobe of lung
51. Left inferior lobe of lung
52. Caudate lobe of liver
53. Segment 1 of liver (caudate)
54. Segment 2 of liver (left lateral superior subsegment)
55. Segment 3 of liver (left lateral inferior subsegment)
56. Segment 4A of liver (left medial superior subsegment)

57. Segment 4B of liver (left medial inferior subsegment)
58. Segment 5 of liver (right anterior inferior subsegment)
59. Segment 6 of liver (right posterior inferior subsegment)
60. Segment 7 of liver (right posterior superior subsegment)
61. Segment 8 of liver (right anterior superior subsegment)

Numbers 1–61 are common to pages 129–130.

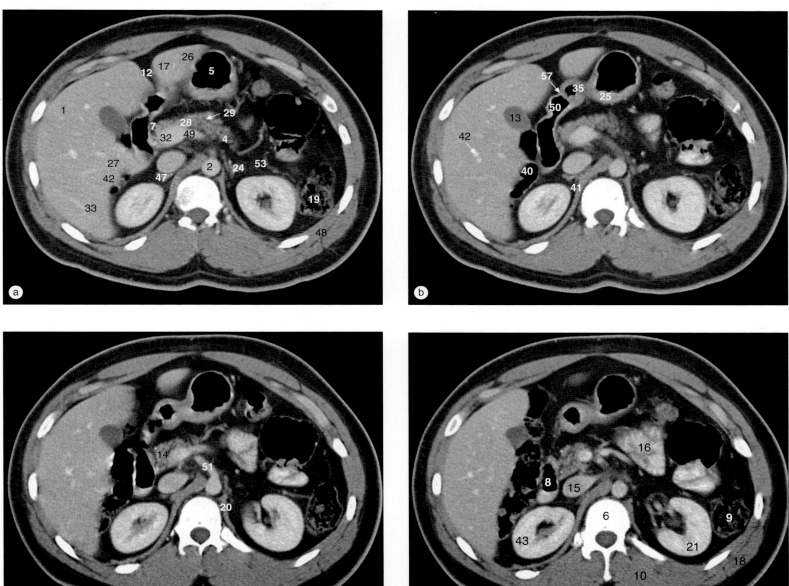

(a)–(h) Abdomen and pelvis in a male, sequential axial CT images, from superior to inferior.

1. Anterior segment of right lobe of liver	**11.** External oblique muscle	**21.** Left kidney
2. Aorta	**12.** Fissure for ligamentum venosum	**22.** Left renal artery
3. Ascending colon	**13.** Gall bladder	**23.** Left renal vein
4. Body of pancreas	**14.** Head of pancreas	**24.** Left suprarenal gland
5. Body of stomach	**15.** Inferior vena cava	**25.** Lesser curvature of stomach
6. Body of vertebra	**16.** Jejunum	**26.** Medial segment of left lobe of liver
7. Common bile duct	**17.** Lateral segment of left lobe of liver	**27.** Middle hepatic vein
8. Descending (second) part of duodenum	**18.** Latissimus dorsi muscle	**28.** Neck of pancreas
9. Descending colon	**19.** Left colic (splenic) flexure	**29.** Pancreatic duct
10. Erector spinae muscle	**20.** Left crus of diaphragm	**30.** Pararenal fat

Numbers 1–57 are common to pages 131–132.

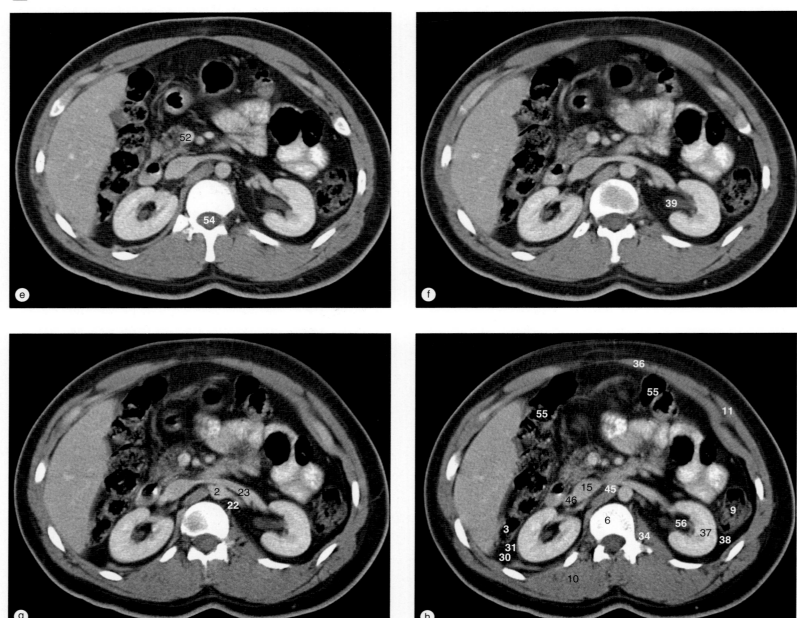

(a)–(h) Abdomen and pelvis in a male, sequential axial CT images, from superior to inferior.

31. Perirenal fat	**40.** Right colic (hepatic) flexure	**49.** Splenic vein
32. Portal vein	**41.** Right crus of diaphragm	**50.** Superior (first) part of duodenum
33. Posterior segment of right lobe of liver	**42.** Right hepatic vein	**51.** Superior mesenteric artery
34. Psoas major muscle	**43.** Right kidney	**52.** Superior mesenteric vein
35. Pyloric part of stomach	**44.** Right lobe of liver	**53.** Tail of pancreas
36. Rectus abdominis muscle	**45.** Right renal artery	**54.** Thecal sac
37. Renal cortex	**46.** Right renal vein	**55.** Transverse colon
38. Renal fascia	**47.** Right suprarenal gland	**56.** Renal sinus fat
39. Renal pelvis	**48.** Serratus anterior muscle	**57.** Pylorus

Numbers 1–57 are common to pages 131–132.

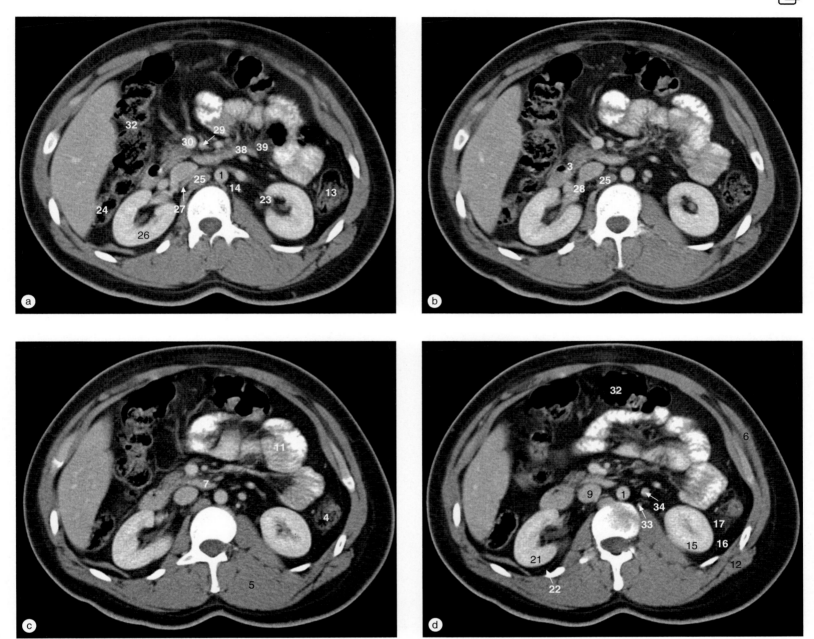

(a)–(h) Abdomen and pelvis in a male, sequential axial CT images, from superior to inferior.

1. Aorta	**8.** Ileum	**15.** Left kidney
2. Ascending colon	**9.** Inferior vena cava	**16.** Pararenal fat
3. Descending (second) part of duodenum	**10.** Internal oblique muscle	**17.** Perirenal fat
4. Descending colon	**11.** Jejunum	**18.** Psoas major muscle
5. Erector spinae muscles	**12.** Latissimus dorsi muscles	**19.** Quadratus lumborum muscle
6. External oblique muscle	**13.** Left colic (splenic) flexure	**20.** Rectus abdominis muscle
7. Horizontal (third) part of duodenum	**14.** Left crus of diaphragm	**21.** Renal cortex

Numbers 1–39 are common to pages 133–134.

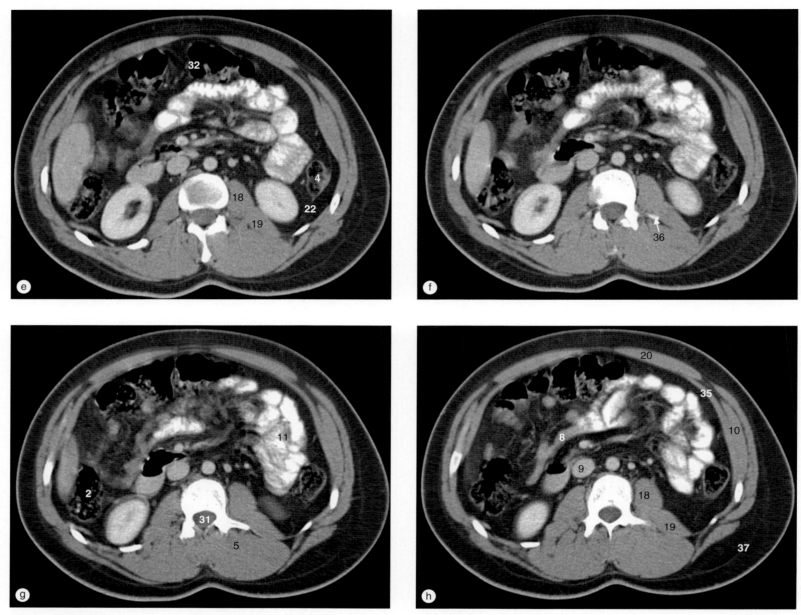

(a)–(h) Abdomen and pelvis in a male, sequential axial CT images, from superior to inferior.

22. Renal fascia	**28.** Right renal vein	**34.** Left testicular vein
23. Renal pelvis	**29.** Superior mesenteric artery	**35.** Transversus abdominis muscle
24. Right colic (hepatic) flexure	**30.** Superior mesenteric vein	**36.** Twelfth rib
25. Right crus of diaphragm	**31.** Thecal sac	**37.** Subcutaneous fascia
26. Right kidney	**32.** Transverse colon	**38.** Fourth (ascending) part of duodenum
27. Right renal artery	**33.** Left testicular artery	**39.** Duodenal–jejunal flexure

Numbers 1–39 are common to pages 133–134.

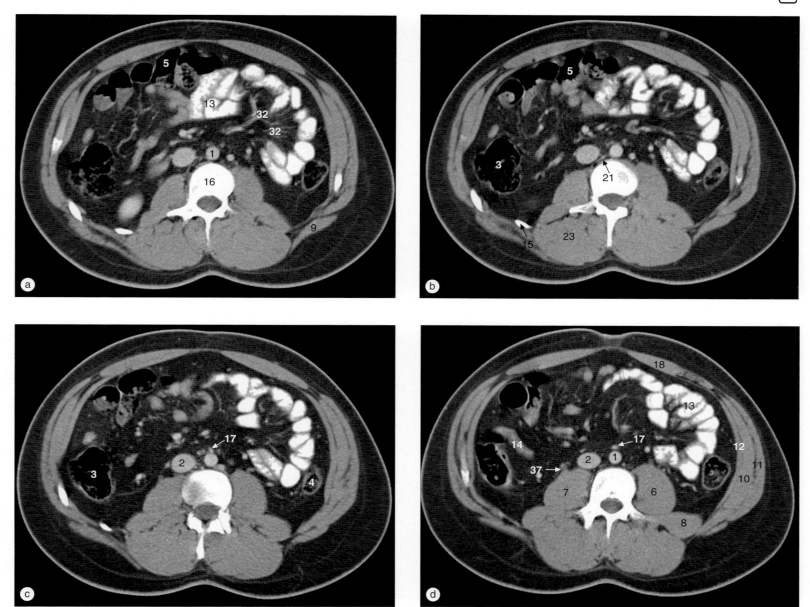

(a)–(h) Abdomen and pelvis in a male, sequential axial CT images, from superior to inferior.

1. Aorta	**8.** Quadratus lumborum muscle	**15.** Twelfth rib
2. Inferior vena cava	**9.** Latissimus dorsi muscle	**16.** Vertebral body
3. Ascending colon	**10.** Internal oblique muscle	**17.** Inferior mesenteric artery
4. Descending colon	**11.** External oblique muscle	**18.** Rectus abdominis muscle
5. Transverse colon	**12.** Transversus abdominis muscle	**19.** Appendicular artery
6. Left psoas muscle	**13.** Jejunum	**20.** Lumbar vein
7. Right psoas muscle	**14.** Ileum	**21.** Lumbar artery

Numbers 1–39 are common to pages 135–136.

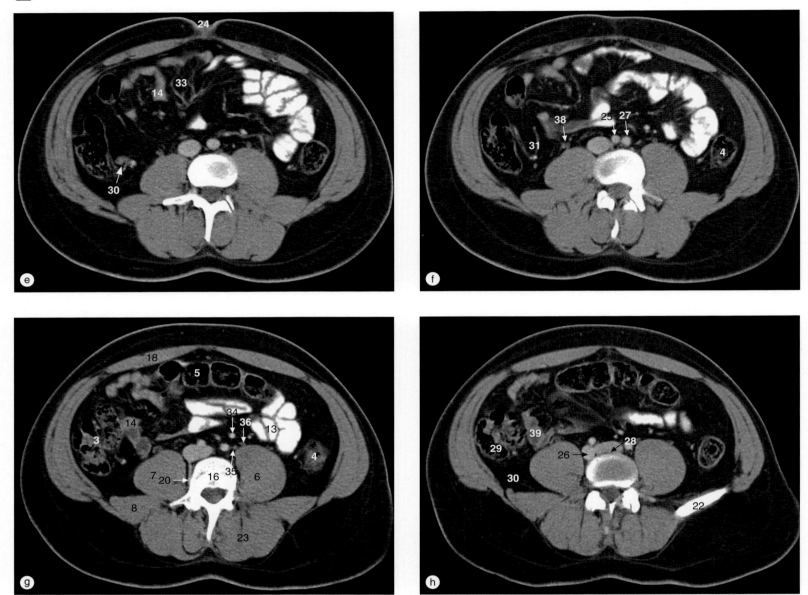

(a)–(h) Abdomen and pelvis in a male, sequential axial CT images, from superior to inferior.

22. Iliac bone	29. Caecum	34. Left testicular artery
23. Erector spinae muscles	30. Appendix	35. Left testicular vein
24. Umbilicus	31. Ileocolic artery	36. Left ureter
25. Right common iliac artery	32. Jejunal branches of superior mesenteric	37. Right ureter
26. Right common iliac vein	artery	38. Right testicular vessels
27. Left common iliac artery	33. Ileal branches of superior mesenteric	39. Terminal ileum
28. Left common iliac vein	artery	

Numbers 1–39 are common to pages 135–136.

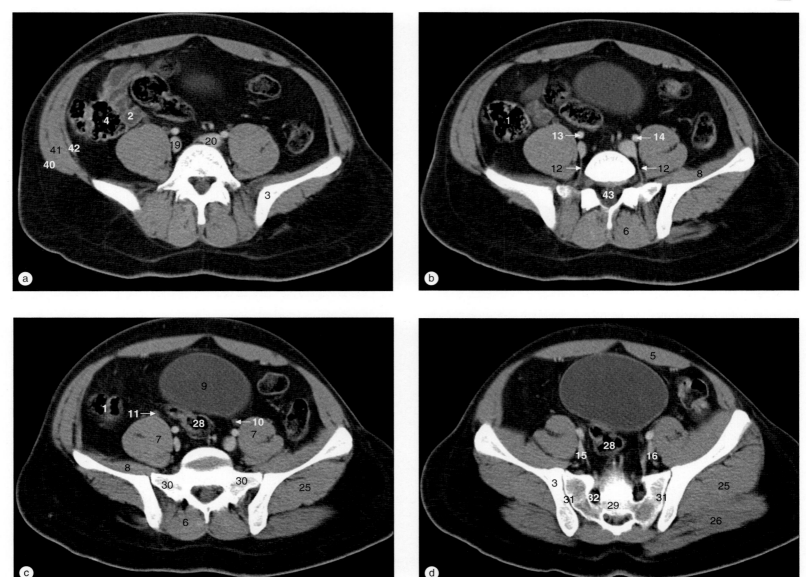

(a)–(h) Abdomen and pelvis in a male, sequential axial CT images, from superior to inferior.

1. Caecum	**9.** Urinary bladder	**17.** Right external iliac artery
2. Terminal ileum	**10.** Left ureter	**18.** Left external iliac artery
3. Iliac bone	**11.** Right ureter	**19.** Right common iliac vein
4. Ascending colon	**12.** Lumbar veins	**20.** Left common iliac vein
5. Rectus abdominis muscle	**13.** Right common iliac artery	**21.** Right internal iliac vein
6. Erector spinae muscles	**14.** Left common iliac artery	**22.** Left internal iliac vein
7. Psoas major muscle	**15.** Right internal iliac artery	**23.** Right external iliac vein
8. Iliacus muscle	**16.** Left internal iliac artery	**24.** Left external iliac vein

Numbers 1–45 are common to pages 137–138.

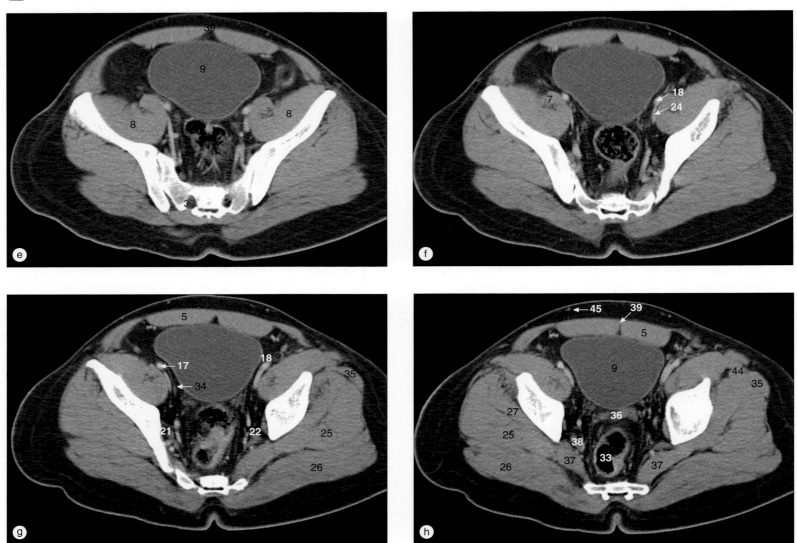

(a)–(h) Abdomen and pelvis in a male, sequential axial CT images, from superior to inferior.

25. Gluteus medius muscle	**32.** Sacral foramen	**39.** Linea alba
26. Gluteus maximus muscle	**33.** Rectum	**40.** External oblique muscle
27. Gluteus minimus muscle	**34.** Vas deferens	**41.** Internal oblique muscle
28. Sigmoid colon	**35.** Tensor fasciae latae muscle	**42.** Transversus abdominis muscle
29. Sacrum	**36.** Seminal vesicle	**43.** Thecal sac
30. Sacral alum	**37.** Piriformis muscle	**44.** Sartorius muscle
31. Sacroiliac joint	**38.** Superior gluteal artery and vein	**45.** Superficial inferior epigastric artery

Numbers 1–45 are common to pages 137–138.

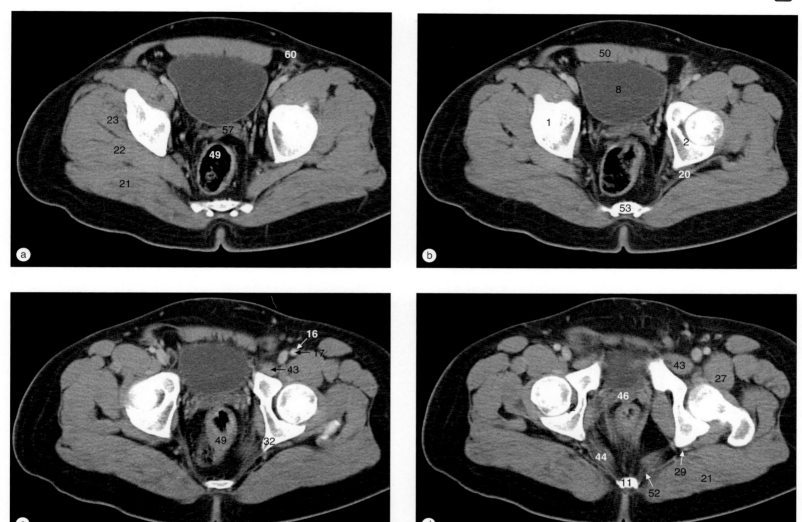

(a)–(h) Abdomen and pelvis in a male, sequential axial CT images, from superior to inferior.

1. Acetabular roof	**12.** Corpus cavernosum	**23.** Gluteus minimus muscle
2. Acetabulum	**13.** Crus of corpus cavernosum	**24.** Gracilis muscle
3. Adductor brevis muscle	**14.** Epididymis	**25.** Greater trochanter of femur
4. Adductor longus muscle	**15.** External anal sphincter	**26.** Head of femur
5. Adductor magnus muscle	**16.** External iliac artery	**27.** Iliopsoas muscle
6. Anal canal	**17.** External iliac vein	**28.** Iliotibial tract
7. Biceps femoris muscle	**18.** Femoral artery	**29.** Inferior gluteal artery and vein
8. Bladder	**19.** Femoral vein	**30.** Inferior ramus of pubis
9. Body of pubis	**20.** Gemellus muscle	**31.** Internal pudendal artery and vein
10. Bulb of penis	**21.** Gluteus maximus muscle	**32.** Ischial spine
11. Coccyx	**22.** Gluteus medius muscle	**33.** Ischio-anal fossa

Numbers 1–66 are common to pages 139–140.

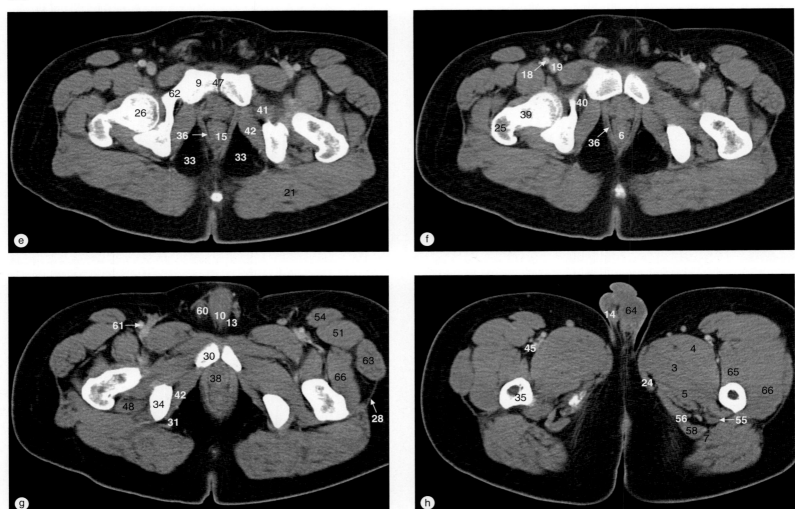

(a)–(h) Abdomen and pelvis in a male, sequential axial CT images, from superior to inferior.

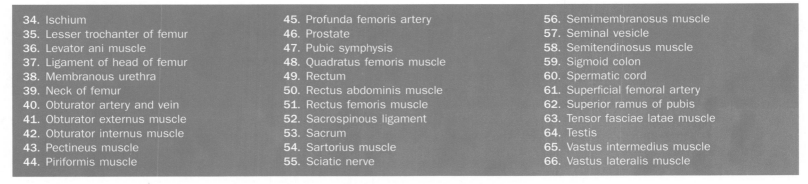

34. Ischium	**45.** Profunda femoris artery	**56.** Semimembranosus muscle
35. Lesser trochanter of femur	**46.** Prostate	**57.** Seminal vesicle
36. Levator ani muscle	**47.** Pubic symphysis	**58.** Semitendinosus muscle
37. Ligament of head of femur	**48.** Quadratus femoris muscle	**59.** Sigmoid colon
38. Membranous urethra	**49.** Rectum	**60.** Spermatic cord
39. Neck of femur	**50.** Rectus abdominis muscle	**61.** Superficial femoral artery
40. Obturator artery and vein	**51.** Rectus femoris muscle	**62.** Superior ramus of pubis
41. Obturator externus muscle	**52.** Sacrospinous ligament	**63.** Tensor fasciae latae muscle
42. Obturator internus muscle	**53.** Sacrum	**64.** Testis
43. Pectineus muscle	**54.** Sartorius muscle	**65.** Vastus intermedius muscle
44. Piriformis muscle	**55.** Sciatic nerve	**66.** Vastus lateralis muscle

Numbers 1–66 are common to pages 139–140.

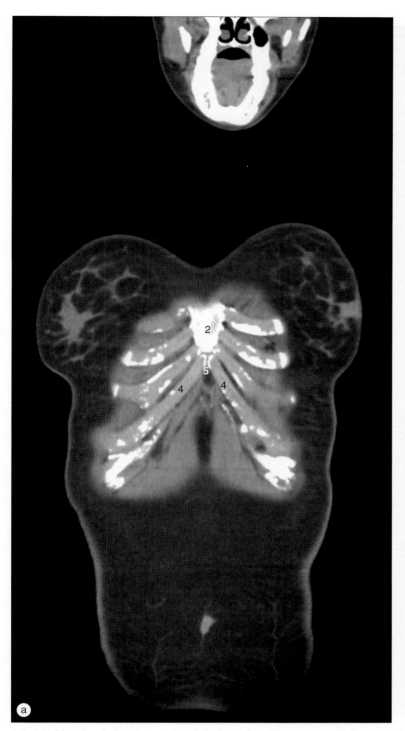

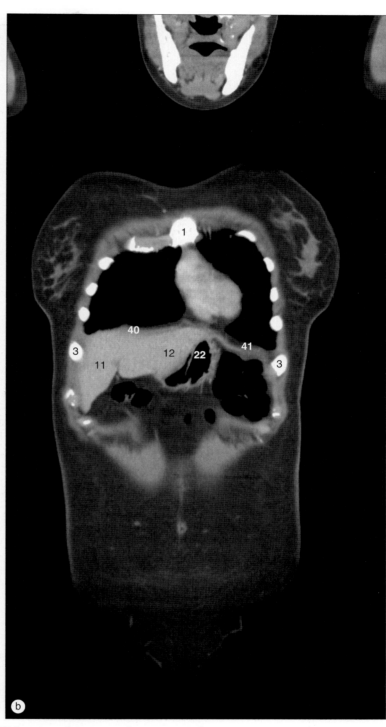

(a)–(d) Chest, abdomen and pelvis in a female, sequential coronal CT images, from anterior to posterior.
Note: Pages 141–150 show sequential images of the same female patient.

1. Manubrium	**8.** Right ventricle	**15.** Rectus abdominis muscle
2. Body of sternum	**9.** Left ventricle	**16.** Internal oblique muscle
3. Rib	**10.** Pulmonary conus	**17.** External oblique muscle
4. Costal cartilage	**11.** Right lobe of liver	**18.** Transversus abdominis muscle
5. Xiphisternum	**12.** Left lobe of liver	**19.** Transverse colon
6. Breast	**13.** Gall bladder	**20.** Left colic flexure
7. Clavicle	**14.** Fissure for falciform ligament	**21.** Right colic flexure

Numbers 1–41 are common to pages 141–142.

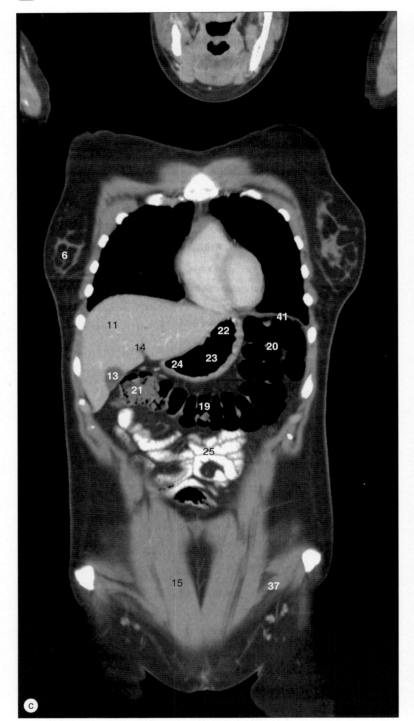

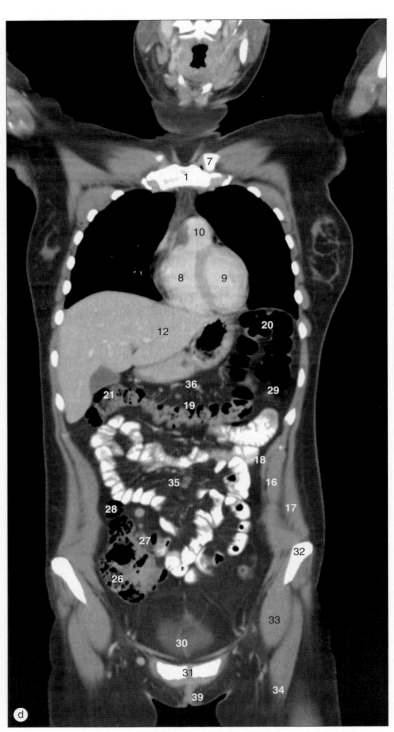

(a)–(d) Chest, abdomen and pelvis in a female, sequential coronal CT images, from anterior to posterior.

22. Fundus of stomach	**29.** Descending colon	**36.** Transverse mesocolon
23. Body of stomach	**30.** Urinary bladder	**37.** Pectineus muscle
24. Antrum of stomach	**31.** Pubic symphysis	**38.** Levator ani muscle
25. Jejunum	**32.** Iliac crest	**39.** Labium majus
26. Caecum	**33.** Iliopsoas muscle	**40.** Right hemidiaphragm
27. Ileum	**34.** Sartorius muscle	**41.** Left hemidiaphragm
28. Ascending colon	**35.** Small bowel mesentery	

Numbers 1–41 are common to pages 141–142.

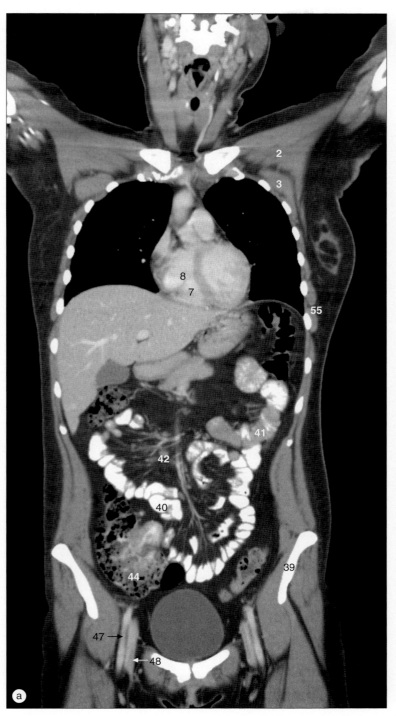

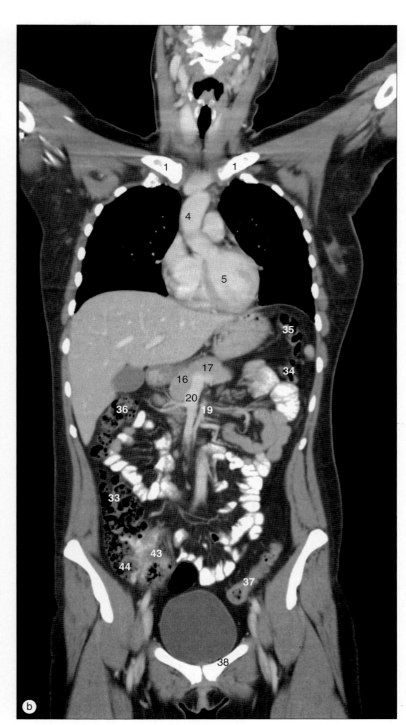

(a)–(d) Chest, abdomen and pelvis in a female, sequential coronal CT images, from anterior to posterior.

1. Clavicle	**11.** Brachiocephalic trunk	**21.** Splenic vein
2. Pectoralis major muscle	**12.** Right lung	**22.** Portal vein
3. Pectoralis minor muscle	**13.** Left lung	**23.** Gall bladder
4. Ascending aorta	**14.** Right lobe of liver	**24.** Inferior vena cava
5. Left ventricle	**15.** Left lobe of liver	**25.** Aorta
6. Pulmonary artery	**16.** Head of pancreas	**26.** Right common iliac artery
7. Right ventricle	**17.** Neck of pancreas	**27.** Left common iliac artery
8. Right atrium	**18.** Body of pancreas	**28.** Psoas muscle
9. Superior vena cava	**19.** Superior mesenteric artery	**29.** Iliacus muscle
10. Left brachiocephalic vein	**20.** Superior mesenteric vein	**30.** Iliopsoas muscle

Numbers 1–55 are common to pages 143–144.

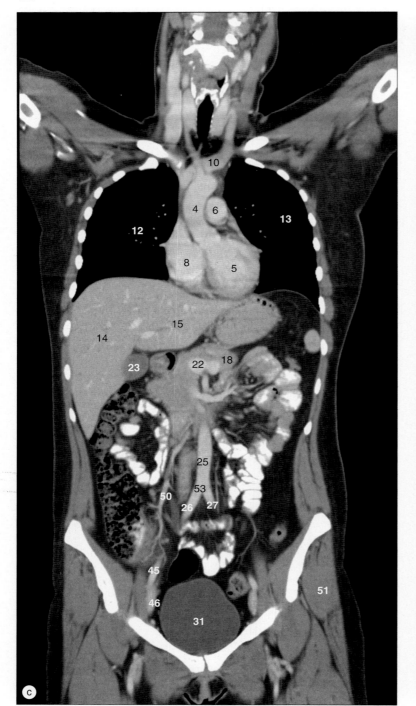

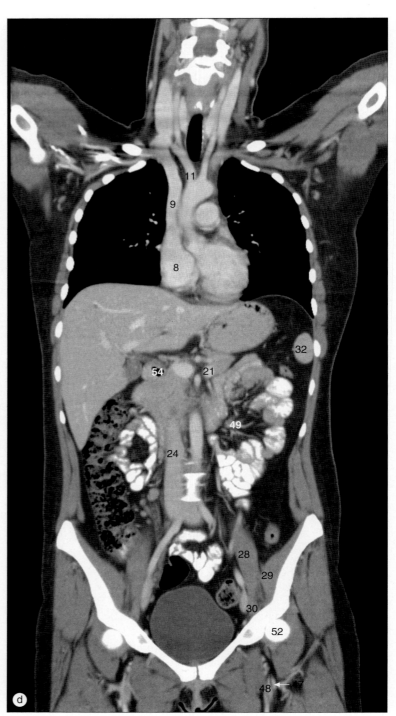

(a)–(d) Chest, abdomen and pelvis in a female, sequential coronal CT images, from anterior to posterior.

31. Urinary bladder	**40.** Ileum	**49.** Jejunal branches of superior mesenteric artery
32. Spleen	**41.** Jejunum	
33. Ascending colon	**42.** Small bowel mesentery	**50.** Ileal branches of superior mesenteric artery
34. Descending colon	**43.** Terminal ileum	
35. Left colic flexure	**44.** Caecum	**51.** Gluteus medius muscle
36. Right colic flexure	**45.** External iliac artery	**52.** Head of femur
37. Sigmoid colon	**46.** External iliac vein	**53.** Aortic bifurcation
38. Superior pubic ramus	**47.** Femoral artery	**54.** First part of duodenum
39. Ilium	**48.** Femoral vein	**55.** Serratus anterior muscle

Numbers 1–55 are common to pages 143–144.

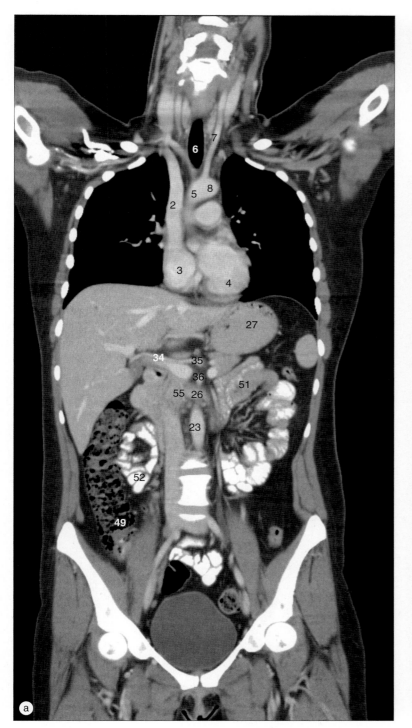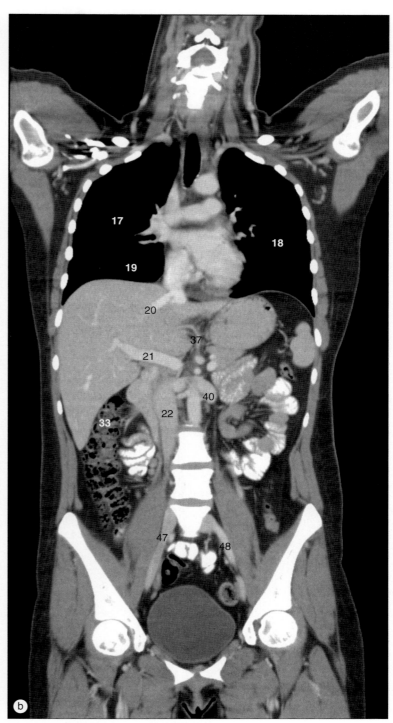

(a)–(d) Chest, abdomen and pelvis in a female, sequential coronal CT images, from anterior to posterior.

1. Oesophagus	12. Right upper lobe bronchus	23. Aorta
2. Superior vena cava	13. Bronchus intermedius	24. Right kidney
3. Right atrium	14. Left main bronchus	25. Right renal artery
4. Left ventricle	15. Left upper lobe bronchus	26. Left renal vein
5. Ascending aorta	16. Left atrium	27. Fundus of stomach
6. Trachea	17. Right lung	28. Spleen
7. Left common carotid artery	18. Left lung	29. Ascending colon
8. Aortic arch	19. Right lower lobe	30. Descending colon
9. Right pulmonary artery	20. Hepatic vein	31. Sigmoid colon
10. Left pulmonary artery	21. Portal vein	32. Left colic flexure
11. Right main bronchus	22. Inferior vena cava	33. Right colic flexure

Numbers 1–60 are common to pages 145–146.

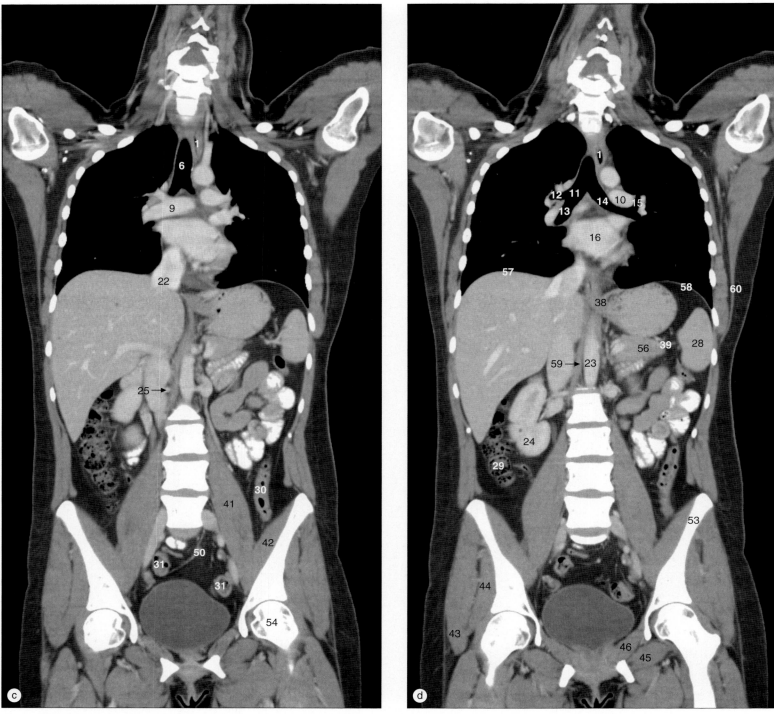

(a)–(d) Chest, abdomen and pelvis in a female, sequential coronal CT images, from anterior to posterior.

34. Common hepatic artery
35. Coeliac axis
36. Superior mesenteric artery
37. Left gastric artery
38. Oesophagogastric junction
39. Splenic artery
40. Left renal artery
41. Psoas muscle
42. Iliacus muscle
43. Gluteus maximus muscle

44. Gluteus medius muscle
45. Obturator externus muscle
46. Obturator internus muscle
47. Right common iliac vein
48. Left common iliac vein
49. Caecum
50. Sigmoid arteries (from inferior mesenteric artery)
51. Jejunum
52. Ileum

53. Iliac bone
54. Head of femur
55. Body of pancreas
56. Tail of pancreas
57. Right hemidiaphragm
58. Left hemidiaphragm
59. Right crus of diaphragm
60. Latissimus dorsi muscle

Numbers 1–60 are common to pages 145–146.

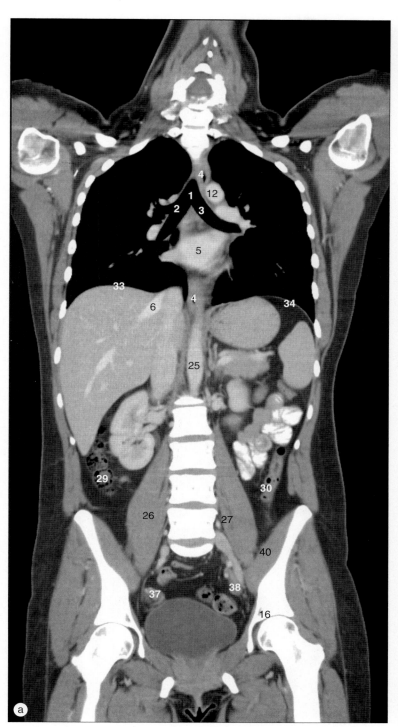
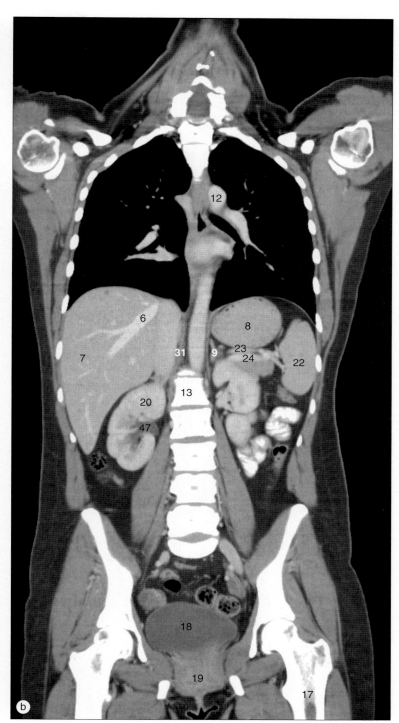

(a)–(d) Chest, abdomen and pelvis in a female, sequential coronal CT images, from anterior to posterior.

1. Carina
2. Right main bronchus
3. Left main bronchus
4. Oesophagus
5. Left atrium
6. Hepatic vein
7. Right lobe of liver
8. Fundus of stomach

9. Left suprarenal gland
10. Right suprarenal gland
11. Descending thoracic aorta
12. Aortic arch (knuckle)
13. Vertebral body of L1
14. Sacrum
15. Sacroiliac joint
16. Acetabulum

17. Femur
18. Urinary bladder
19. Vagina
20. Right kidney
21. Left kidney
22. Spleen
23. Splenic artery
24. Splenic vein

Numbers 1–47 are common to pages 147–148.

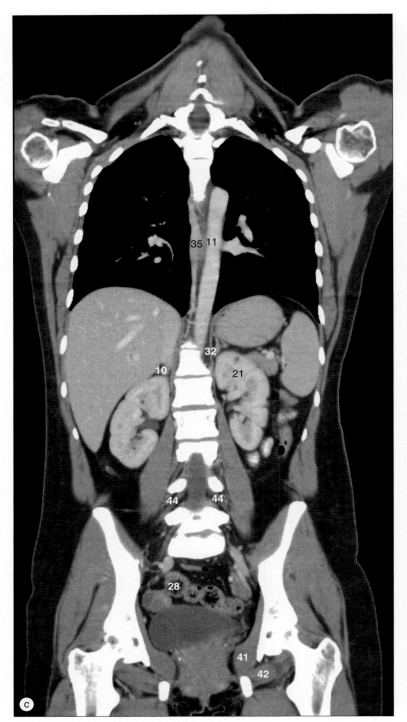
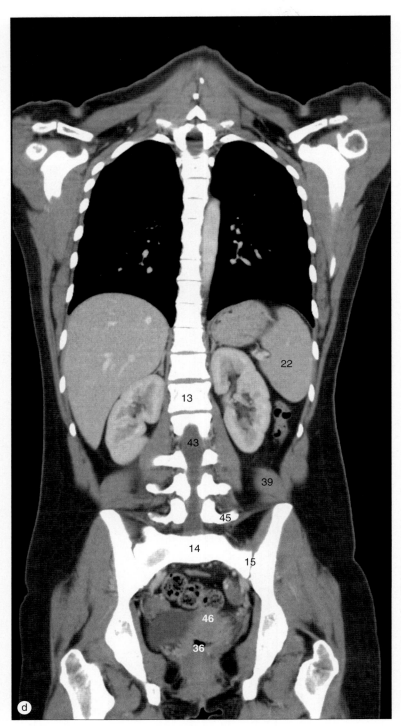

(a)–(d) Chest, abdomen and pelvis in a female, sequential coronal CT images, from anterior to posterior.

25. Abdominal aorta	**33.** Right hemidiaphragm	**41.** Obturator internus muscle
26. Psoas major muscle	**34.** Left hemidiaphragm	**42.** Obturator externus muscle
27. Psoas minor muscle	**35.** Azygos vein	**43.** Spinal canal
28. Sigmoid colon	**36.** Rectum	**44.** Lumbar nerve roots
29. Ascending colon	**37.** Right internal iliac vessels	**45.** Transverse process of L5
30. Descending colon	**38.** Left internal iliac vessels	**46.** Uterus
31. Right crus of diaphragm	**39.** Quadratus lumborum muscle	**47.** Renal pelvis
32. Left crus of diaphragm	**40.** Iliacus muscle	

Numbers 1–47 are common to pages 147–148.

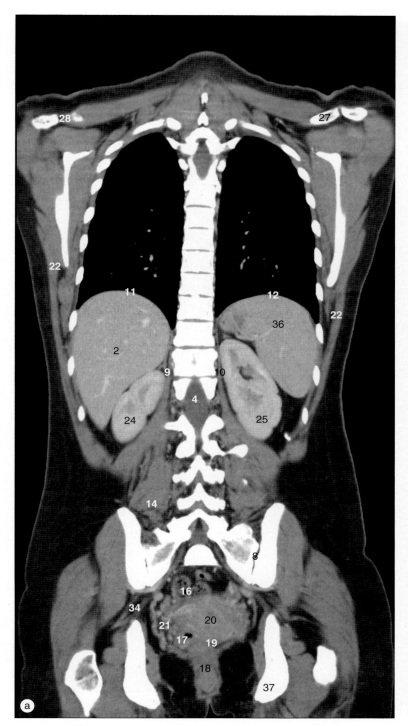
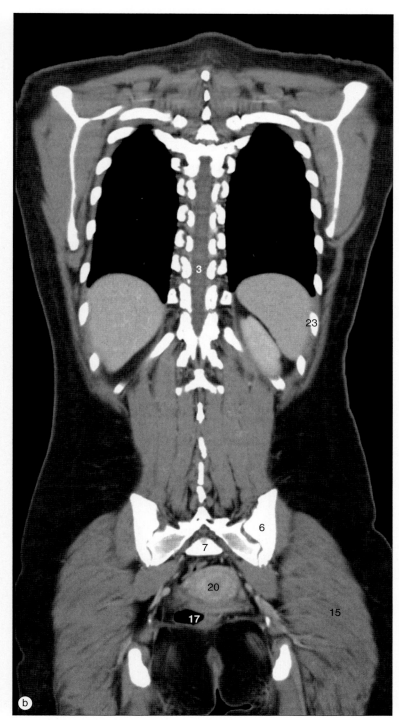

(a)–(d) Chest, abdomen and pelvis in a female, sequential coronal CT images, from anterior to posterior.

1. Twelfth rib	**8.** Sacroiliac joint	**15.** Gluteus maximus muscle
2. Liver	**9.** Right crus of diaphragm	**16.** Sigmoid colon
3. Spinal cord	**10.** Left crus of diaphragm	**17.** Rectum
4. Spinal canal	**11.** Right hemidiaphragm	**18.** Vagina
5. Spinous process	**12.** Left hemidiaphragm	**19.** Cervix
6. Iliac bone	**13.** Erector spinae muscles	**20.** Uterus
7. Sacrum	**14.** Quadratus lumborum muscle	**21.** Uterine veins

Numbers 1–37 are common to pages 149–150.

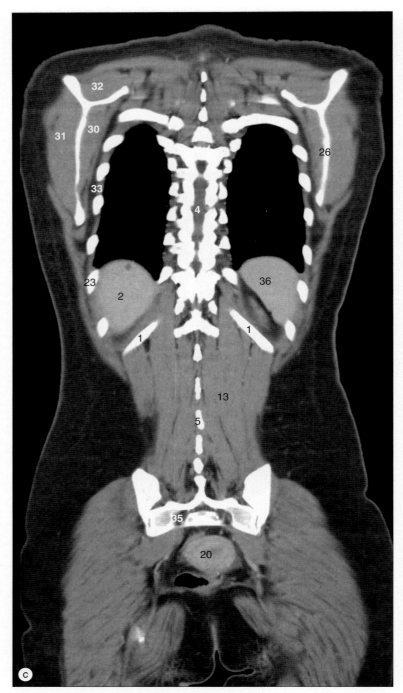

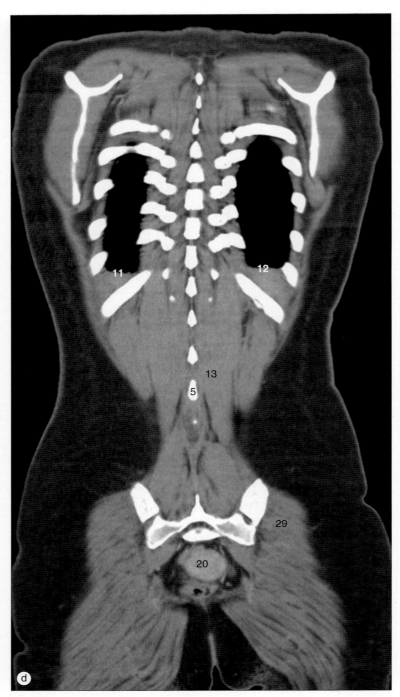

(a)–(d) Chest, abdomen and pelvis in a female, sequential coronal CT images, from anterior to posterior.

22. Latissimus dorsi muscle	**28.** Acromioclavicular joint	**34.** Sciatic nerve
23. Tenth rib	**29.** Gluteus maximus muscle	**35.** Sacral nerve foramen
24. Right kidney	**30.** Subscapularis muscle	**36.** Spleen
25. Left kidney	**31.** Infraspinatus muscle	**37.** Ischium
26. Scapula	**32.** Supraspinatus muscle	
27. Clavicle	**33.** Intercostal muscle	

Numbers 1–37 are common to pages 149–150.

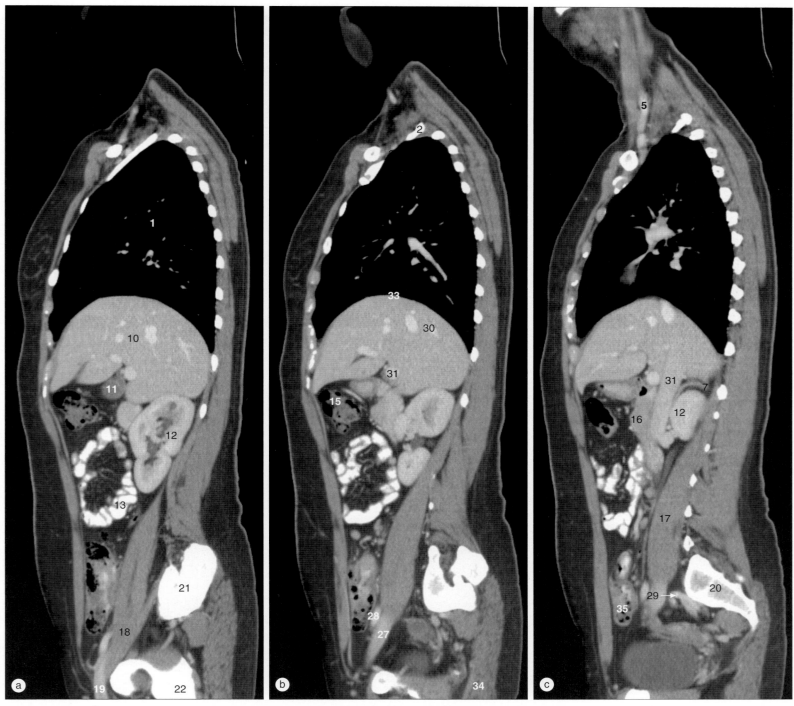

(a)–(h) Chest, abdomen and pelvis in a female, sequential sagittal CT images, from right to left.
Note: Pages 151–153 show sequential images of the same female patient.

1. Right lung	13. Jejunum	25. Sigmoid colon
2. Right first rib	14. Ileum	26. Right common iliac artery
3. Right clavicle	15. Right colic flexure	27. Right external iliac vein
4. Manubrium	16. Pancreas	28. Right external iliac artery
5. Right internal jugular vein	17. Psoas major muscle	29. Right common iliac vein
6. Aorta	18. Iliopsoas muscle	30. Hepatic vein
7. Inferior vena cava	19. Common femoral vessels	31. Portal vein
8. Superior vena cava	20. Sacrum	32. Pubic bone
9. Right atrium	21. Ilium	33. Right hemidiaphragm
10. Right lobe of liver	22. Ischium	34. Gluteus maximus muscle
11. Gall bladder	23. Urinary bladder	35. Caecum
12. Right kidney	24. Rectum	

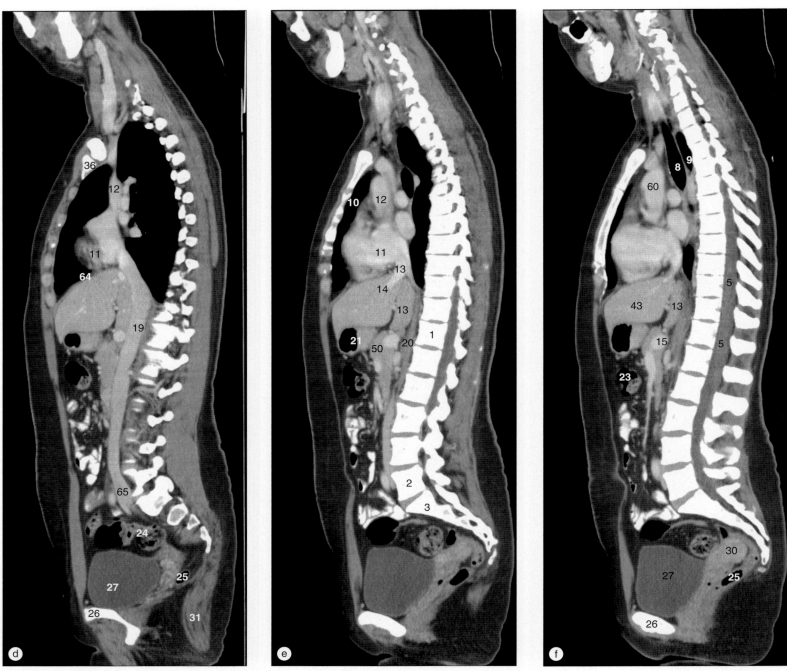

(a)–(h) Chest, abdomen and pelvis in a female, sequential sagittal CT images, from right to left.

1. Body of T12 vertebra	10. Right lung	19. Aorta	28. Cervix
2. Body of L5 vertebra	11. Right atrium	20. Right crus of diaphragm	29. Vagina
3. Sacrum	12. Superior vena cava	21. Stomach	30. Uterus
4. Coccyx	13. Inferior vena cava	22. Descending colon	31. Gluteus maximus muscle
5. Spinal cord	14. Hepatic vein	23. Transverse colon	32. Iliac bone
6. Spinal canal	15. Splenic vein	24. Sigmoid colon	33. Head of femur
7. Filum terminale	16. Superior mesenteric vein	25. Rectum	34. Ischium
8. Trachea	17. Superior mesenteric artery	26. Pubic bone	35. Sternum
9. Oesophagus	18. Coeliac axis	27. Urinary bladder	36. Manubrium

Numbers 1–65 are common to pages 152–153.

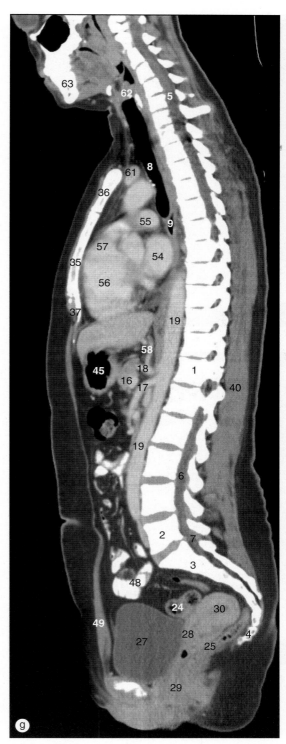

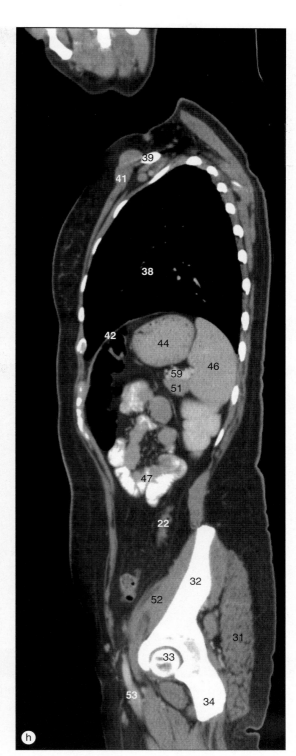

(a)–(h) Chest, abdomen and pelvis in a female, sequential sagittal CT images, from right to left.

37. Xiphisternum	**47.** Jejunum	**57.** Pulmonary outflow tract
38. Left lung	**48.** Ileum	**58.** Common hepatic artery
39. Left clavicle	**49.** Rectus abdominis muscle	**59.** Splenic artery
40. Erector spinae muscles	**50.** Body of pancreas	**60.** Ascending thoracic aorta
41. Left pectoralis major muscle	**51.** Tail of pancreas	**61.** Left brachiocephalic vein
42. Left hemidiaphragm	**52.** Iliacus muscle	**62.** Larynx
43. Liver	**53.** Left femoral vessels	**63.** Mandible
44. Fundus of stomach	**54.** Left atrium	**64.** Right hemidiaphragm
45. Body of stomach	**55.** Right pulmonary artery	**65.** Right common iliac artery
46. Spleen	**56.** Right ventricle	

Numbers 1–65 are common to pages 152–153.

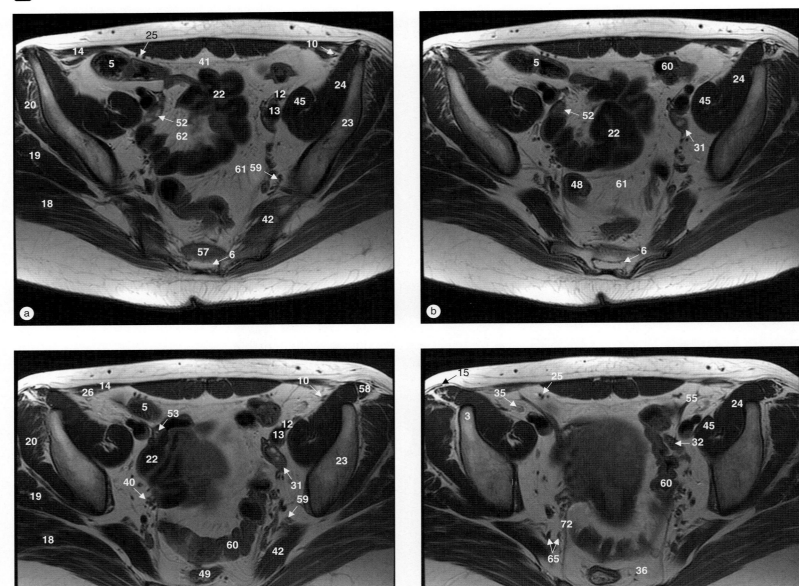

(a)–(p) Female pelvis, sequential axial T2-weighted MR images, from superior to inferior.

1. Acetabular labrum (posterior)	13. External iliac vein	24. Iliacus muscle
2. Anterior vaginal fornix	14. External oblique aponeurosis	25. Inferior epigastric vessels
3. Anterior inferior iliac spine	15. Fascia lata	26. Inguinal ligament
4. Bladder	16. Femoral head	27. Internal cervical os
5. Caecal pole	17. Femoral nerve	28. Ischial spine
6. Central sacral canal	18. Gluteus maximus muscle	29. Ischio-anal fossa
7. Cervical wall	19. Gluteus medius muscle	30. Ischium
8. Common femoral artery	20. Gluteus minimus muscle	31. Left ovary
9. Common femoral vein	21. Hip joint capsule (with iliofemoral	32. Left uterine tube
10. Deep circumflex iliac vessels	ligament)	33. Levator ani muscle (puborectalis)
11. External cervical os	22. Ileum	34. Ligamentum teres
12. External iliac artery	23. Iliac bone	35. Lymph node

Numbers 1-72 are common to pages 154-155.

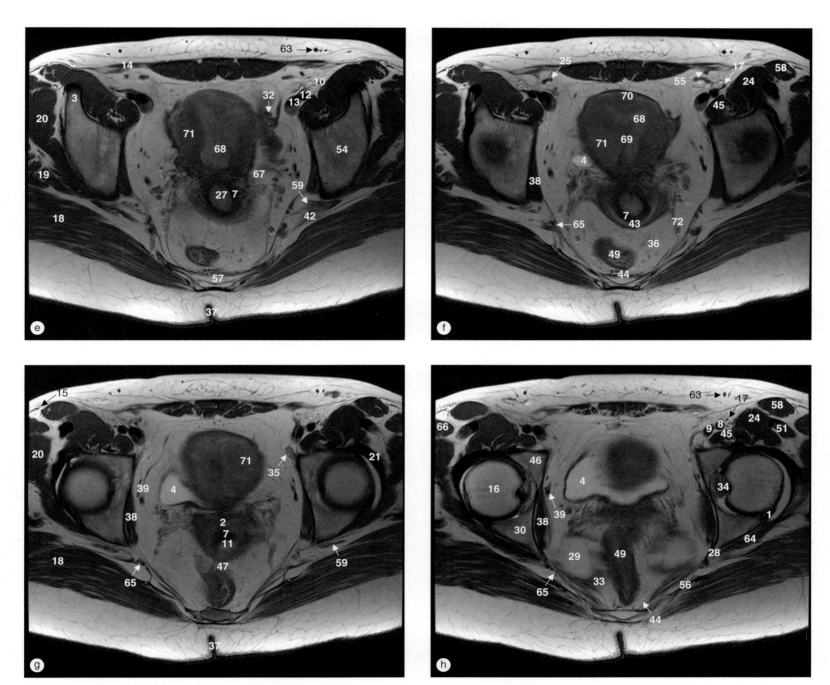

(a)–(p) Female pelvis, sequential axial T2-weighted MR images, from superior to inferior.

36. Mesorectum	49. Rectum	62. Small bowel mesentery
37. Natal cleft	50. Rectus abdominis muscle	63. Superficial epigastric vessels
38. Obturator internus muscle	51. Rectus femoris muscle	64. Superior gemellus muscle
39. Obturator vessels	52. Right ovary	65. Superior gluteal vessels
40. Ovarian vessels	53. Right uterine tube	66. Tensor fascia latae muscle
41. Parietal peritoneum	54. Roof of acetabulum	67. Transverse cervical ligament
42. Piriformis muscle	55. Round ligament of uterus	68. Uterine cavity
43. Posterior vaginal fornix	56. Sacrospinous ligament	69. Uterine endometrium
44. Presacral (Waldeyer's) fascia	57. Sacrum	70. Uterine fundus
45. Psoas muscle	58. Sartorius muscle	71. Uterine myometrium
46. Pubic bone	59. Sciatic nerve	72. Uterosacral ligament
47. Recto-uterine pouch (of Douglas)	60. Sigmoid colon	
48. Rectosigmoid junction	61. Sigmoid mesentery	

Numbers 1-72 are common to pages 154-155.

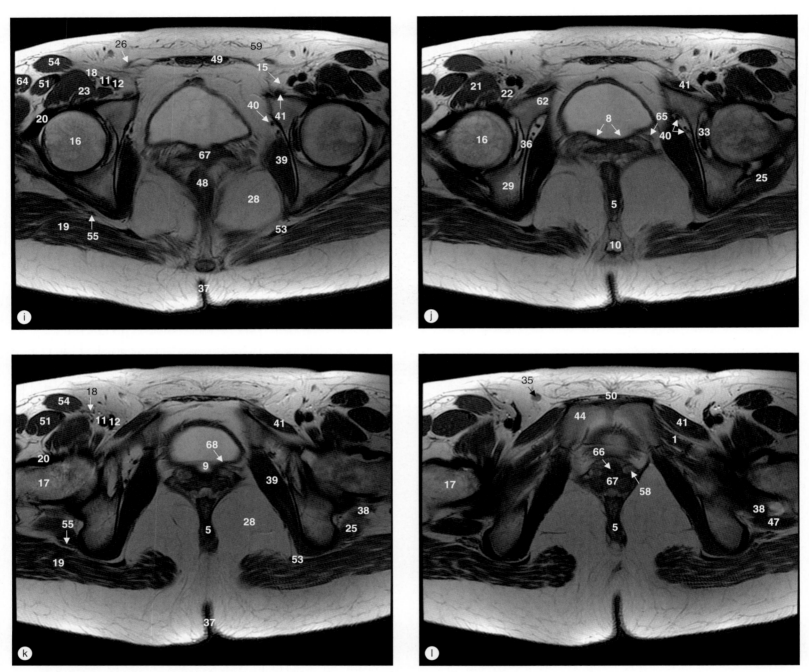

(a)–(p) Female pelvis, sequential axial T2-weighted MR images, from superior to inferior.

1. Adductor brevis muscle	13. External anal sphincter	24. Iliopsoas tendon
2. Adductor longus muscle	14. Extraperitoneal fat (cave of Retzius)	25. Inferior gemellus muscle
3. Adductor magnus muscle	15. Femoral canal	26. Inguinal ligament
4. Anal canal	16. Femoral head	27. Ischial tuberosity
5. Anococcygeal ligament	17. Femoral neck	28. Ischio-anal fossa
6. Anorectal junction	18. Femoral nerve branches	29. Ischium
7. Biceps femoris tendon	19. Gluteus maximus muscle	30. Labia minora
8. Bladder base	20. Hip joint capsule (with the iliofemoral ligament)	31. Labium majus
9. Bladder neck		32. Lesser trochanter of femur
10. Coccyx	21. Iliacus muscle	33. Ligamentum teres
11. Common femoral artery	22. Iliocapsularis muscle	34. Long saphenous vein
12. Common femoral vein	23. Iliopsoas muscle complex	35. Lymph node

Numbers 1-68 are common to pages 156-157.

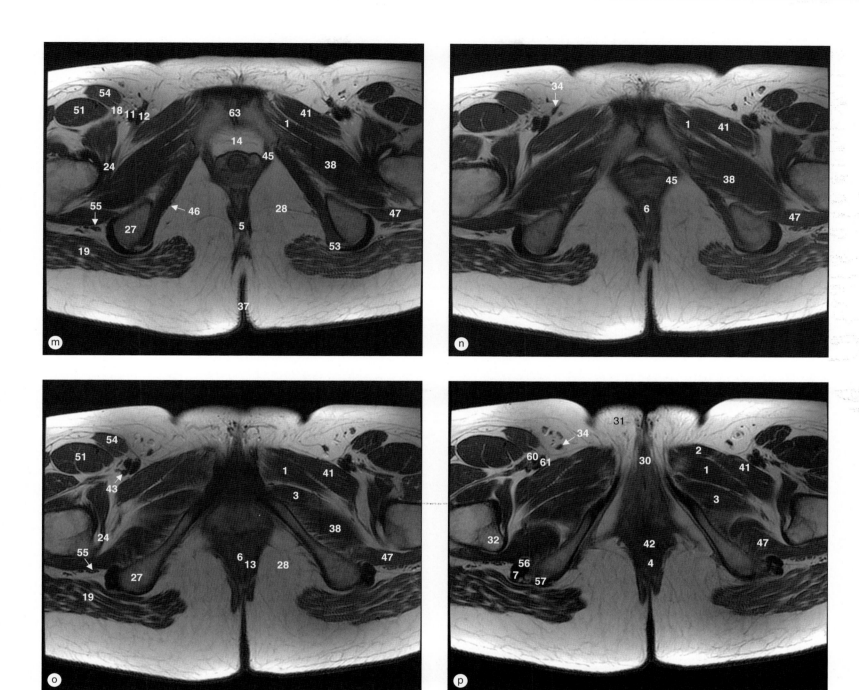

(a)–(p) Female pelvis, sequential axial T2-weighted MR images, from superior to inferior.

36. Medial wall of the acetabulum	47. Quadratus femoris muscle	59. Superficial fascial layer (Camper's fascia)
37. Natal cleft	48. Rectum	60. Superficial femoral artery
38. Obturator externus muscle	49. Rectus abdominis muscle	61. Superficial femoral vein
39. Obturator internus muscle	50. Rectus abdominis tendon	62. Superior pubic ramus
40. Obturator vessels and nerve	51. Rectus femoris muscle	63. Symphysis pubis
41. Pectineus muscle	52. Round ligament of the uterus	64. Tensor fascia latae muscle
42. Perineal body	53. Sacrotuberous ligament	65. Ureter
43. Profunda femoris artery	54. Sartorius muscle	66. Urethra
44. Pubic body	55. Sciatic nerve	67. Vagina
45. Puborectalis muscle	56. Semimembranosus tendon	68. Vesicoureteric junction
46. Pudendal neurovascular bundle (Alcock's canal)	57. Semitendinosus tendon	
	58. Skene's glands	

Numbers 1-68 are common to pages 156-157.

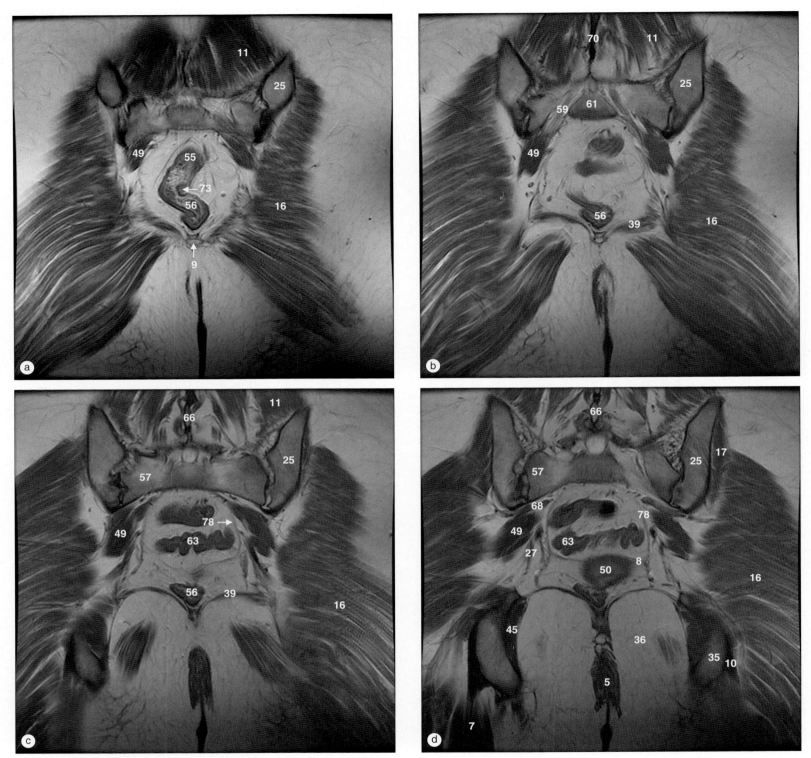

(a)–(p) Female pelvis, sequential coronal T2-weighted MR images, from posterior to anterior.

1. Acetabulum	13. External cervical os	25. Iliac bone
2. Adductor brevis muscle	14. Femoral head	26. Inferior gemellus muscle
3. Adductor longus muscle	15. Femoral neck	27. Inferior gluteal vessels
4. Adductor magnus muscle	16. Gluteus maximus muscle	28. Inferior pubic ramus
5. Anal canal	17. Gluteus medius muscle	29. Inferior rectal neurovascular bundle
6. Anterior fornix of vagina	18. Gluteus minimus muscle	30. Internal cervical os
7. Biceps femoris muscle	19. Gracilis muscle	31. Internal iliac vessels
8. Broad ligament of uterus	20. Greater trochanter of femur	32. Internal pudendal neurovascular bundle (Alcock's canal)
9. Coccyx	21. Ileum	
10. Common hamstring origin	22. Iliac crest	33. Intertrochanteric region of femur
11. Erector spinae muscle	23. Iliacus muscle	34. Intervertebral disc at L5/S1 (posterior margin)
12. External anal sphincter	24. Iliopsoas tendon	

Numbers 1-79 are common to pages 158-159.

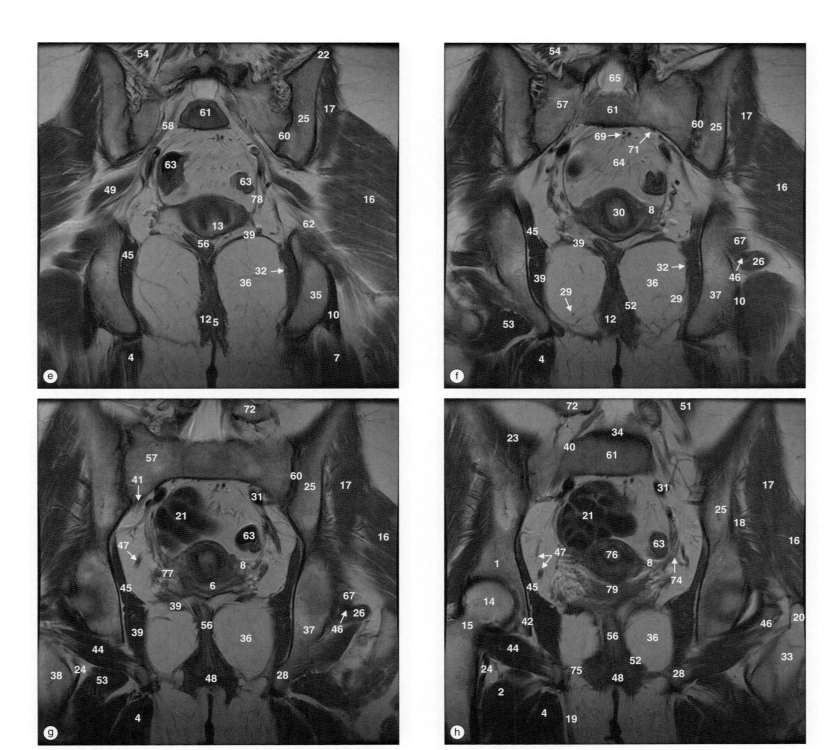

(a)–(p) Female pelvis, sequential coronal T2-weighted MR images, from posterior to anterior.

35. Ischial tuberosity	**50.** Posterior fornix of vagina	**65.** Spinal canal
36. Ischio-anal fossa	**51.** Psoas major muscle	**66.** Spinous process of L5
37. Ischium	**52.** Puborectalis muscle	**67.** Superior gemellus muscle
38. Lesser trochanter of femur	**53.** Quadratus femoris muscle	**68.** Superior gluteal vessels
39. Levator ani muscle	**54.** Quadratus lumborum muscle	**69.** Superior rectal vessels
40. Lumbar nerve (L5)	**55.** Rectosigmoid junction	**70.** Supraspinous ligament
41. Lumbosacral trunk	**56.** Rectum	**71.** Sympathetic chain
42. Medial wall of acetabulum	**57.** Sacral ala	**72.** Transverse process of L5
43. Middle rectal vessels	**58.** Sacral nerve (S1)	**73.** Transverse rectal fold (of Houston)
44. Obturator externus muscle	**59.** Sacral nerve (S2)	**74.** Ureter
45. Obturator internus muscle	**60.** Sacroiliac joint	**75.** Urogenital diaphragm
46. Obturator internus tendon	**61.** Sacrum	**76.** Uterine cavity
47. Obturator neurovascular bundle	**62.** Sciatic nerve	**77.** Uterine vessels
48. Perineal body	**63.** Sigmoid colon	**78.** Uterosacral ligament
49. Piriformis muscle	**64.** Sigmoid mesentery	**79.** Vagina

Numbers 1-79 are common to pages 158-159.

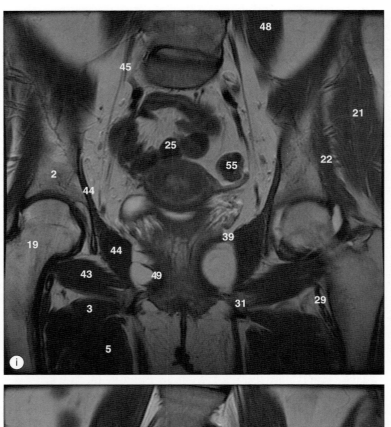

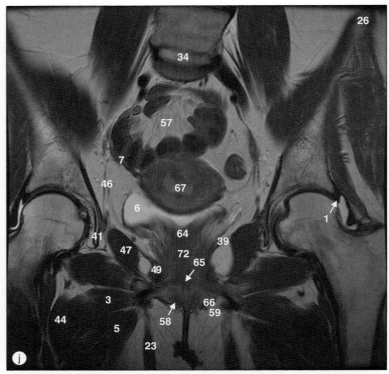

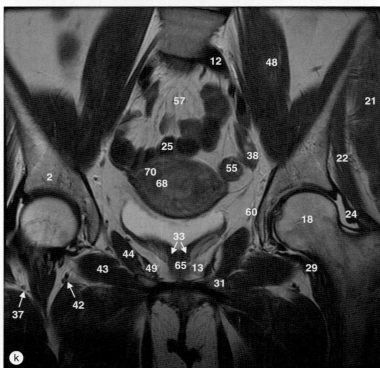

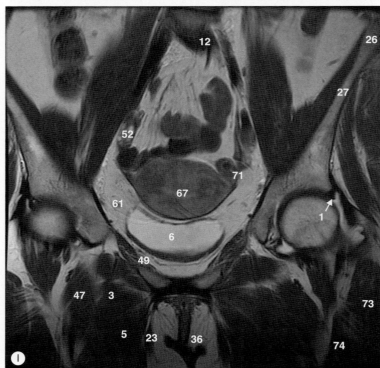

(a)–(p) Female pelvis, sequential coronal T2-weighted MR images, from posterior to anterior.

1. Acetabular labrum	13. Deep perineal pouch	25. Ileum
2. Acetabular roof	14. Descending colon	26. Iliac crest
3. Adductor brevis muscle	15. External iliac artery	27. Iliac wing
4. Adductor longus muscle	16. External oblique muscle	28. Iliacus muscle
5. Adductor magnus muscle	17. Femoral canal	29. Iliopsoas tendon
6. Bladder	18. Femoral head	30. Inferior epigastric vessels
7. Broad ligament of the uterus	19. Femoral neck	31. Inferior pubic ramus
8. Caecum	20. Femoral nerve	32. Internal oblique muscle
9. Common femoral artery	21. Gluteus medius muscle	33. Internal sphincter of bladder
10. Common femoral vein	22. Gluteus minimus muscle	34. Intervertebral disc at L5/S1
11. Common iliac artery	23. Gracilis muscle	35. Labia minora
12. Common iliac vein	24. Hip joint capsule	36. Labium majorum

Numbers 1-74 are common to pages 160-161.

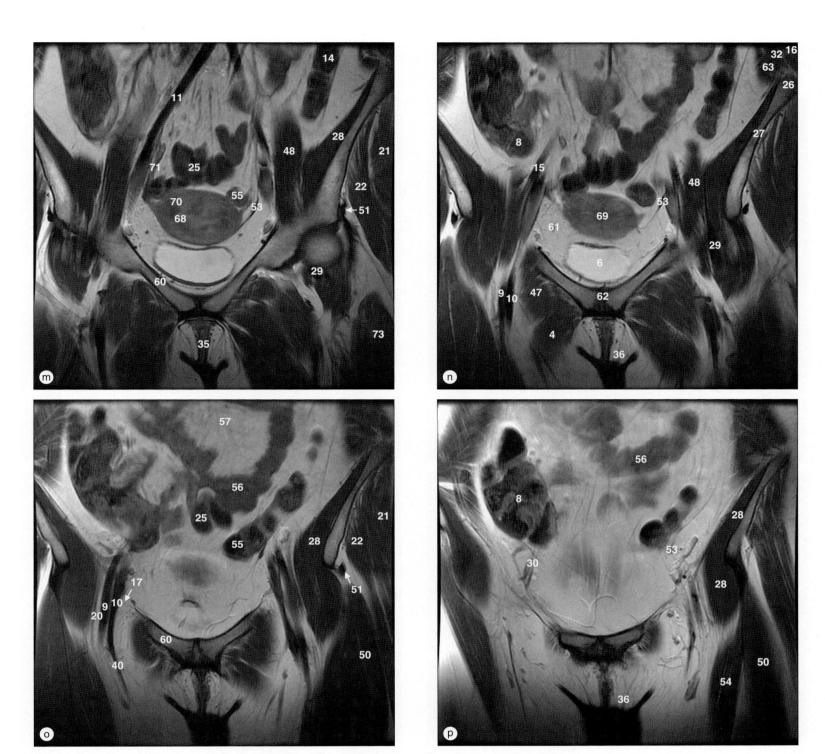

(a)–(p) Female pelvis, sequential coronal T2-weighted MR images, from posterior to anterior.

37. Lateral circumflex femoral vessels	**50.** Rectus femoris muscle	**63.** Transversus abdominis muscle
38. Left ovary	**51.** Reflected head of rectus femoris muscle	**64.** Trigone of bladder
39. Levator ani muscle	**52.** Right ovary	**65.** Urethra
40. Long saphenous vein	**53.** Round ligament of the uterus	**66.** Urogenital diaphragm
41. Medial acetabulum	**54.** Sartorius muscle	**67.** Uterine cavity
42. Medial circumflex femoral vessels	**55.** Sigmoid colon	**68.** Uterine endometrium
43. Obturator externus muscle	**56.** Small bowel	**69.** Uterine fundus
44. Obturator internus muscle	**57.** Small bowel mesentery	**70.** Uterine myometrium
45. Obturator nerve	**58.** Sphincter urethralis	**71.** Uterine tube
46. Obturator neurovascular bundle	**59.** Superficial perineal pouch	**72.** Vagina
47. Pectineus muscle	**60.** Superior pubic ramus	**73.** Vastus lateralis muscle
48. Psoas major muscle	**61.** Superior vesical vessels	**74.** Vastus intermedius muscle
49. Puborectalis muscle	**62.** Symphysis pubis	

Numbers 1-74 are common to pages 160-161.

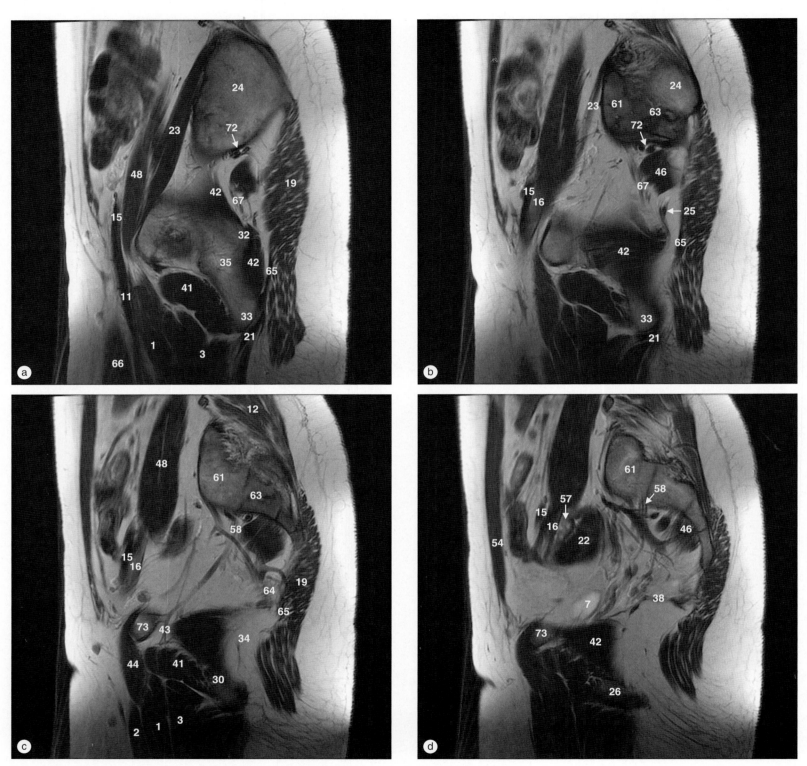

(a)–(p) Female pelvis, sequential sagittal T2-weighted MR images, from right to left.

1. Adductor brevis muscle	**9.** Cervix	**17.** Extraperitoneal fat
2. Adductor longus muscle	**10.** Coccyx	**18.** Filum terminale
3. Adductor magnus muscle	**11.** Common femoral vein	**19.** Gluteus maximus muscle
4. Anococcygeal raphe	**12.** Erector spinae muscles	**20.** Gracilis muscle
5. Anterior fornix of vagina	**13.** External anal sphincter	**21.** Hamstring origin
6. Anus	**14.** External cervical os	**22.** Ileum
7. Bladder	**15.** External iliac artery	**23.** Iliacus muscle
8. Broad ligament of the uterus	**16.** External iliac vein	**24.** Ilium

Numbers 1–88 are common to pages 162–165.

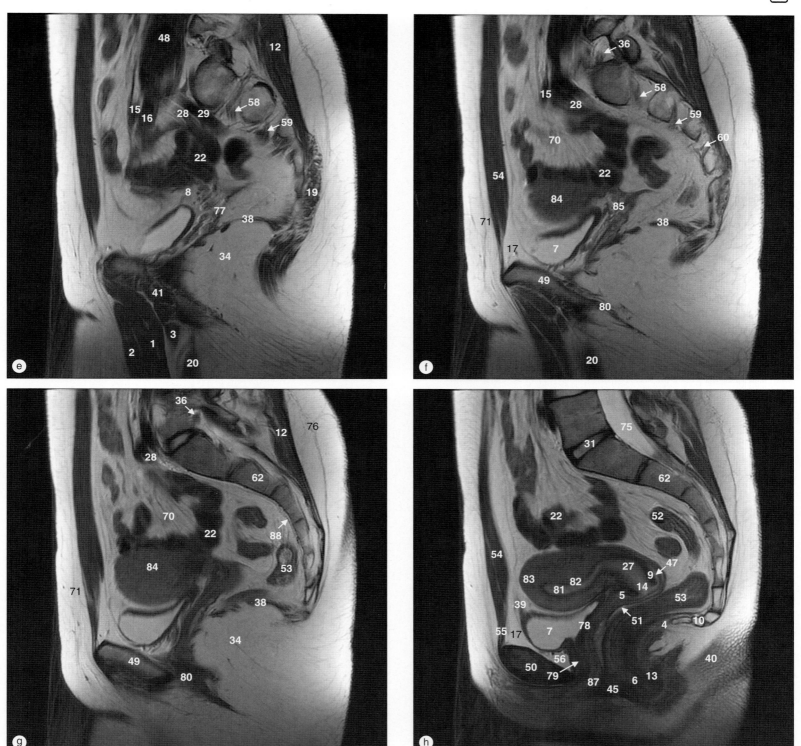

(a)–(p) Female pelvis, sequential sagittal T2-weighted MR images, from right to left.

25. Inferior gluteal vessels	**32.** Ischial spine	**40.** Natal cleft
26. Inferior pubic ramus	**33.** Ischial tuberosity	**41.** Obturator externus muscle
27. Internal cervical os	**34.** Ischioanal fossa	**42.** Obturator internus muscle
28. Internal iliac artery	**35.** Ischium	**43.** Obturator neurovascular bundle
29. Internal iliac vein	**36.** L5 nerve root	**44.** Pectineus muscle
30. Internal pudendal neurovascular bundle (Alcock's canal)	**37.** Left ovary	**45.** Perineal body
	38. Levator ani	**46.** Piriformis muscle
31. Intervertebral disc at L5/S1	**39.** Median umbilical ligament	**47.** Posterior fornix of vagina

Numbers 1–88 are common to pages 162–165.

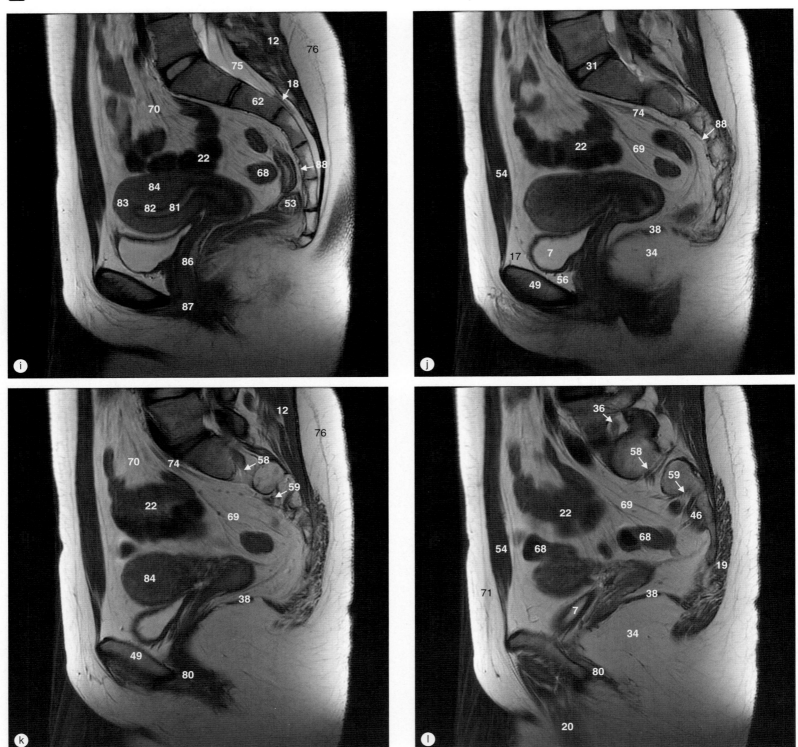

(a)–(p) Female pelvis, sequential sagittal T2-weighted MR images, from right to left.

48. Psoas major muscle	55. Rectus sheath	61. Sacral ala
49. Pubic body	56. Retropubic space (cave of Retzius,	62. Sacral body
50. Pubic symphysis	extraperitoneal fat)	63. Sacroiliac joint
51. Recto-uterine pouch (of Douglas)	57. Right ovary	64. Sacrospinous ligament
52. Rectosigmoid junction	58. S1 nerve root	65. Sacrotuberous ligament
53. Rectum	59. S2 nerve root	66. Sartorius muscle
54. Rectus abdominis muscle	60. S3 nerve root	67. Sciatic nerve

Numbers 1–88 are common to pages 162–165.

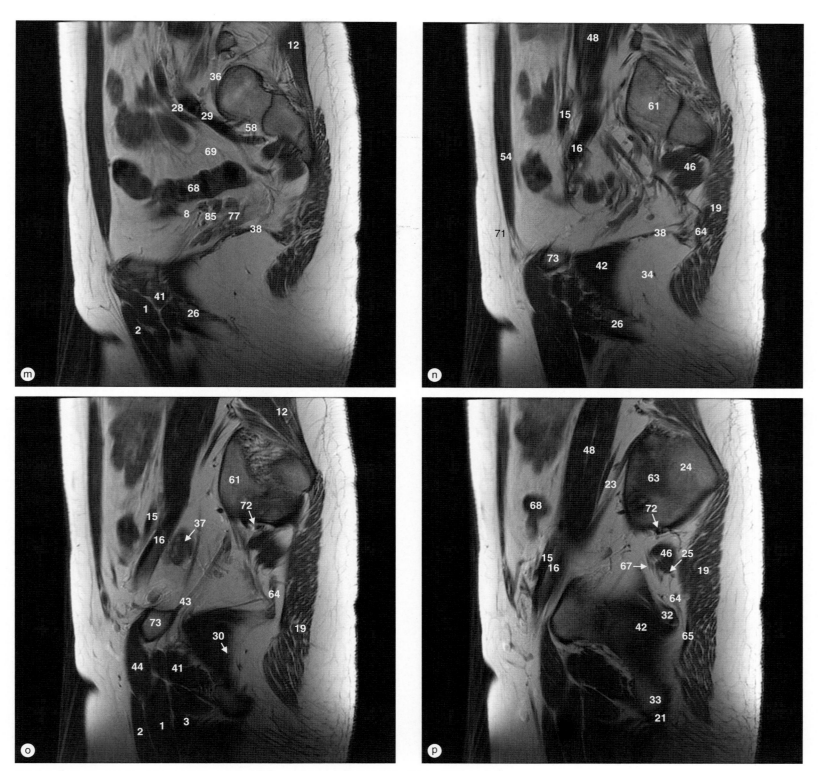

(a)–(p) Female pelvis, sequential sagittal T2-weighted MR images, from right to left.

68. Sigmoid colon	75. Thecal sac	82. Uterine endometrium
69. Sigmoid mesentery	76. Thoracolumbar fascia	83. Uterine fundus
70. Small bowel mesentery	77. Transverse cervical ligament	84. Uterine myometrium
71. Superficial fascia of the abdomen	78. Trigone of the bladder	85. Uterine vessels
72. Superior gluteal vessels	79. Urethra	86. Vagina
73. Superior pubic ramus	80. Urogenital diaphragm	87. Vaginal introitus
74. Superior rectal vessels	81. Uterine cavity	88. Waldeyer's (presacral) fascia

Numbers 1–88 are common to pages 162–165.

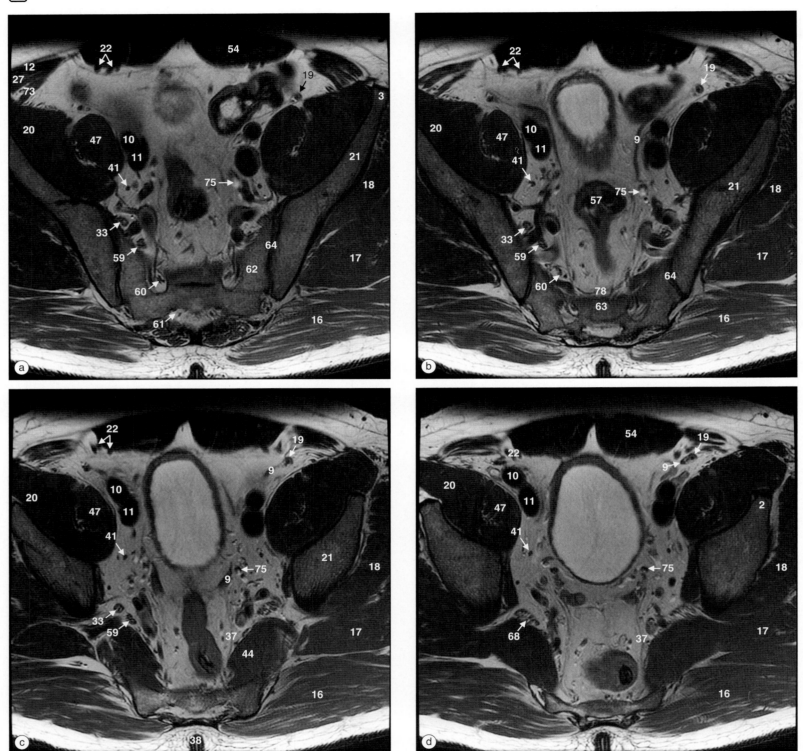

(a)–(w) Male pelvis, sequential axial T2-weighted MR images, from superior to inferior.

1. Acetabulum	**7.** Common femoral vein	**13.** Femoral canal
2. Anterior inferior iliac spine	**8.** Common hamstring origin	**14.** Femoral head
3. Anterior superior iliac spine	**9.** Ductus (vas) deferens	**15.** Femoral nerve branches
4. Bladder	**10.** External iliac artery	**16.** Gluteus maximus muscle
5. Coccyx	**11.** External iliac vein	**17.** Gluteus medius muscle
6. Common femoral artery	**12.** External oblique muscle	**18.** Gluteus minimus muscle

Numbers 1–78 are common to pages 166–169.

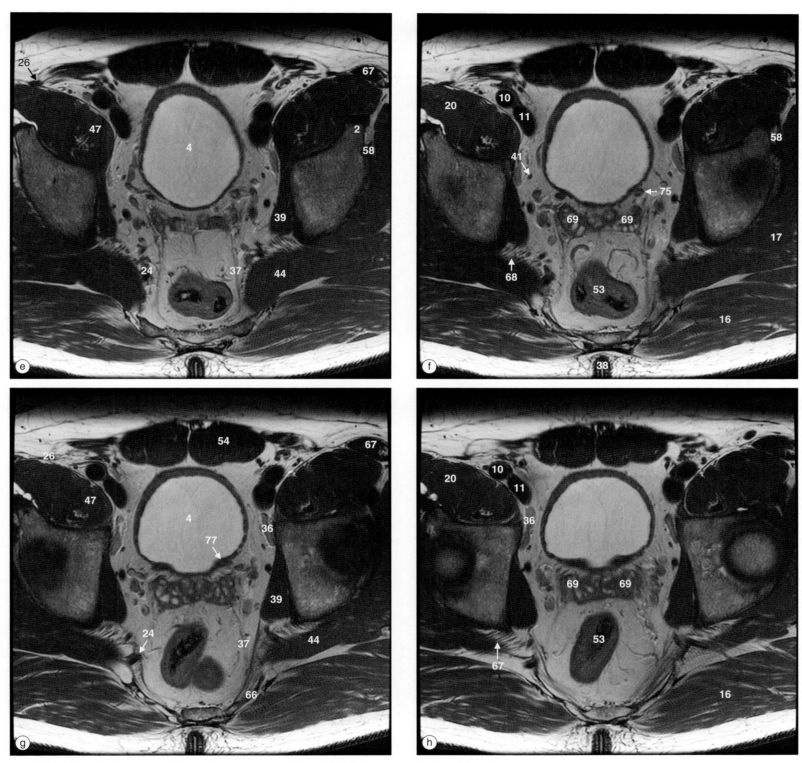

(a)–(w) Male pelvis, sequential axial T2-weighted MR images, from superior to inferior.

19. Gonadal vessels	26. Inguinal ligament	33. L5 nerve root
20. Iliacus muscle	27. Internal oblique muscle	34. Levator ani
21. Ilium	28. Internal urethral meatus	35. Ligamentum teres
22. Inferior epigastric vessels	29. Ischial spine	36. Lymph node
23. Inferior gemellus muscle	30. Ischial tuberosity	37. Mesorectum
24. Inferior gluteal vessels	31. Ischioanal fossa	38. Natal cleft
25. Inferior rectal vessels and nerve	32. Ischium	39. Obturator internus muscle

Numbers 1–78 are common to pages 166–169.

(a)–(w) Male pelvis, sequential axial T2-weighted MR images, from superior to inferior.

40. Obturator internus tendon	46. Prostate (peripheral zone)	52. Quadratus femoris muscle
41. Obturator nerve	47. Psoas major muscle	53. Rectum
42. Obturator neurovascular bundle	48. Psoas tendon	54. Rectus abdominis muscle
43. Pectineus muscle	49. Pubic symphysis	55. Rectus femoris muscle
44. Piriformis muscle	50. Pubic tubercle	56. Rectus sheath
45. Prostate (central and transitional zones)	51. Puborectalis	57. Rectosigmoid junction

Numbers 1–78 are common to pages 166–169.

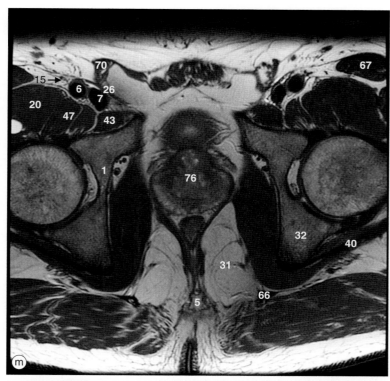

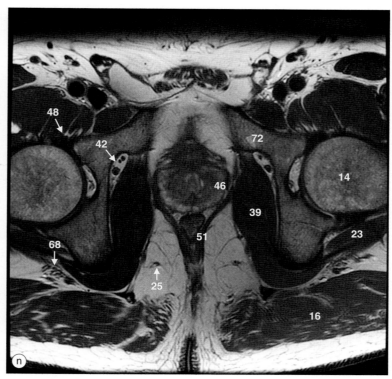

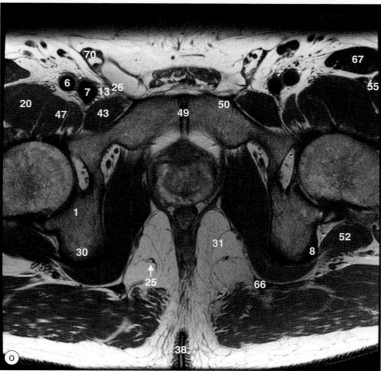

(a)–(w) Male pelvis, sequential axial T2-weighted MR images, from superior to inferior.

58. Reflected head of rectus femoris
59. S1 nerve root
60. S2 nerve root
61. S3 nerve root
62. Sacral ala
63. Sacral body
64. Sacro-iliac joint
65. Sacrospinous ligament
66. Sacrotuberous ligament
67. Sartorius muscle
68. Sciatic nerve
69. Seminal vesicles
70. Spermatic cord
71. Superior gemellus muscle
72. Superior pubic ramus
73. Transversus abdominis muscle
74. Trigone
75. Ureter
76. Verumontanum
77. Vesicoureteric junction
78. Waldeyer's (presacral) fascia

Numbers 1–78 are common to pages 166–169.

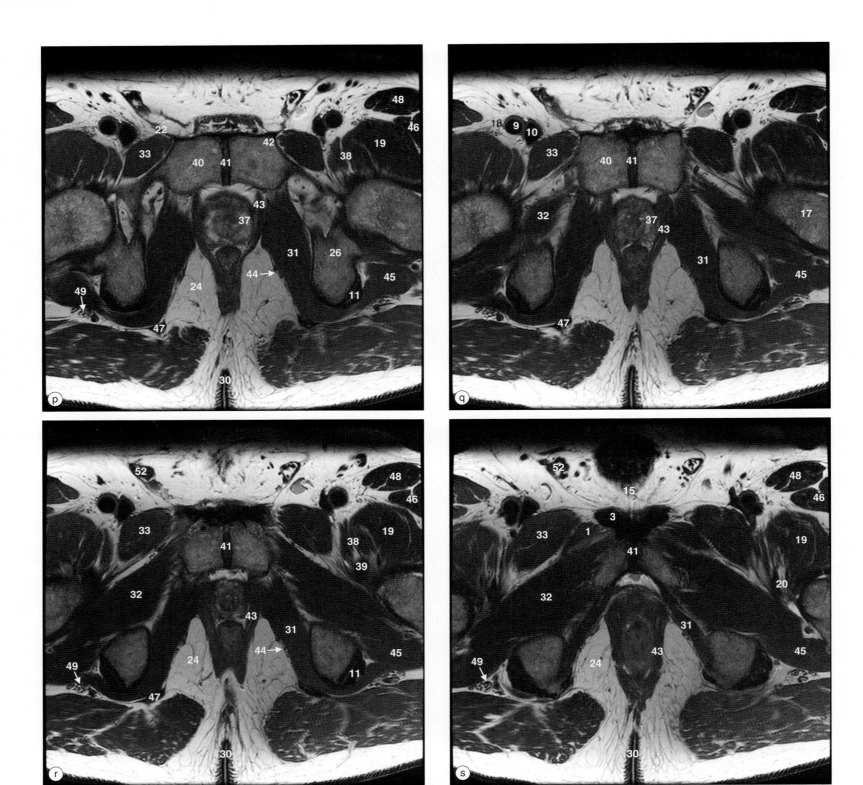

(a)–(w) Male pelvis, sequential axial T2-weighted MR images, from superior to inferior.

1. Adductor brevis muscle	**9.** Common femoral artery
2. Adductor longus muscle	**10.** Common femoral vein
3. Adductor longus tendon	**11.** Common hamstring origin
4. Adductor magnus muscle	**12.** Corpus cavernosum
5. Anal canal	**13.** Corpus spongiosum
6. Biceps femoris tendon	**14.** Crus of penis
7. Bulb of penis	**15.** Dorsal penile vessels
8. Bulbospongiosus muscle	**16.** External anal sphincter

17. Femoral neck
18. Femoral nerve branches
19. Iliacus muscle
20. Iliopsoas tendon
21. Inferior pubic ramus
22. Inguinal ligament
23. Ischial tuberosity
24. Ischioanal fossa

Numbers 1-54 are common to pages 170-171.

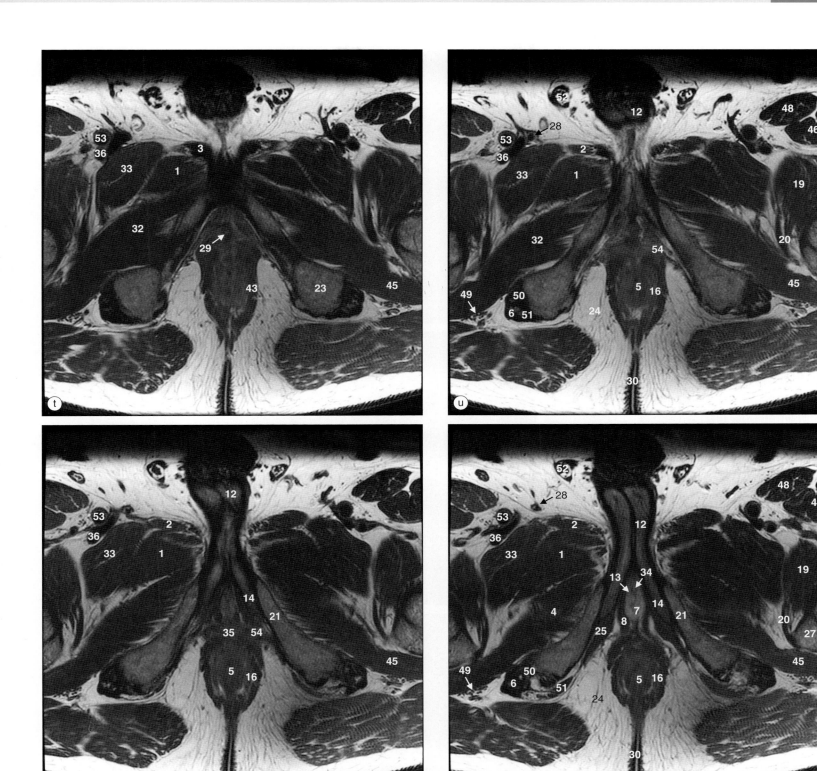

(a)–(w) Male pelvis, sequential axial T2-weighted MR images, from superior to inferior.

25. Ischiocavernosus muscle
26. Ischium
27. Lesser trochanter of the femur
28. Long saphenous vein
29. Membranous urethra
30. Natal cleft
31. Obturator internus muscle
32. Obturator externus muscle
33. Pectineus muscle
34. Penile urethra
35. Perineal body

36. Profunda femoris artery
37. Prostate (peripheral zone)
38. Psoas muscle
39. Psoas tendon
40. Pubic body
41. Pubic symphysis
42. Pubic tubercle
43. Puborectalis
44. Pudendal neurovascular bundle (Alcock's canal)
45. Quadratus femoris muscle

46. Rectus femoris muscle
47. Sacrotuberous ligament
48. Sartorius muscle
49. Sciatic nerve
50. Semimembranosus tendon
51. Semitendinosus tendon
52. Spermatic cord
53. Superficial femoral artery
54. Transverse perinei (urogenital diaphragm)

Numbers 1-54 are common to pages 170-171.

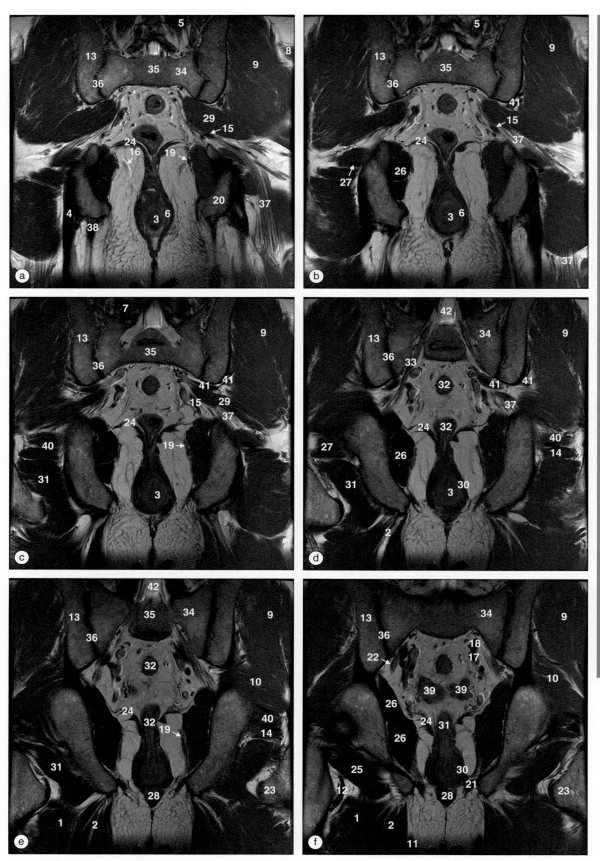

1. Adductor brevis muscle
2. Adductor magnus muscle
3. Anal canal
4. Common hamstring tendon
5. Erector spinae muscles
6. External anal sphincter
7. Facet joint (L5/S1)
8. Gluteus maximus muscle
9. Gluteus medius muscle
10. Gluteus minimus muscle
11. Gracilis muscle
12. Iliopsoas tendon
13. Ilium
14. Inferior gemellus muscle
15. Inferior gluteal vessels
16. Inferior rectal neurovascular bundle
17. Internal iliac artery
18. Internal iliac vein
19. Internal pudendal neurovascular bundle (Alcock's canal)
20. Ischial tuberosity
21. Ischiocavernosus muscle
22. L5 nerve root
23. Lesser trochanter of the femur
24. Levator ani muscle
25. Obturator externus muscle
26. Obturator internus muscle
27. Obturator internus tendon
28. Perineal body
29. Piriformis muscle
30. Puborectalis muscle
31. Quadratus femoris muscle
32. Rectum
33. S1 nerve root
34. Sacral ala
35. Sacral body
36. Sacroiliac joint
37. Sciatic nerve
38. Semitendinosus tendon
39. Seminal vesicles
40. Superior gemellus muscle
41. Superior gluteal vessels
42. Thecal sac

(a)–(x) Male pelvis, sequential coronal T2-weighted MR images, from posterior to anterior.

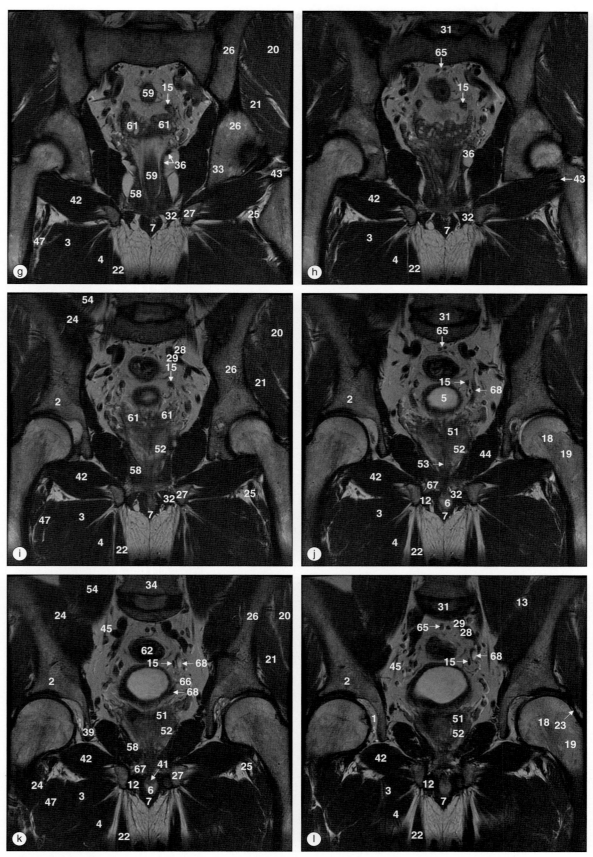

1. Acetabular fossa
2. Acetabular roof
3. Adductor brevis muscle
4. Adductor magnus muscle
5. Bladder
6. Bulb of the penis
7. Bulbospongiosus muscle
8. Common iliac artery
9. Common iliac vein
10. Corpus cavernosum
11. Corpus spongiosum
12. Crus of the penis

(a)–(x) Male pelvis, sequential coronal T2-weighted MR images, from posterior to anterior.

Numbers 1–69 are common to pages 173–174.

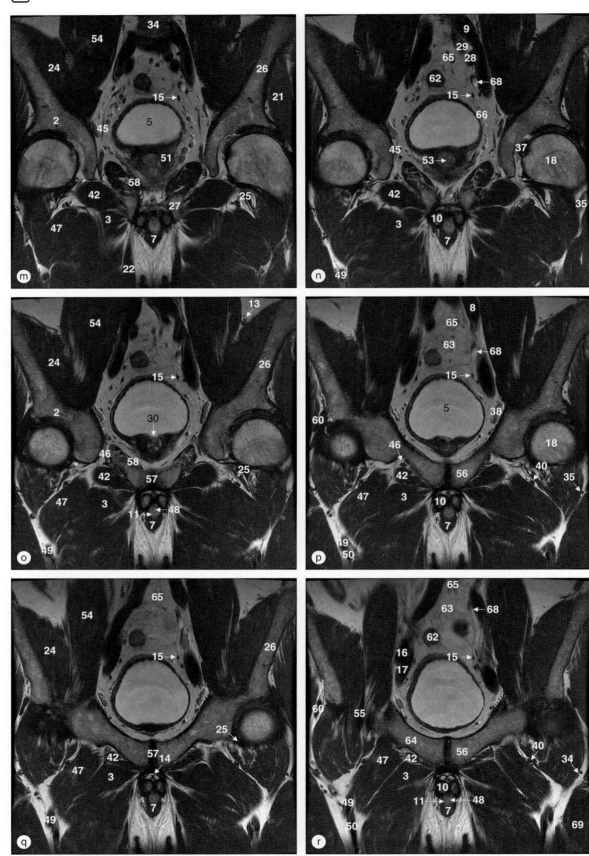

13. Deep circumflex iliac vessels
14. Dorsal vessels of the penis
15. Ductus (vas) deferens
16. External iliac artery
17. External iliac vein
18. Femoral head
19. Femoral neck
20. Gluteus medius muscle
21. Gluteus minimus muscle
22. Gracilis muscle
23. Hip joint capsule
24. Iliacus muscle
25. Iliopsoas tendon
26. Ilium
27. Inferior pubic ramus
28. Internal iliac artery
29. Internal iliac vein
30. Internal urethral meatus
31. Intervertebral disc (L5/S1)
32. Ischiocavernosus muscle
33. Ischium
34. L5 vertebral body
35. Lateral circumflex femoral vessels
36. Levator ani
37. Ligamentum teres
38. Lymph node
39. Medial acetabulum
40. Medial circumflex femoral vessels
41. Membranous urethra
42. Obturator externus muscle
43. Obturator externus tendon
44. Obturator internus muscle
45. Obturator nerve
46. Obturator neurovascular bundle
47. Pectineus muscle
48. Penile urethra
49. Profunda femoris artery
50. Profunda femoris vein
51. Prostate (central and transitional zone)
52. Prostate (peripheral zone)
53. Prostatic urethra
54. Psoas major muscle
55. Psoas major tendon
56. Pubic body
57. Pubic symphysis
58. Puborectalis muscle
59. Rectum
60. Reflected head of rectus femoris
61. Seminal vesicles
62. Sigmoid colon
63. Sigmoid mesentery
64. Superior pubic ramus
65. Superior rectal vessels
66. Superior vesical vessels
67. Transverse perinei (urogenital diaphragm)
68. Ureter
69. Vastus lateralis muscle

(a)–(x) Male pelvis, sequential coronal T2-weighted MR images, from posterior to anterior.

Numbers 1–69 are common to pages 173–174.

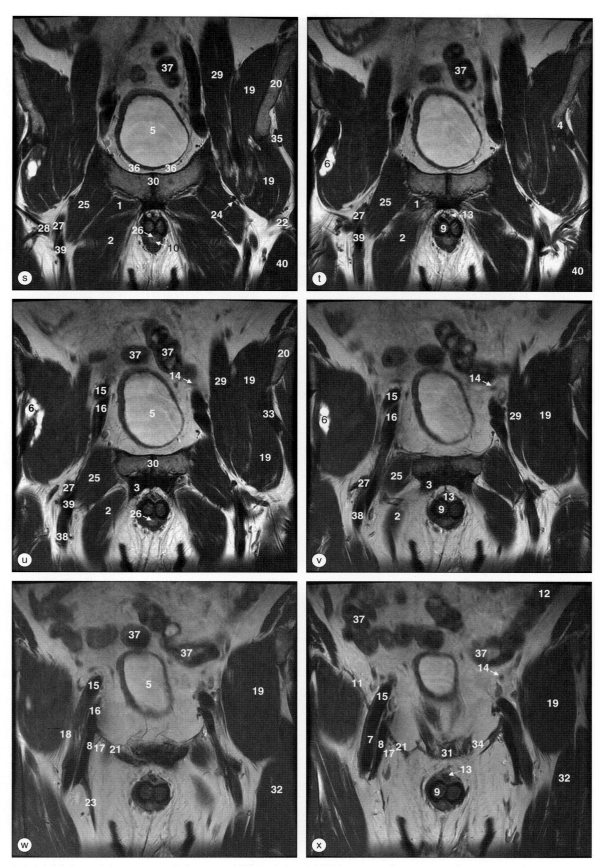

1. Adductor brevis muscle
2. Adductor longus muscle
3. Adductor longus tendon
4. Anterior inferior iliac spine
5. Bladder
6. Bursa around rectus femoris tendon (straight head)
7. Common femoral artery
8. Common femoral vein
9. Corpus cavernosum
10. Corpus spongiosum
11. Deep circumflex iliac vessels
12. Descending colon
13. Dorsal vessels of the penis
14. Ductus (vas) deferens
15. External iliac artery
16. External iliac vein
17. Femoral canal
18. Femoral nerve
19. Iliacus muscle
20. Ilium
21. Inguinal ligament
22. Lateral circumflex femoral vessels
23. Long saphenous vein
24. Medial circumflex femoral vessels
25. Pectineus muscle
26. Penile urethra
27. Profunda femoris artery
28. Profunda femoris vein
29. Psoas major muscle
30. Pubic symphysis
31. Rectus abdominis muscle
32. Rectus femoris muscle
33. Rectus femoris tendon (straight head)
34. Rectus sheath
35. Reflected head of rectus femoris
36. Retropubic space (cave of Retzius)
37. Sigmoid colon
38. Superficial femoral artery
39. Superficial femoral vein
40. Vastus lateralis muscle

(a)–(x) Male pelvis, sequential coronal T2-weighted MR images, from posterior to anterior.

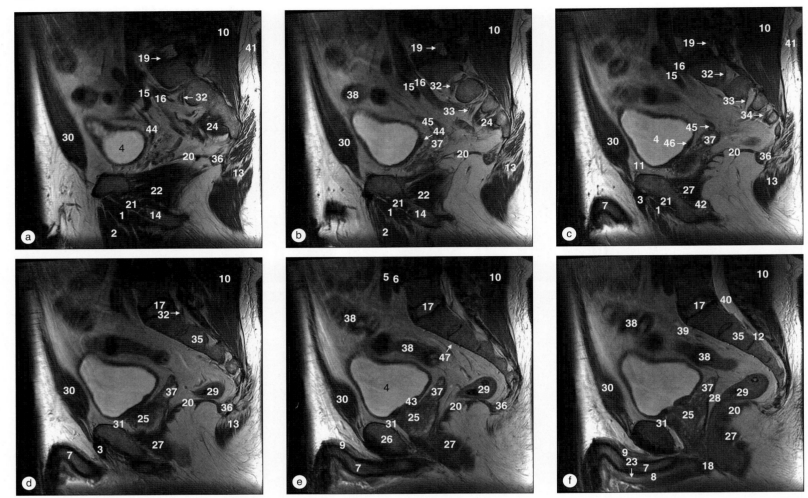

(a)–(l) Male pelvis, sequential sagittal T2-weighted MR images, from right to left.

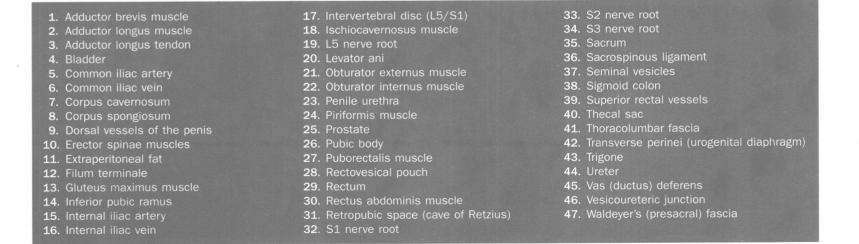

1. Adductor brevis muscle	17. Intervertebral disc (L5/S1)	33. S2 nerve root
2. Adductor longus muscle	18. Ischiocavernosus muscle	34. S3 nerve root
3. Adductor longus tendon	19. L5 nerve root	35. Sacrum
4. Bladder	20. Levator ani	36. Sacrospinous ligament
5. Common iliac artery	21. Obturator externus muscle	37. Seminal vesicles
6. Common iliac vein	22. Obturator internus muscle	38. Sigmoid colon
7. Corpus cavernosum	23. Penile urethra	39. Superior rectal vessels
8. Corpus spongiosum	24. Piriformis muscle	40. Thecal sac
9. Dorsal vessels of the penis	25. Prostate	41. Thoracolumbar fascia
10. Erector spinae muscles	26. Pubic body	42. Transverse perinei (urogenital diaphragm)
11. Extraperitoneal fat	27. Puborectalis muscle	43. Trigone
12. Filum terminale	28. Rectovesical pouch	44. Ureter
13. Gluteus maximus muscle	29. Rectum	45. Vas (ductus) deferens
14. Inferior pubic ramus	30. Rectus abdominis muscle	46. Vesicoureteric junction
15. Internal iliac artery	31. Retropubic space (cave of Retzius)	47. Waldeyer's (presacral) fascia
16. Internal iliac vein	32. S1 nerve root	

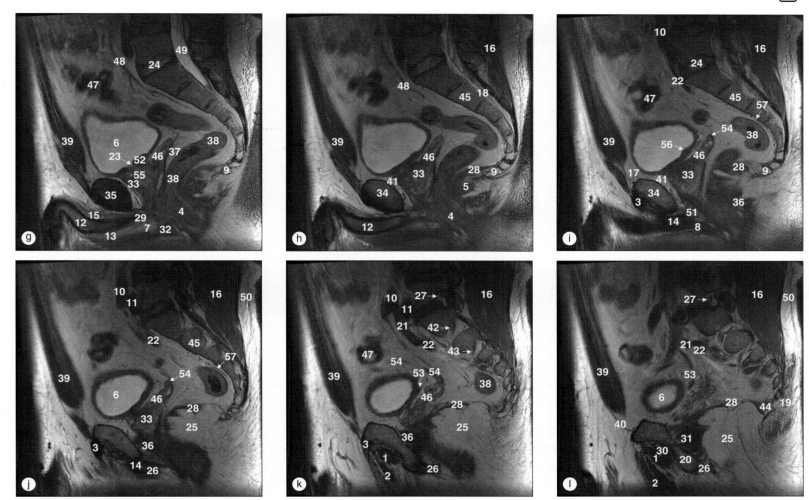

(a)–(l) Male pelvis, sequential sagittal T2-weighted MR images, from right to left.

1. Adductor brevis muscle	20. Inferior pubic ramus	39. Rectus abdominis muscle
2. Adductor longus muscle	21. Internal iliac artery	40. Rectus sheath
3. Adductor longus tendon	22. Internal iliac vein	41. Retropubic space (cave of Retzius)
4. Anal canal	23. Internal urethral meatus	42. S1 nerve root
5. Anococcygeal raphe	24. Intervertebral disc (L5/S1)	43. S2 nerve root
6. Bladder	25. Ischioanal fossa	44. Sacrospinous ligament
7. Bulb of the penis	26. Ischiocavernosus muscle	45. Sacrum
8. Bulbospongiosus muscle	27. L5 nerve root	46. Seminal vesicles
9. Coccyx	28. Levator ani	47. Sigmoid colon
10. Common iliac artery	29. Membranous urethra	48. Superior rectal vessels
11. Common iliac vein	30. Obturator externus muscle	49. Thecal sac
12. Corpus cavernosum	31. Obturator internus muscle	50. Thoracolumbar fascia
13. Corpus spongiosum	32. Perineal body	51. Transverse perinei (urogenital diaphragm)
14. Crus of the penis	33. Prostate	52. Trigone
15. Dorsal vessels of the penis	34. Pubic body	53. Ureter
16. Erector spinae muscles	35. Pubic symphysis	54. Vas (ductus) deferens
17. Extraperitoneal fat	36. Puborectalis muscle	55. Verumontanum
18. Filum terminale	37. Rectovesical pouch	56. Vesicoureteric junction
19. Gluteus maximus muscle	38. Rectum	57. Waldeyer's (presacral) fascia

Bonus e-materials

Cross-sectional image stack slideshows: Axial CT of the upper abdomen with intravenous contrast medium taken in the portal venous phase and oral contrast medium, Axial CT of the lower abdomen with intravenous contrast medium taken in the portal venous phase and oral contrast medium, Axial CT of the pelvis with intravenous contrast medium taken in the portal venous phase and oral contrast medium

Multi-tier labelling in slideshow/test yourself: T2-weighted midline sagittal MRI through the female pelvis, T2-weighted midline sagittal MRI through the male pelvis

Selected pages from Imaging Atlas 4e

Tutorials: Tutorials 6a, 6b, 6c, 6d, 6e, 6f, 6g, 6h, 6i, 7a, 7b, 7c

Single best answer (SBA) self-assessment questions

Table of Variations

Variant	Frequency	Clinical implications
Pelvic appendix	30%	Symptoms confused with acute cystitis on presentation.
Right hepatic artery arising from the proximal super mesenteric artery	20%	Access for arterial embolisation of liver lesions, e.g. primary tumour, metastases.
Pancreas divisum	<10%	Association with pancreatitis; variant anatomy to navigate at ERCP.
Meckel's diverticulum	1%	Site of ectopic gastric mucosa; source of occult gastrointestinal haemorrhage; Meckel's diverticulitis.
Duplex kidney	<1%	Obstruction of the upper pole moiety; vesicoureteric reflux in the lower pole moiety; increased risk of infection.
Left-sided inferior vena cava	<0.5%	Implications for planning surgical vascular procedures and IVC filter placement.
Annular pancreas	<0.5%	Duodenal obstruction; increased risk of chronic pancreatitis.
Horseshoe kidney	<0.25%	Increased risk of traumatic injury, infection, hydronephrosis, renal calculi and malignancy.
Pelvic kidney	<0.05%	Can be asymptomatic; presentation as pelvic mass; increased risk of infection and secondary hypertension; should be considered instead of renal agenesis; other associated renal, vascular and genital developmental abnormalities.
Intestinal malrotation	0.01%	Risk of midgut volvulus; association with other developmental anomalies; look for reversed relationship of superior mesenteric artery and vein in addition to abnormal positioning of duodenojejunal flexure, small and large bowel.

ERCP, *Endoscopic retrograde cholangiopancreatography;* IVC, *inferior vena cava.*

10 Abdomen and pelvis: non cross-sectional

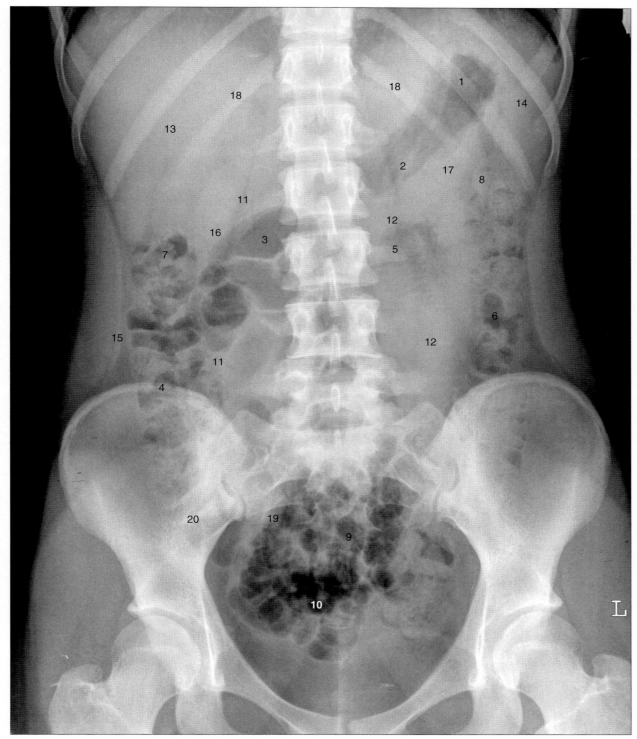

Supine abdominal radiograph.

1. Gas in fundus of stomach
2. Gas in body of stomach
3. Gas in first part of duodenum (duodenal cap)
4. Ascending colon
5. Transverse colon
6. Descending colon
7. Hepatic flexure of colon
8. Splenic flexure of colon
9. Sigmoid colon
10. Rectum
11. Right psoas margin
12. Left psoas margin
13. Liver
14. Spleen
15. Properitoneal fat line
16. Right kidney
17. Left kidney
18. Twelfth rib
19. Gas in ileum
20. Gas in caecum

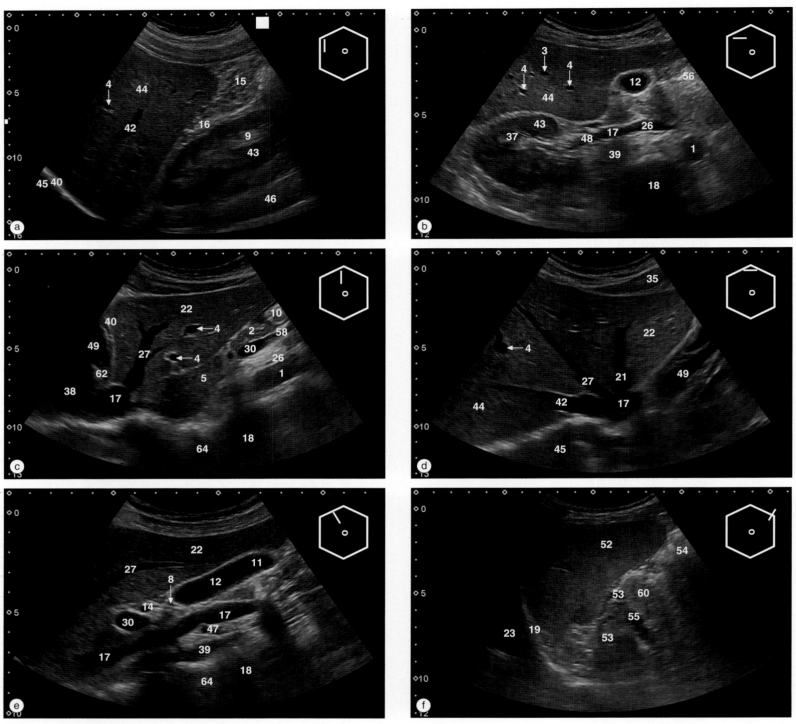

(a)–(f) Upper abdomen, ultrasound images.

1. Abdominal aorta	11. Fundus of gall bladder	21. Left hepatic vein
2. Body of pancreas	12. Gall bladder	22. Left lobe of liver
3. Branch of hepatic vein	13. Head of pancreas	23. Left lung base
4. Branch of portal vein*	14. Hepatic artery	24. Left psoas muscle
5. Caudate lobe of liver	15. Hepatic flexure of colon (right colic)	25. Left renal artery
6. Coeliac trunk	16. Hepatorenal recess	26. Left renal vein
7. Common bile duct	17. Inferior vena cava	27. Middle hepatic vein
8. Cystic duct	18. Intervertebral disc	28. Neck of pancreas
9. Fat in renal sinus	19. Left dome of diaphragm	29. Pancreatic duct
10. First part of duodenum	20. Left gastric vessels	30. Portal vein

Numbers 1–64 are common to pages 180–183.

—————————

*Accompanied by branch of hepatic artery and bile duct

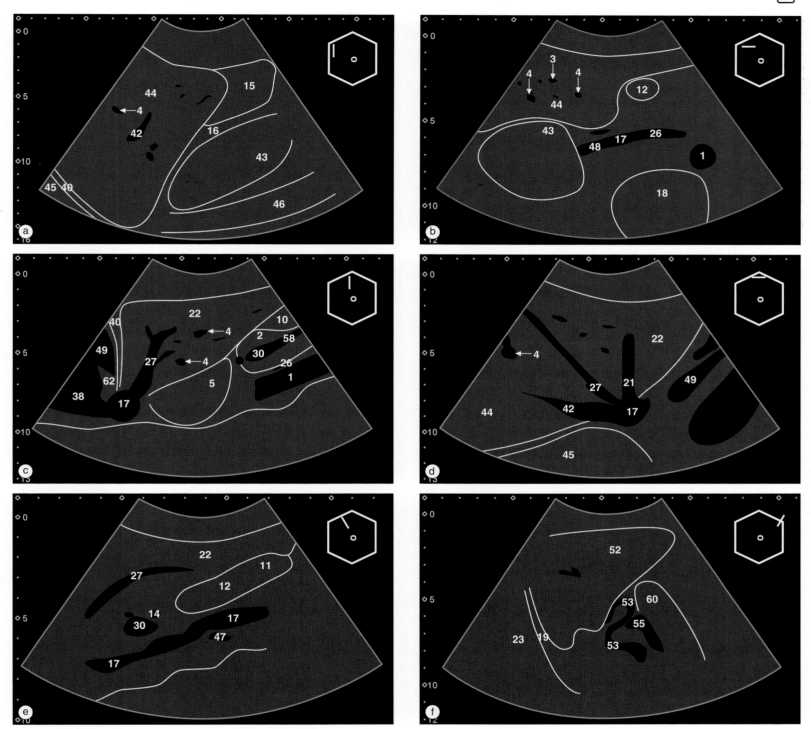

(a)–(f) Line diagrams of ultrasound images opposite.

31. Prostate gland	43. Right kidney	55. Splenic vein
32. Pubic symphysis	44. Right lobe of liver	56. Stomach
33. Puborectalis	45. Right lung base	57. Superior mesenteric artery
34. Rectum	46. Right psoas muscle	58. Superior mesenteric vein
35. Rectus abdominis muscle	47. Right renal artery	59. Superior pubic ramus
36. Rectus abdominis tendon	48. Right renal vein	60. Tail of pancreas
37. Renal papilla	49. Right ventricle	61. Transverse colon
38. Right atrium	50. Seminal vesicles	62. Tricuspid valve
39. Right crus of diaphragm	51. Small bowel	63. Urinary bladder
40. Right dome of diaphragm	52. Spleen	64. Vertebral body
41. Right hepatic artery	53. Splenic artery	
42. Right hepatic vein	54. Splenic flexure of colon (left colic)	

Numbers 1–64 are common to pages 180–183.

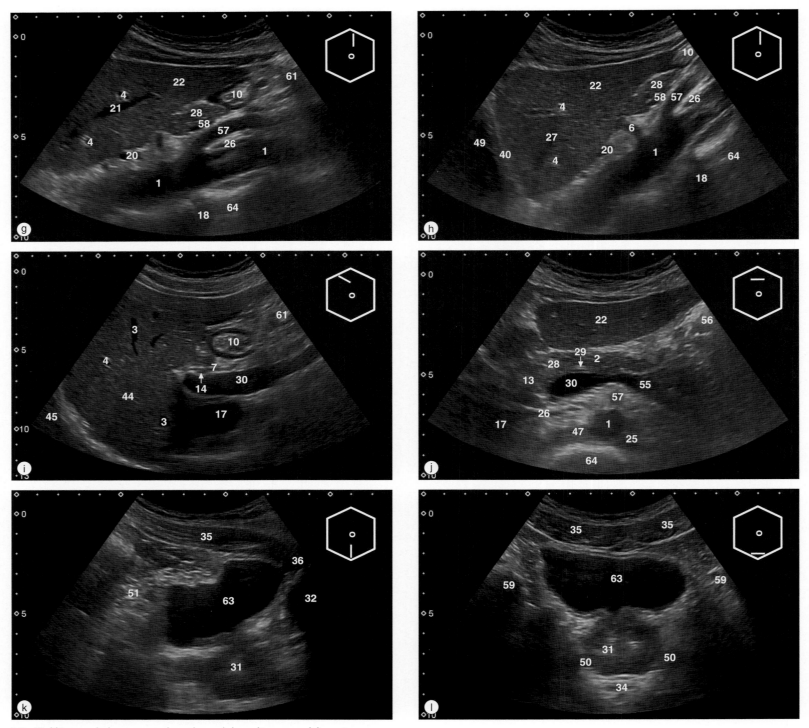

(g)–(l) Upper abdomen and male pelvis, ultrasound images.

1. Abdominal aorta	12. Gall bladder	23. Left lung base
2. Body of pancreas	13. Head of pancreas	24. Left psoas muscle
3. Branch of hepatic vein	14. Hepatic artery	25. Left renal artery
4. Branch of portal vein*	15. Hepatic flexure of colon (right colic)	26. Left renal vein
5. Caudate lobe of liver	16. Hepatorenal recess	27. Middle hepatic vein
6. Coeliac trunk	17. Inferior vena cava	28. Neck of pancreas
7. Common bile duct	18. Intervertebral disc	29. Pancreatic duct
8. Cystic duct	19. Left dome of diaphragm	30. Portal vein
9. Fat in renal sinus	20. Left gastric vessels	31. Prostate gland
10. First part of duodenum	21. Left hepatic vein	32. Pubic symphysis
11. Fundus of gall bladder	22. Left lobe of liver	33. Puborectalis

Numbers 1–64 are common to pages 180–183.

*Accompanied by branch of hepatic artery and bile duct

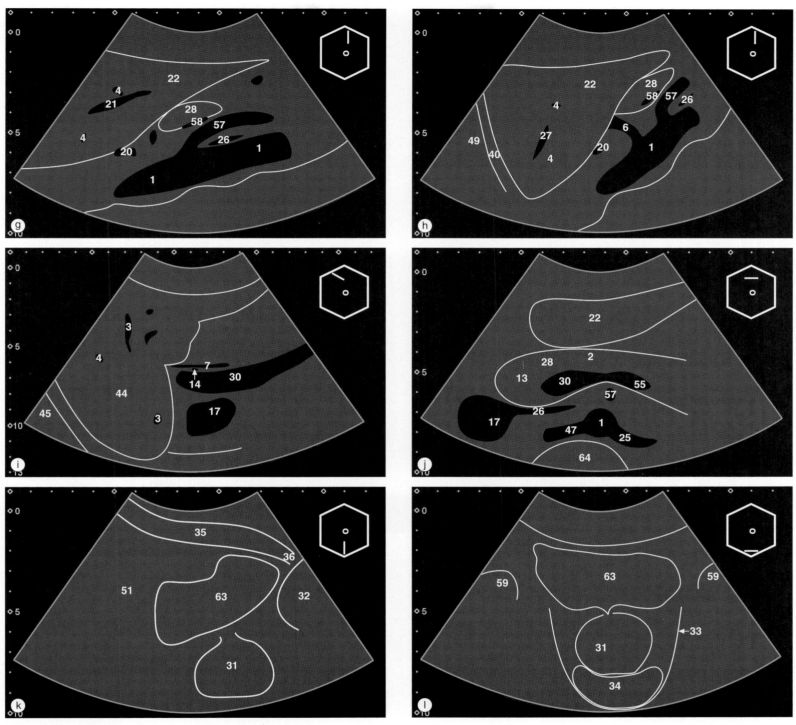

(g)–(l) Line diagrams of ultrasound images opposite.

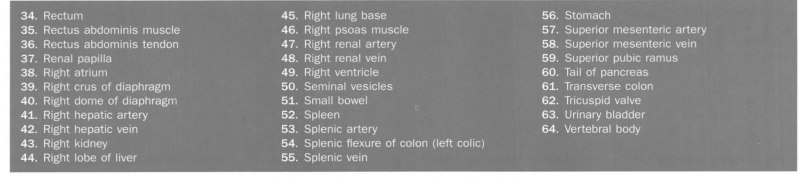

34. Rectum	45. Right lung base	56. Stomach
35. Rectus abdominis muscle	46. Right psoas muscle	57. Superior mesenteric artery
36. Rectus abdominis tendon	47. Right renal artery	58. Superior mesenteric vein
37. Renal papilla	48. Right renal vein	59. Superior pubic ramus
38. Right atrium	49. Right ventricle	60. Tail of pancreas
39. Right crus of diaphragm	50. Seminal vesicles	61. Transverse colon
40. Right dome of diaphragm	51. Small bowel	62. Tricuspid valve
41. Right hepatic artery	52. Spleen	63. Urinary bladder
42. Right hepatic vein	53. Splenic artery	64. Vertebral body
43. Right kidney	54. Splenic flexure of colon (left colic)	
44. Right lobe of liver	55. Splenic vein	

Numbers 1–64 are common to pages 180–183.

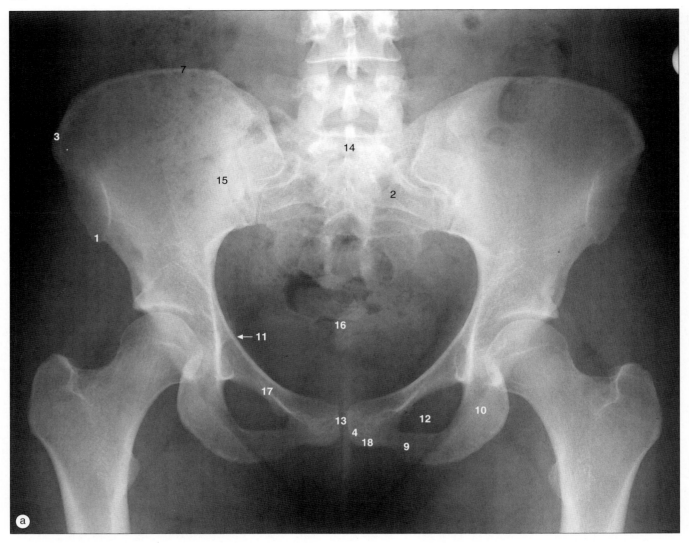

(a) Pelvis and hips of an adult female, anteroposterior radiograph.
(b) and (c) Pelvis of a 17-year-old male, anteroposterior radiographs.

1. Anterior inferior iliac spine	7. Iliac crest	13. Pubic symphysis
2. Anterior sacral foramen	8. Ilium	14. Sacral crest
3. Anterior superior iliac spine	9. Inferior ramus of pubis	15. Sacroiliac joint (anterior margin)
4. Body of pubis	10. Ischial ramus	16. Segment of coccyx
5. Ossification centre for iliac crest	11. Ischial spine	17. Superior ramus of pubis
6. Ossification centre for ischial tuberosity	12. Obturator foramen	18. Tubercle of pubis

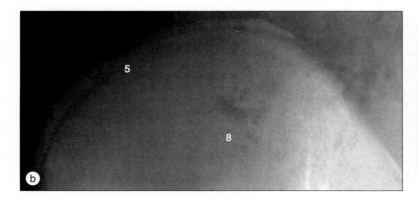

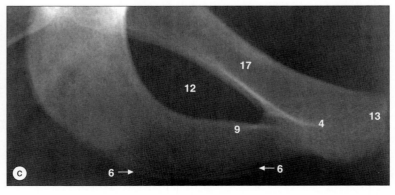

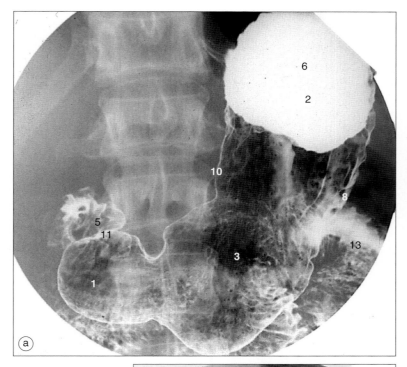

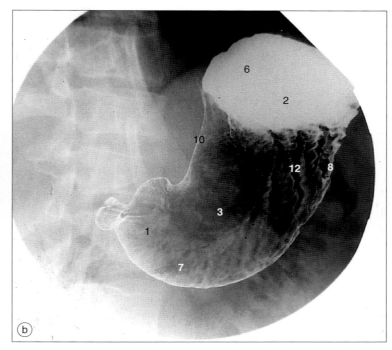

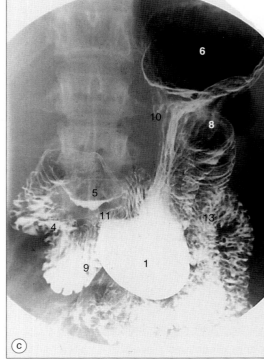

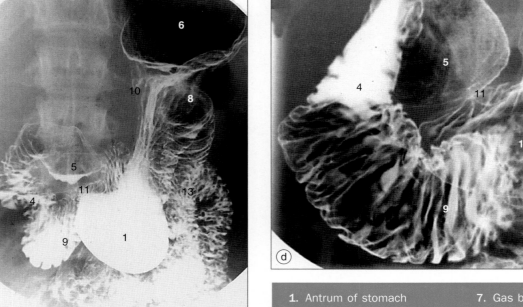

Abdomen. Double-contrast barium meals of stomach and duodenum, (a) and (b) with the patient supine (to show the mucosa of the stomach), (c) with the patient erect, (d) with the patient in a supine oblique position (to show the duodenum).

1. Antrum of stomach
2. Barium pooling in fundus of stomach
3. Body of stomach
4. Descending (second) part of duodenum
5. Duodenal cap (superior or first part of duodenum)
6. Fundus of stomach
7. Gas bubbles
8. Greater curvature of stomach
9. Horizontal (third) part of duodenum
10. Lesser curvature of stomach
11. Region of pyloric canal
12. Rugae of stomach
13. Small bowel (jejunum)

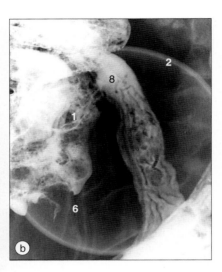

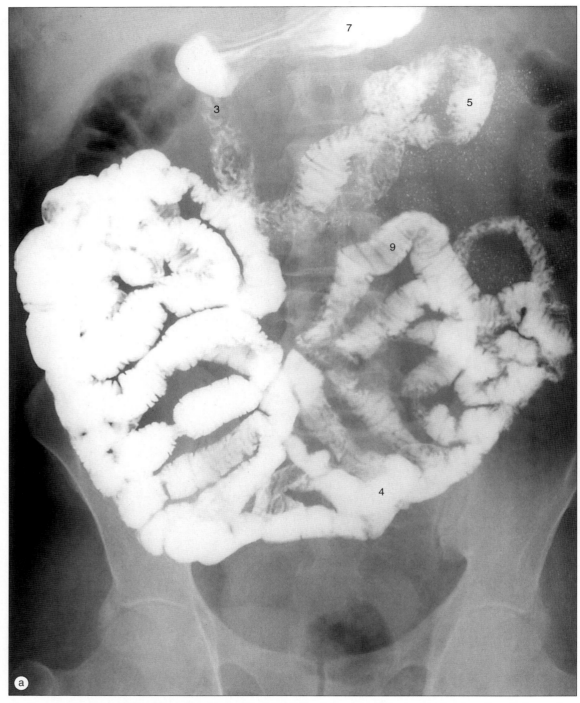

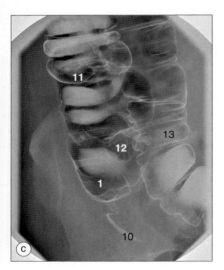

Abdomen, barium follow-throughs, (a) with the patient supine, (b) showing a localised view of the terminal ileum and (c) ileocaecal valve. Anteroposterior radiographs.

1. Caecum	8. Terminal ileum
2. Compression device	9. Valvulae conniventes (plicae circulares) of
3. Descending (second) part of duodenum	jejunum
4. Proximal ileum	10. Appendix
5. Proximal jejunum	11. Ascending colon
6. Right sacroiliac joint	12. Ileocaecal valve
7. Stomach	13. Transverse colon

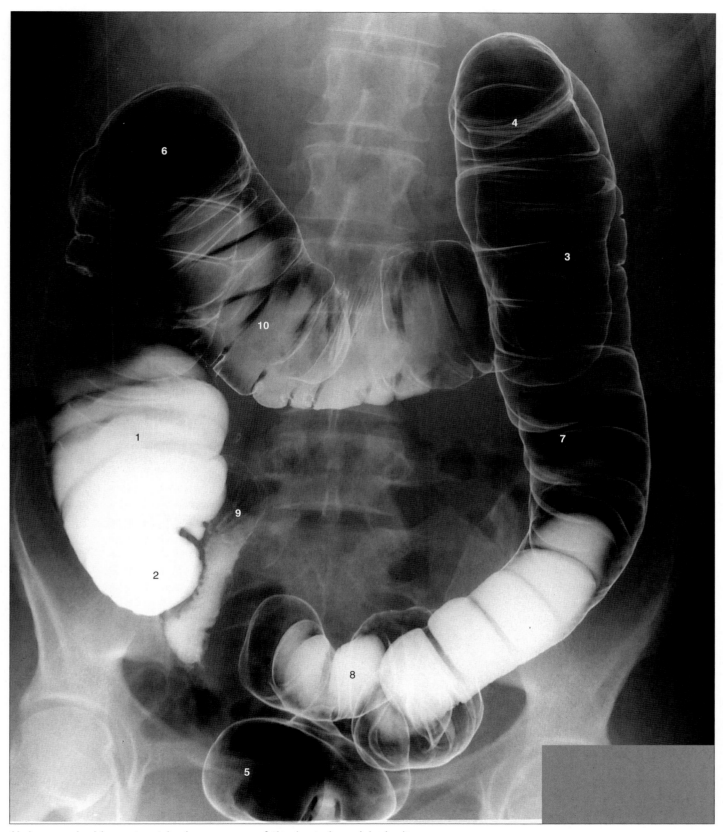

Abdomen, double-contrast barium enema of the large bowel (colon).

1. Ascending portion of colon
2. Caecum
3. Descending portion of colon
4. Left colic (splenic) flexure of colon
5. Rectum
6. Right colic (hepatic) flexure of colon
7. Sacculations (haustrations) of colon
8. Sigmoid colon
9. Terminal ileum
10. Transverse colon

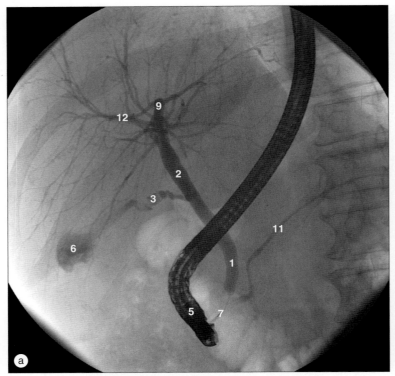

(a) Endoscopic retrograde cholangiopancreatogram (ERCP).

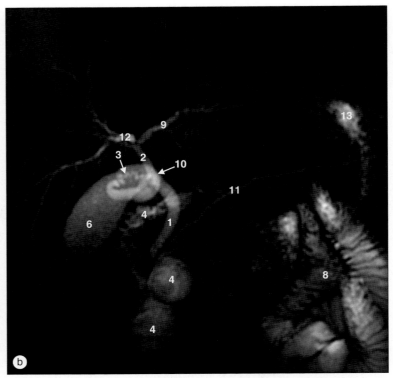

(b) Magnetic resonance cholangiopancreatogram (MRCP).

1. Common bile duct
2. Common hepatic duct
3. Cystic duct
4. Duodenum
5. Endoscope in duodenum

6. Gall bladder
7. Hepatopancreatic (Vater's) ampulla
8. Jejunum
9. Left hepatic duct
10. Neck of gall bladder

11. Pancreatic duct
12. Right hepatic duct
13. Stomach

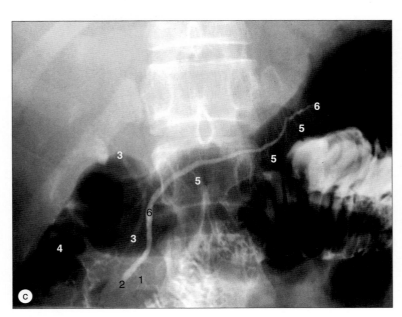

(c) ERCP.

1. Accessory pancreatic duct (Santorini's)
2. Ampullary part of pancreatic duct
3. Common bile duct
4. Contrast and gas in descending (second) part of duodenum
5. Intralobular ducts
6. Main pancreatic duct

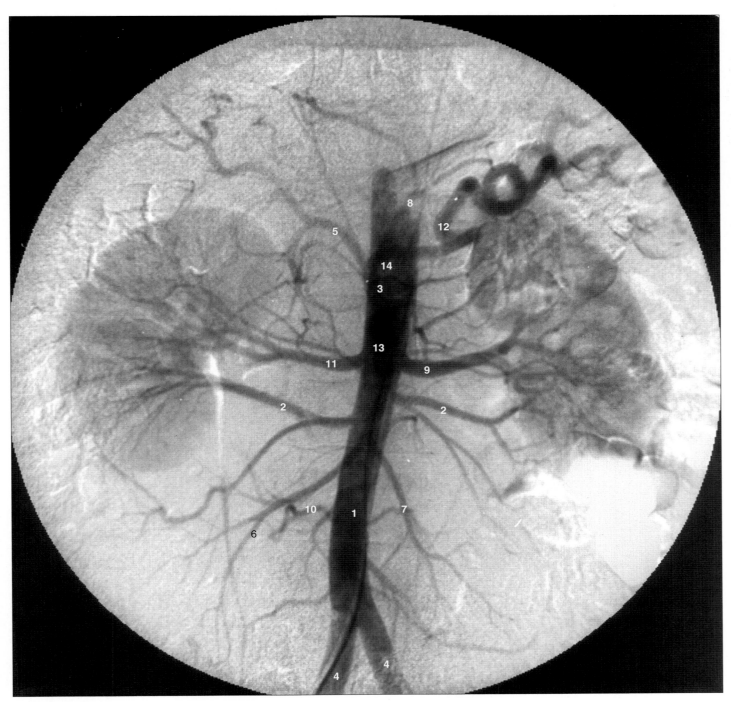

Abdominal aortogram.

1. Abdominal aorta
2. Accessory renal arteries
3. Coeliac trunk
4. Common iliac arteries
5. Hepatic artery
6. Ileocolic artery
7. Jejunal branches of superior mesenteric artery
8. Left gastric artery
9. Left renal artery
10. Lumbar arteries
11. Right renal artery
12. Splenic artery
13. Superior mesenteric artery
14. Tip of pigtail catheter in abdominal aorta

(a) and (b) Subtracted coeliac trunk arteriograms.

1. Dorsal pancreatic artery
2. Gastroduodenal artery
3. Hepatic artery
4. Left gastric artery
5. Left gastro-epiploic artery
6. Left hepatic artery
7. Pancreatica magna artery
8. Phrenic artery
9. Right gastro-epiploic artery
10. Right hepatic artery
11. Splenic artery
12. Superior pancreaticoduodenal artery
13. Tip of catheter in coeliac trunk
14. Transverse pancreatic artery

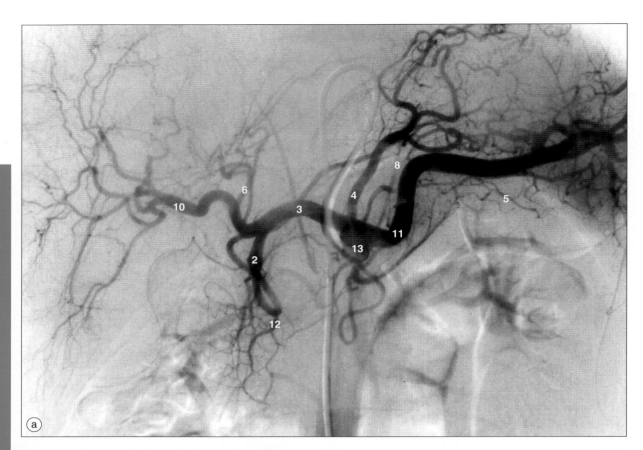

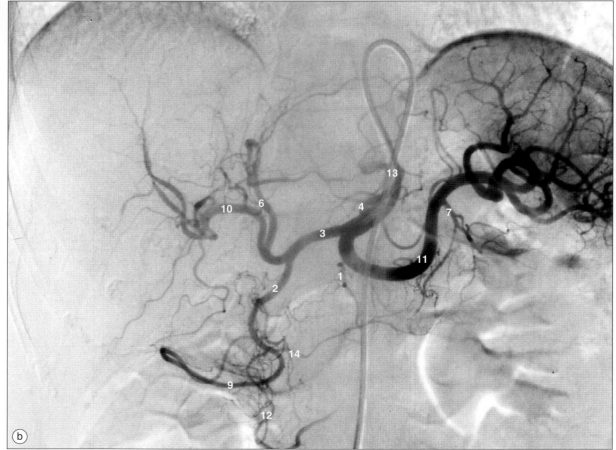

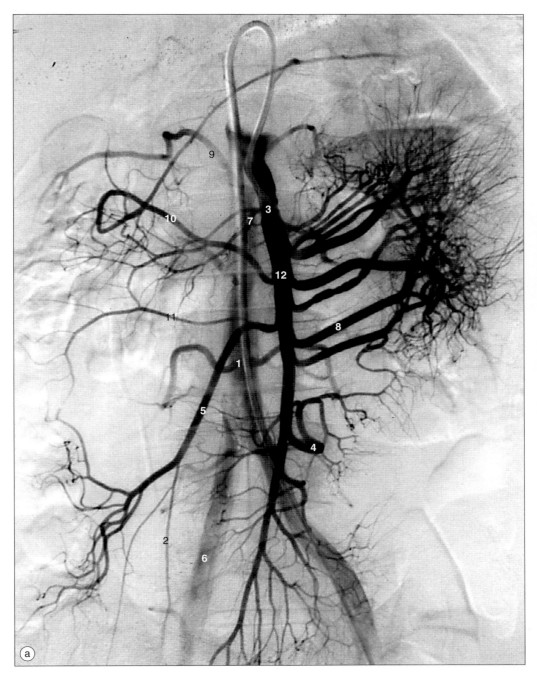

(a) Subtracted superior mesenteric arteriogram.

1. Aorta
2. Appendicular artery
3. Catheter with tip selectively in superior mesenteric artery
4. Ileal branches of superior mesenteric artery
5. Ileocolic artery
6. Right common iliac artery
7. Inferior pancreaticoduodenal artery
8. Jejunal branches of superior mesenteric artery
9. Lumbar arteries arising from abdominal aorta
10. Middle colic artery
11. Right colic artery
12. Superior mesenteric artery

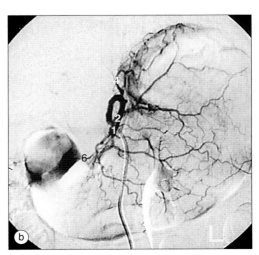 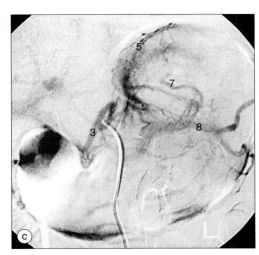

(b) Gastric arteries, (c) gastric veins.

1. Catheter in origin of left gastric artery
2. Left gastric artery
3. Left gastric vein
4. Oesophageal branch of left gastric artery
5. Oesophageal branches of left gastric vein
6. Right gastric artery
7. Short gastric veins
8. Splenic vein

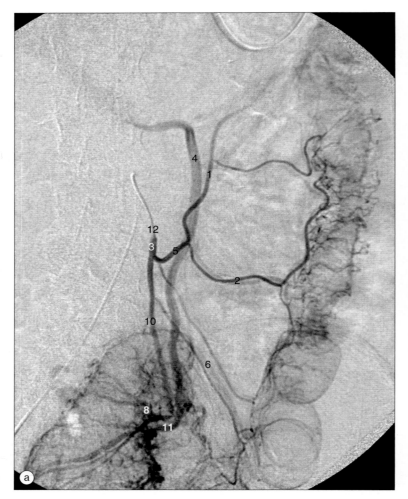

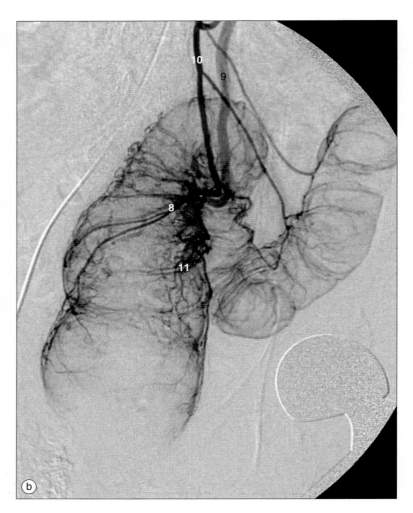

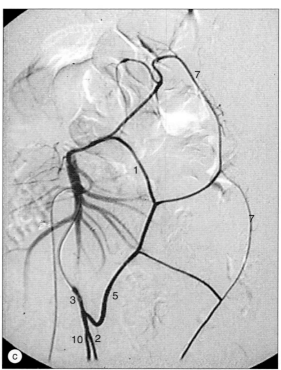

1. Ascending branch of left colic artery
2. Descending branch of left colic artery
3. Inferior mesenteric artery
4. Inferior mesenteric vein
5. Left colic artery
6. Left colic vein
7. Marginal artery of Drummond
8. Sigmoid arteries
9. Sigmoid vein
10. Superior rectal artery
11. Superior rectal vein
12. Tip of catheter in inferior mesenteric artery

(a)–(c) Inferior mesenteric arteriograms.

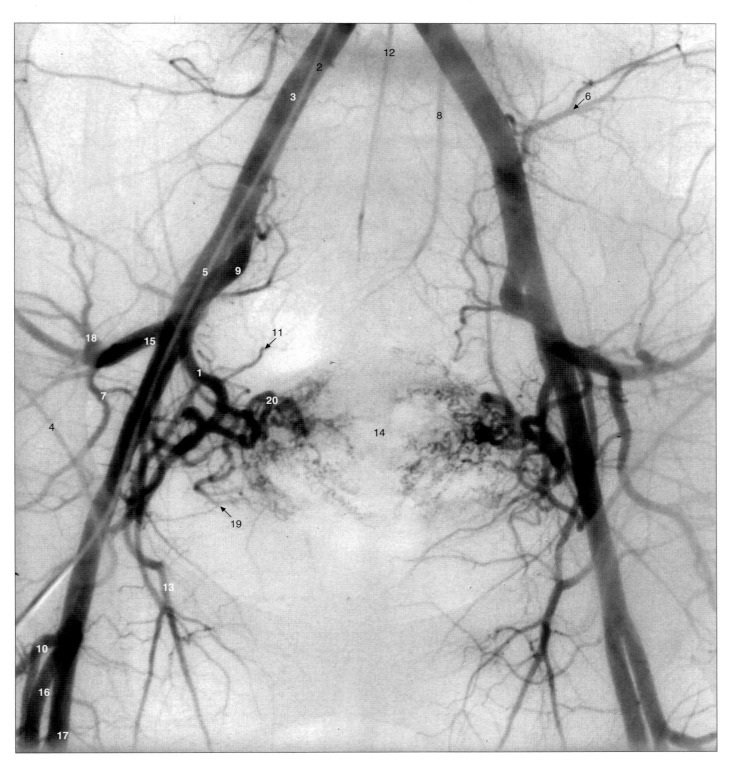

Subtracted pelvic arteriogram.

This anteroposterior film of the pelvis demonstrates both the internal and the external iliac arteries and their branches. Many of the vessels are superimposed; to see them more clearly, oblique projections could be obtained. The contrast medium injected into the arteries is excreted by the kidneys, and a full bladder may obscure the branches. Selective catheterisation of the internal and external iliac arteries using a preshaped catheter gives better detail without superimposition of the vessels.

1. Anterior trunk of internal iliac artery
2. Catheter introduced into distal abdominal aorta via right femoral artery
3. Common iliac artery
4. Deep circumflex iliac artery
5. External iliac artery
6. Iliolumbar artery
7. Inferior gluteal artery
8. Inferior mesenteric artery
9. Internal iliac artery
10. Lateral circumflex femoral artery
11. Lateral sacral artery
12. Median sacral artery
13. Obturator artery
14. Position of uterus
15. Posterior trunk of internal iliac artery
16. Profunda femoris artery
17. Superficial femoral artery
18. Superior gluteal artery
19. Superior vesical artery
20. Uterine artery

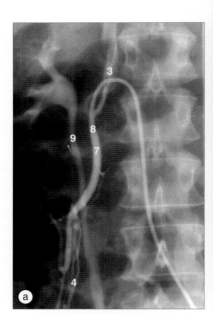

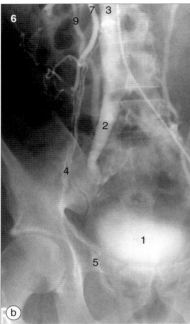

(a) and **(b)** Right testicular venograms.

The gonadal veins drain into one or two main veins via a venous plexus. On the left, the main vein drains into the left renal vein. It may occasionally communicate with the inferior mesenteric vein and drain into the portal venous system. On the right, the main vein usually drains into the inferior vena cava directly (as in the case illustrated), but it can drain into the right renal vein.

1. Bladder
2. Common iliac veins
3. Inferior vena cava
4. Pampiniform plexus of veins
5. Pampiniform plexus of veins (undescended testis in inguinal canal)
6. Renal capsular veins
7. Right testicular vein
8. Tip of catheter in right testicular vein, introduced via left femoral vein
9. Ureter

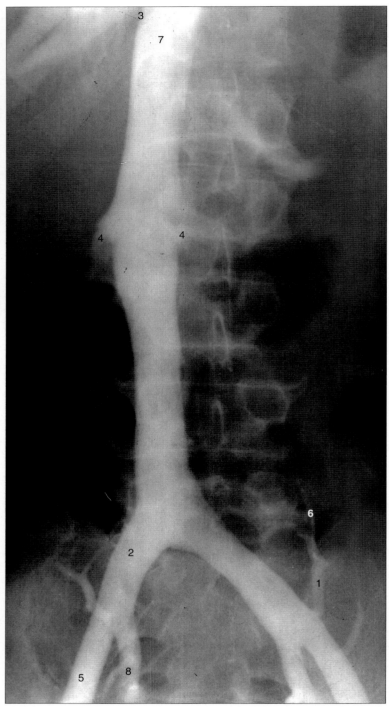

(c) Inferior vena cavogram.

1. Ascending lumbar vein
2. Common iliac vein
3. Entrance of hepatic veins
4. Entrance of renal veins
5. External iliac vein
6. Iliolumbar vein
7. Inferior vena cava
8. Internal iliac vein

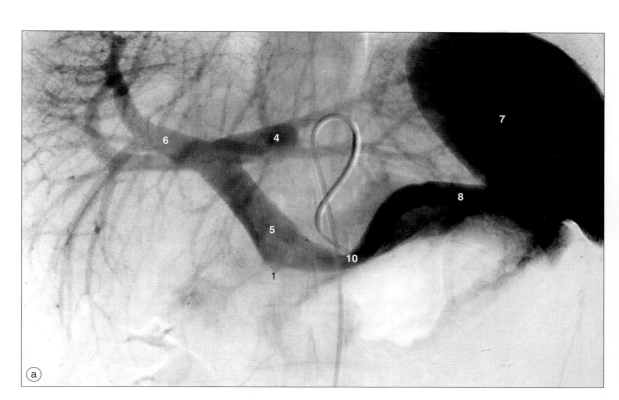

(a) Indirect splenoportogram.

(b) and (c) Venous phase of superior mesenteric arteriogram.

1. Entry of superior mesenteric vein
2. Ileocolic vein
3. Jejunal vein
4. Left branch of portal vein
5. Portal vein
6. Right branch of portal vein
7. Spleen
8. Splenic vein
9. Superior mesenteric vein
10. Tip of catheter in splenic artery
11. Tip of catheter in superior mesenteric artery

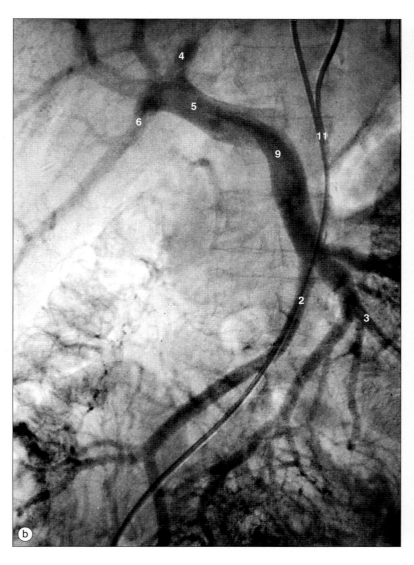

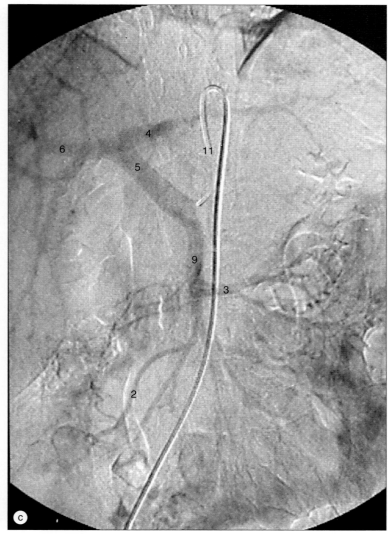

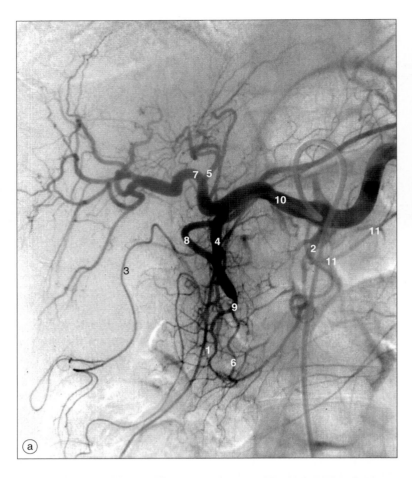

(a) Subtracted hepatic arteriogram.

1. Anterior branch of inferior pancreaticoduodenal artery
2. Dorsal pancreatic artery
3. Epiploic artery
4. Gastroduodenal artery
5. Left branch of hepatic artery
6. Posterior branch of superior pancreaticoduodenal artery
7. Right branch of hepatic artery
8. Right gastro-epiploic artery
9. Superior pancreaticoduodenal artery
10. Tip of catheter in hepatic artery
11. Transverse pancreatic artery

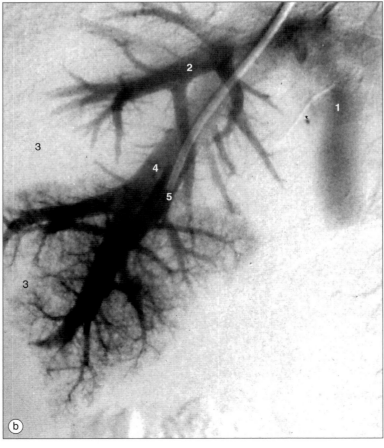

(b) Subtracted hepatic venogram.

1. Inferior vena cava
2. Middle hepatic vein
3. Parenchyma of liver
4. Right hepatic vein
5. Tip of catheter in hepatic vein

(a) Selective gastroduodenal arteriogram.

(b) Subtracted pancreatic arteriogram.

1. Anterior branch of inferior pancreaticoduodenal artery
2. Anterior branch of superior pancreaticoduodenal artery
3. Gastroduodenal artery
4. Left gastro-epiploic artery
5. Posterior branch of inferior pancreaticoduodenal artery
6. Posterior branch of superior pancreaticoduodenal artery
7. Right gastro-epiploic artery
8. Superior mesenteric artery
9. Tip of catheter in dorsal pancreatic artery
10. Transverse pancreatic artery

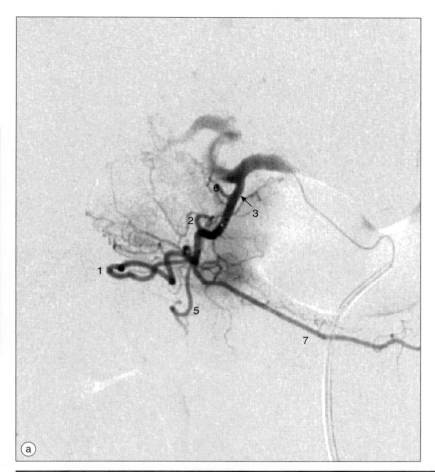

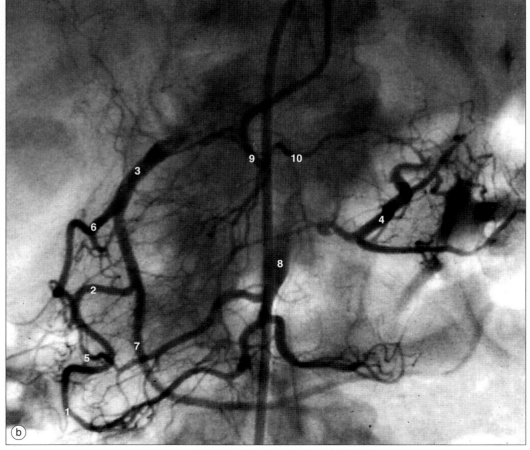

(a) Renal arteriogram.

1. Arcuate arteries
2. Interlobar arteries
3. Lobar arteries
4. Main renal artery
5. Tip of catheter in renal artery
6. Interlobular artery

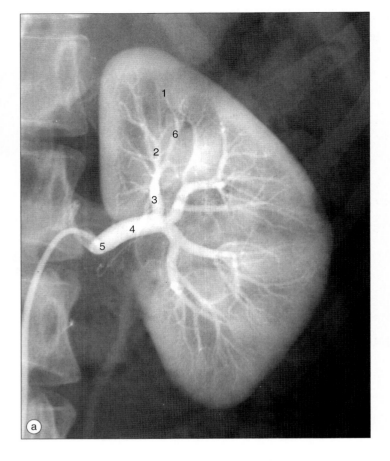

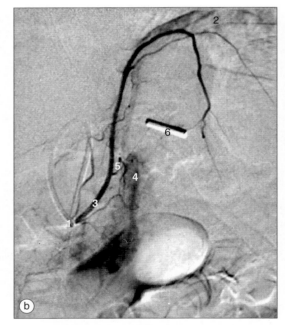

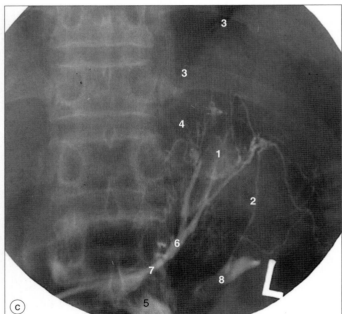

(b) Left suprarenal arteriogram.

(c) Left suprarenal venogram.

1. Catheter in origin of inferior phrenic artery
2. Diaphragm
3. Inferior phrenic artery
4. Left suprarenal gland
5. Superior suprarenal arteries
6. Tip of nasogastric tube

1. Adenoma in suprarenal gland
2. Capsular veins
3. Diaphragm
4. Inferior phrenic vein
5. Left renal vein
6. Left suprarenal vein
7. Tip of catheter in left suprarenal vein
8. Upper pole calyx

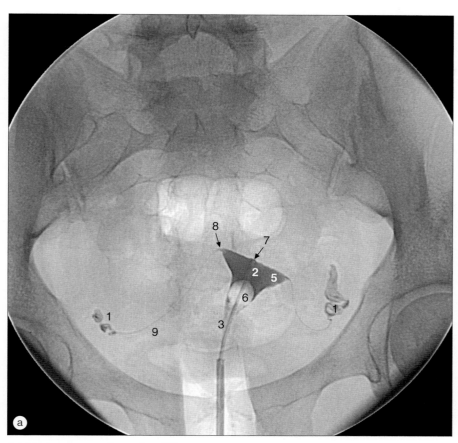

(a) Early phase of uterine filling.

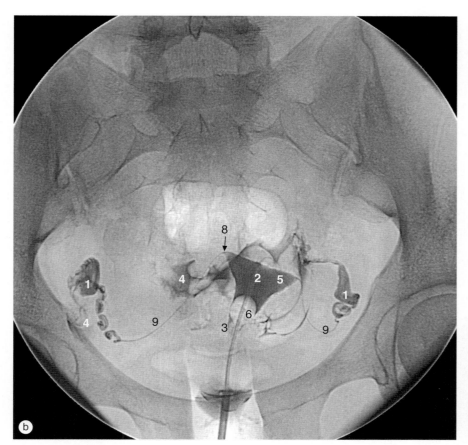

(b) Late phase with peritoneal spill.

1. Ampulla of uterine tube
2. Body of uterus
3. Cervix of uterus
4. Contrast spillage into peritoneal cavity
5. Cornu of uterus
6. Foley balloon catheter in uterus
7. Fundus of uterus
8. Isthmus of uterine tube
9. Uterine tube (fallopian tube)

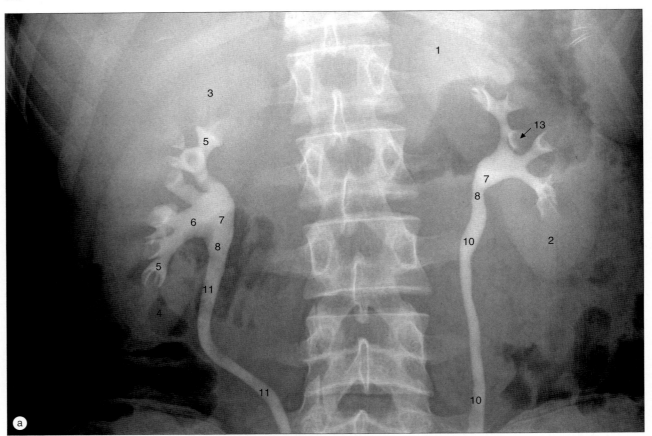

(a) 10 minutes intravenous urogram (IVU) with abdominal compression.

(b) Full-length 15 minutes IVU after release of compression.

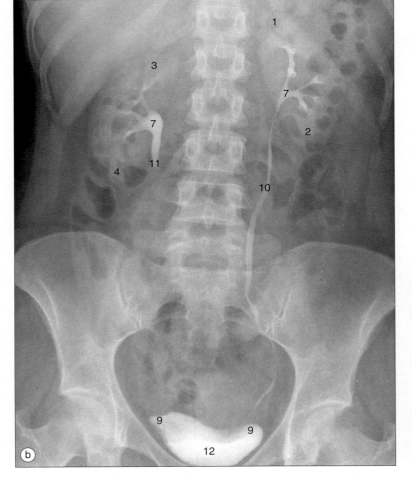

1.	Upper pole of left kidney
2.	Lower pole of left kidney
3.	Upper pole of right kidney
4.	Lower pole of right kidney
5.	Minor calyx
6.	Major calyx
7.	Renal pelvis
8.	Pelvi-ureteric junction
9.	Vesico-ureteric junction
10.	Left ureter
11.	Right ureter
12.	Urinary bladder
13.	Renal papilla

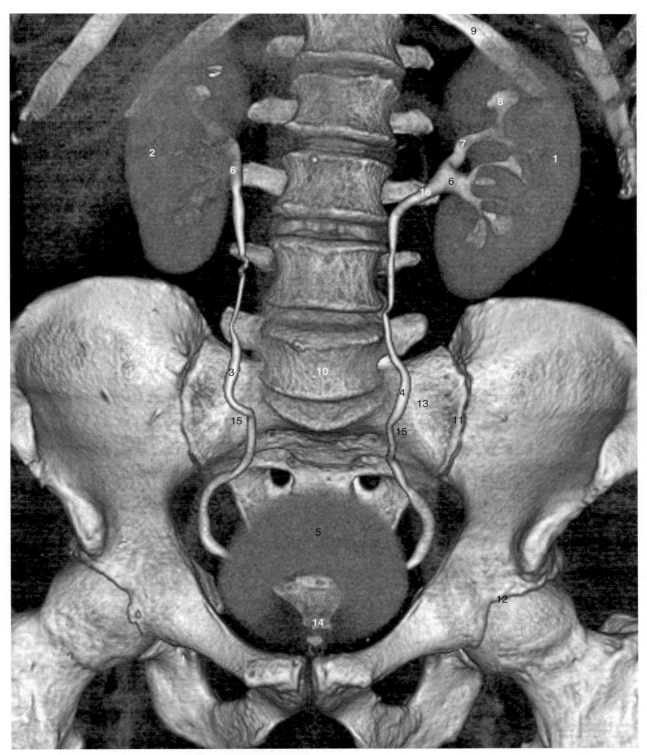

3D CT urogram at 10 minutes post intravenous injection.

1. Left kidney
2. Right kidney
3. Right ureter
4. Left ureter
5. Urinary bladder
6. Renal pelvis
7. Major calyx
8. Minor calyx
9. Twelfth rib
10. Body of L5 vertebra
11. Sacroiliac joint
12. Hip joint
13. Sacral ala
14. Coccyx
15. Point of ureteric crossover of common iliac vessels
16. Pelvi-ureteric junction

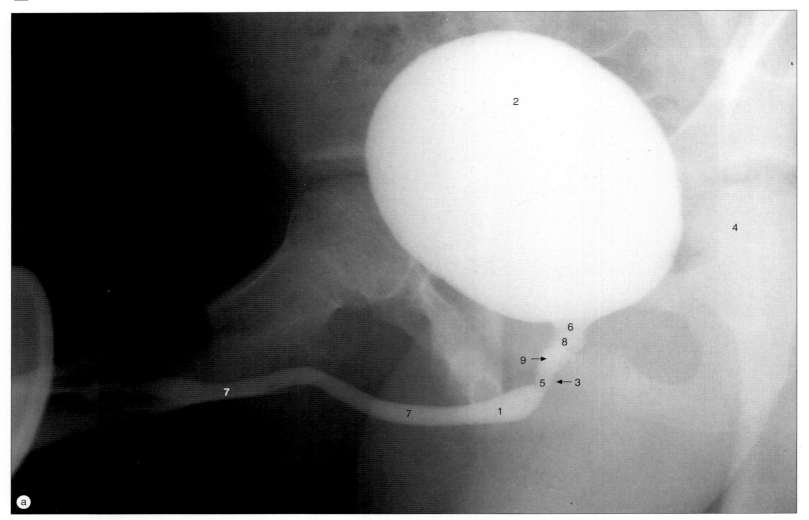

(a) Male urethrogram, oblique image.

(b) Penile arteriogram.

(c) Cavernosogram.

1. Bulbous urethra	6. Neck of urinary bladder
2. Contrast in urinary bladder	7. Penile urethra
3. External sphincter (sphincter urethrae)	8. Prostatic urethra
	9. Seminal colliculus (verumontanum)
4. Head of femur	
5. Membranous urethra	

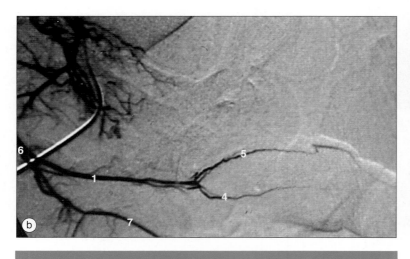

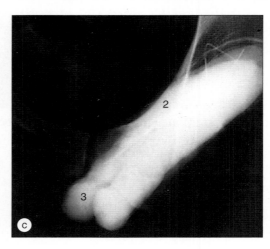

1. Artery of the penis	5. Dorsal artery of the penis
2. Corpus cavernosum	6. Internal pudendal artery
3. Crus of corpus cavernosum	7. Perineal artery
4. Deep artery of the penis	

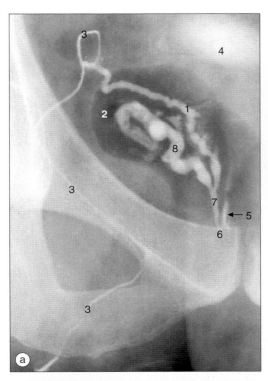

(a) Seminal vesiculogram.

1. Ampulla of ductus deferens
2. Colonic gas
3. Ductus deferens (vas deferens)
4. Full urinary bladder
5. Left ejaculatory duct
6. Position of seminal colliculus (verumontanum)
7. Right ejaculatory duct
8. Seminal vesicle

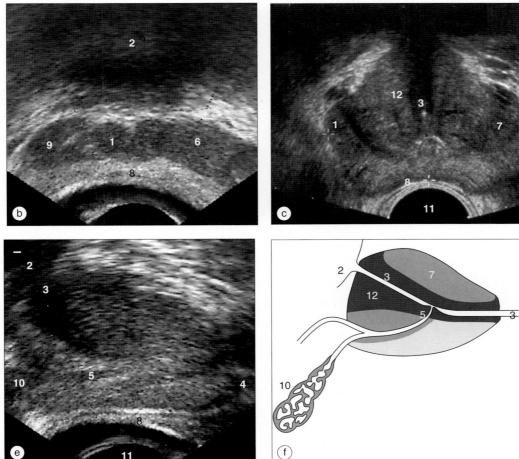

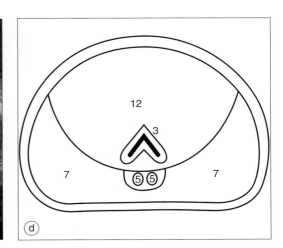

1. Ampulla of ductus deferens
2. Bladder
3. Course of urethra
4. Distal urethra
5. Ejaculatory duct (passing through central zone)
6. Left seminal vesicle
7. Peripheral zone of prostate
8. Rectal wall
9. Right seminal vesicle
10. Seminal vesicle
11. Transducer
12. Transitional zone of prostate

Rectal ultrasound of the prostate, **(b)** axial scan through bladder base, **(c)** axial scan through mid prostate, **(d)** line drawing of axial scan prostate, **(e)** sagittal midline scan, **(f)** line drawing of midline sagittal scan.

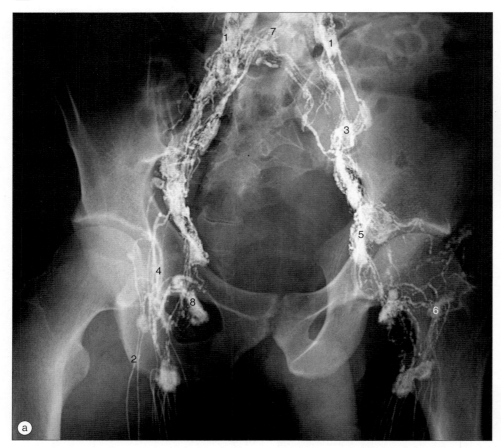

(a) Lymphangiogram pelvis, early filling phase.

(b) Lymphangiogram pelvis, late filling phase.

1. Ascending lumbar chains
2. Afferent inguinal lymphatics
3. Common iliac nodes
4. Efferent inguinal lymphatics
5. External iliac nodes
6. Superficial inguinal nodes
7. Lumbar crossover
8. Deep inguinal nodes

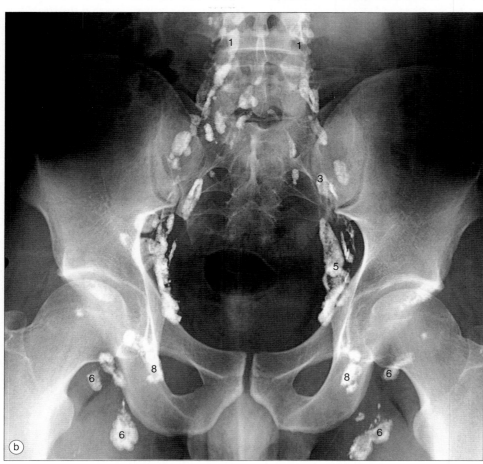

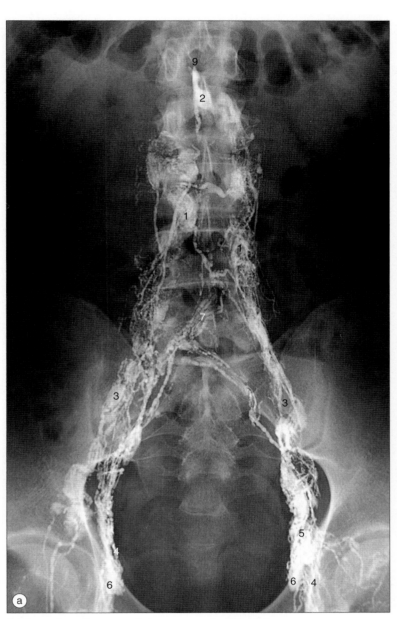

(a) Lymphangiogram abdomen, early filling phase.

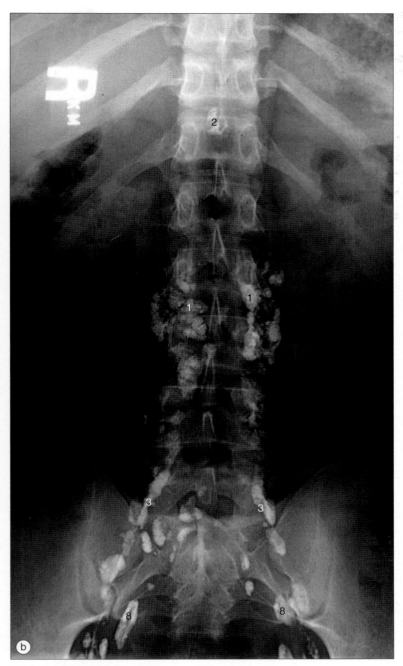

(b) Lymphangiogram abdomen, late filling phase.

1. Ascending lumbar chains
2. Cisterna chyli
3. Common iliac nodes
4. Efferent inguinal lymphatics
5. External iliac nodes (early filling)
6. Inguinal nodes (early filling)
7. Lumbar crossover
8. Deep inguinal nodes
9. Thoracic duct

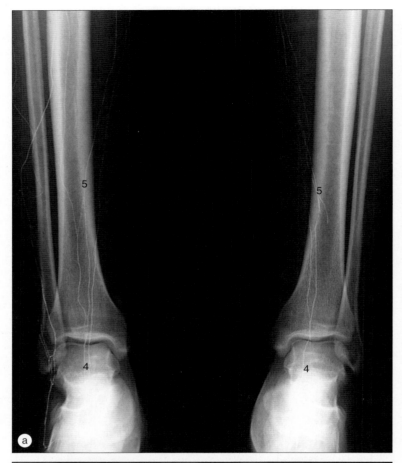

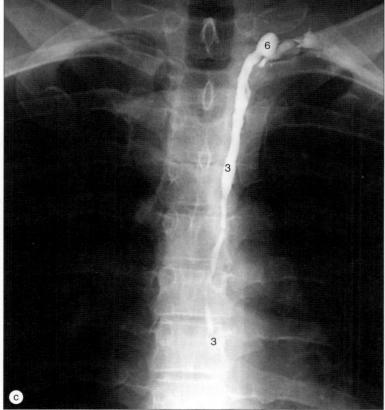

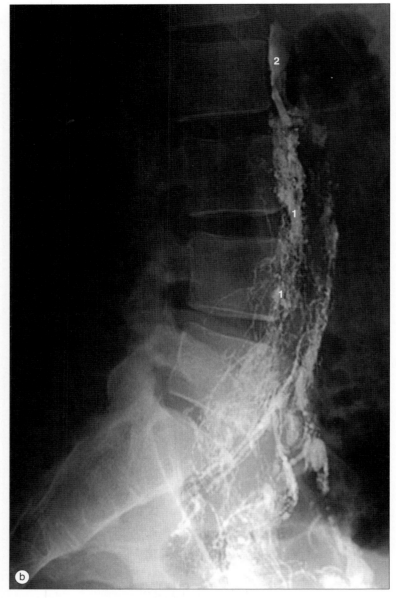

(a) Lymphangiogram calf, following cannulation of lymphatic vessels in the feet.

(b) Lymphangiogram abdomen lateral, early phase filling.

(c) Lymphangiogram thoracic duct, following cannulation of lymphatic vessels in abdomen and pelvis.

1. Ascending lumbar chains of lymph nodes
2. Cisterna chyli
3. Thoracic duct
4. Peripheral foot lymphatic channels
5. Peripheral lower leg lymphatic channels
6. Terminal ampulla

Bonus e-materials

Slidelines for radiograph features: Supine radiograph of the abdomen, Anteroposterior radiograph of the pelvis (female)

Selected pages from Imaging Atlas 4e

Tutorials: Tutorials 6a, 6b, 6c, 6d, 6e, 6f, 6g, 6h, 6i, 7a, 7b, 7c

Single best answer (SBA) self-assessment questions

Table of Variations

Variant	Frequency	Clinical implications
Pelvic appendix	30%	Symptoms confused with cystitis on presentation.
Right hepatic artery arising from the proximal super mesenteric artery	20%	Access for arterial embolisation of liver lesions, e.g. primary tumour, metastases.
Long cystic duct parallel to the extrahepatic bile duct	10%	Mistaken ligation or transection of the extrahepatic bile duct instead of the cystic duct at cholecystectomy; variant anatomy to navigate at ERCP.
Pancreas divisum	<10%	Association with pancreatitis; variant anatomy to navigate at ERCP.
Meckel's diverticulum	1%	Site of ectopic gastric mucosa; source of occult gastrointestinal haemorrhage; Meckel's diverticulitis.
Duplex kidney	<1%	Obstruction of the upper pole moiety; vesicoureteric reflux in the lower pole moiety; increased risk of infection.
Left-sided IVC	<0.5%	Implications for planning surgical vascular procedures and IVC filter placement.
Annular pancreas	<0.5%	Duodenal obstruction; increased risk of chronic pancreatitis.
Horseshoe kidney	<0.25%	Increased risk of traumatic injury, infection, hydronephrosis, renal calculi and malignancy.
Pelvic kidney	<0.05%	Can be asymptomatic; presentation as pelvic mass; increased risk of infection and secondary hypertension; should be considered instead of renal agenesis; other associated renal, vascular and genital developmental abnormalities.
Intestinal malrotation	0.01%	Risk of midgut volvulus; association with other developmental anomalies.

ERCP, *Endoscopic retrograde cholangiopancreatography*; IVC, *inferior vena cava*.

11 Lower limb

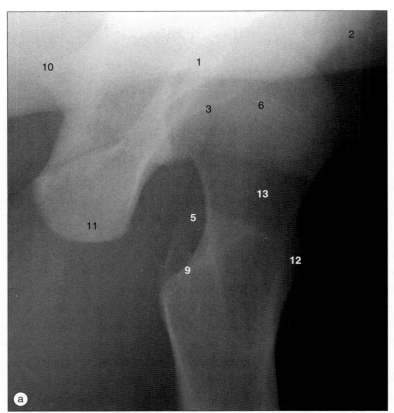

(a) Hip (for neck of femur), lateral film.

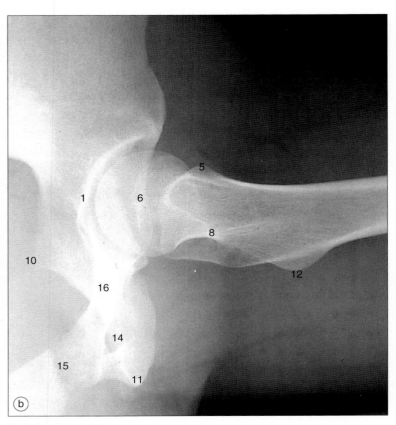

(b) Hip, lateral film.

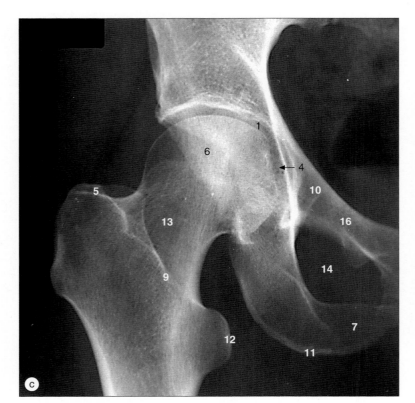

(c) Hip, anteroposterior film.

1. Acetabulum
2. Anterior inferior iliac spine
3. Epiphysial line
4. Fovea
5. Greater trochanter of femur
6. Head of femur
7. Inferior ramus of pubis
8. Intertrochanteric crest of femur
9. Intertrochanteric line
10. Ischial spine
11. Ischial tuberosity
12. Lesser trochanter of femur
13. Neck of femur
14. Obturator foramen
15. Pubic symphysis
16. Superior ramus of pubis

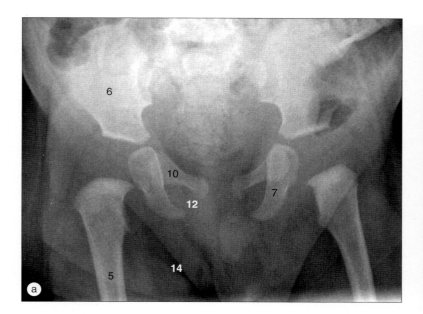

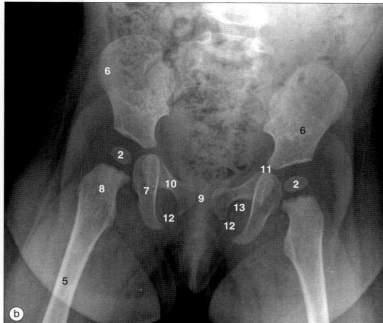

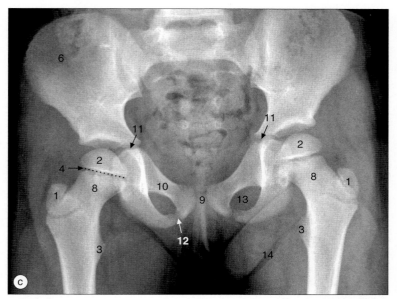

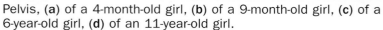

Pelvis, (a) of a 4-month-old girl, (b) of a 9-month-old girl, (c) of a 6-year-old girl, (d) of an 11-year-old girl.

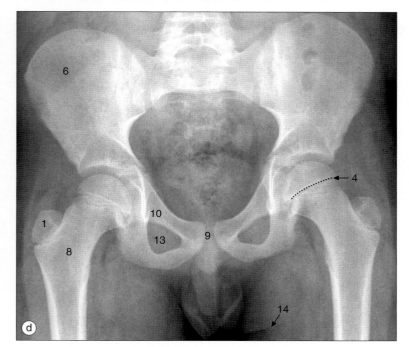

1. Centre for greater trochanter
2. Centre for head of femur (femoral capital epiphysis)
3. Centre for lesser trochanter
4. Epiphysial line
5. Femur
6. Ilium
7. Ischium
8. Neck of femur
9. Pubic symphysis
10. Pubis
11. Triradiate cartilage
12. Unossified junction between ischium and pubis
13. Obturator foramen
14. Fat creases

Innominate (Hip)	Appears	Fused
Ilium	2–3 miu	7–9 yrs
Ischium	4 miu	7–9 yrs
Pubis	4 miu	7–9 yrs
Acetabulum	11–14 yrs	15–25 yrs
Ant. sup. iliac spine	Puberty	15–25 yrs
Iliac crest/sup. spines	Puberty	15–25 yrs
Ischial tuberosity	Puberty +	15–25 yrs
Femur (c)		
Shaft	7 wiu	
Head	4–6 mths	14–18 yrs
Greater trochanter	2–4 yrs	14–18 yrs
Lesser trochanter	10–12 yrs	14–18 yrs
Distal end	9 miu	17–19 yrs

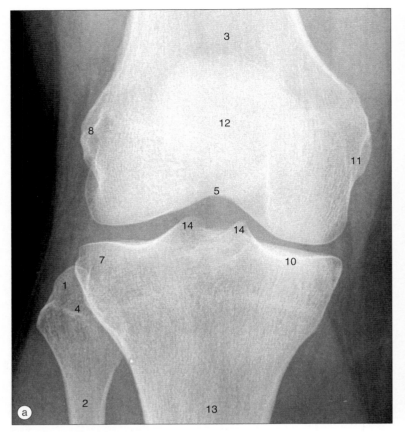

(a) Anteroposterior film.

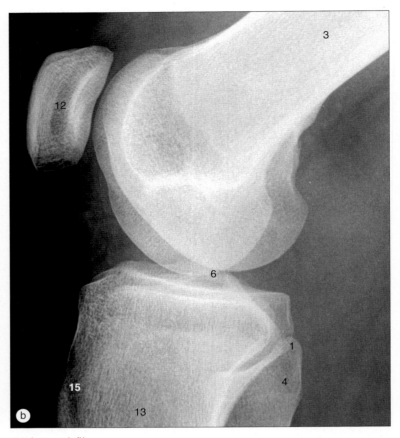

(b) Lateral film.

1. Apex (styloid process) of fibula
2. Fibula neck
3. Femur
4. Head of fibula
5. Intercondylar fossa
6. Lateral condyle of femur
7. Lateral condyle of tibia
8. Lateral epicondyle of femur
9. Medial condyle of femur
10. Medial condyle of tibia
11. Medial epicondyle of femur
12. Patella
13. Tibia
14. Tubercles of intercondylar eminence
15. Tuberosity of tibia

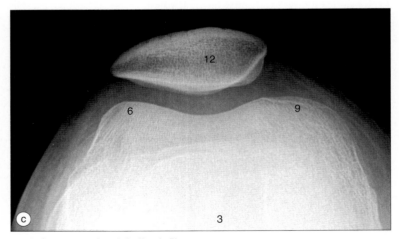

(c) Inferosuperior (skyline) film.

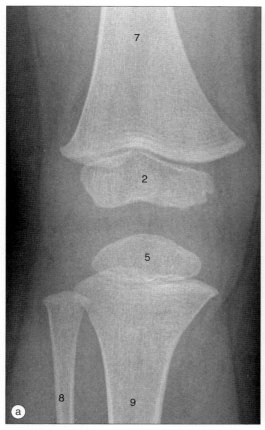

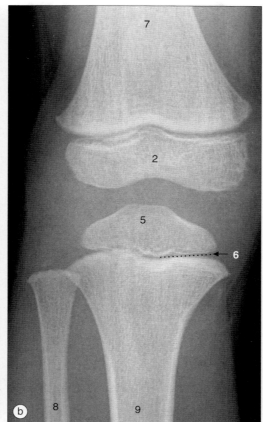

(a) 2-year-old girl.

(b) and (c) 5-year-old girl.

1. Antero-inferior extension of proximal tibial centre for tuberosity of tibia
2. Centre for distal femur
3. Centre for head of fibula
4. Patella
5. Centre for proximal tibia
6. Epiphysial line
7. Femur
8. Fibula
9. Tibia

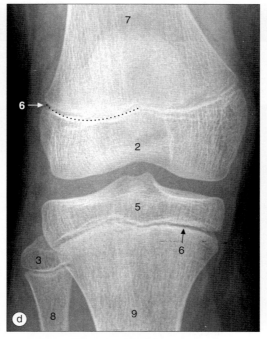

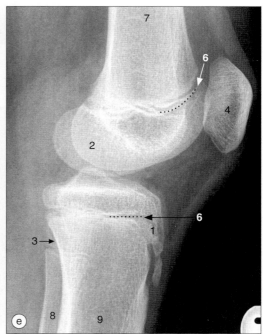

Patella (c)	Appears	Fused
1–3 centres	3–5 yrs	Puberty
Tibia (c)		
Shaft	7 wiu	
Proximal/plateau	9 miu	16–18 yrs
Tuberosity	10–12 yrs	12–14 yrs
Distal end	4 mths–1 yr	15–17 yrs
Fibula (c)		
Shaft	8 wiu	
Proximal end/head	2–4 yrs	17–19 yrs
Distal end	6 mths–1 yr	15–17 yrs

(d) and (e) 12-year-old girl.

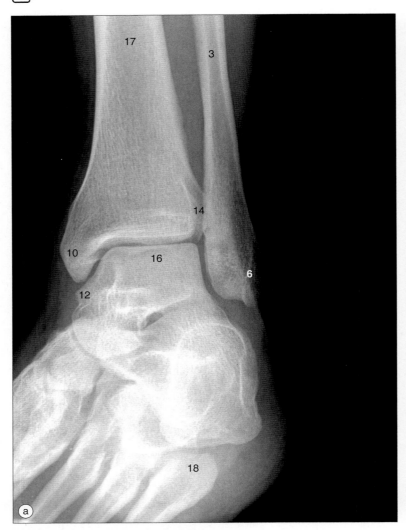

(a) Ankle joint, anteroposterior film.

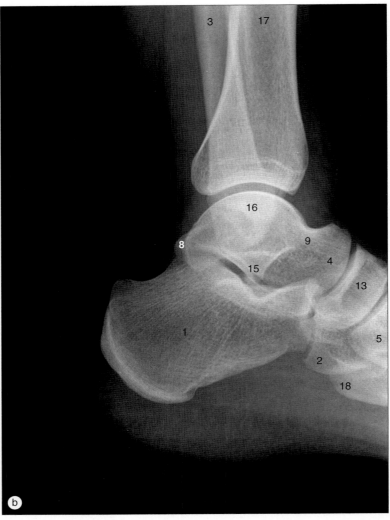

(b) Ankle joint, lateral film.

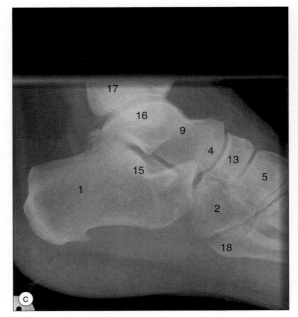

(c) Calcaneus, lateral film.

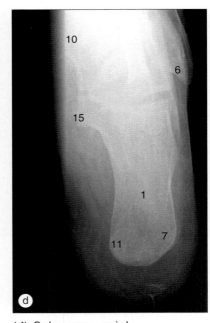

(d) Calcaneus, axial (caudocranial) film.

1. Calcaneus
2. Cuboid
3. Fibula
4. Head of talus
5. Lateral cuneiform
6. Lateral malleolus of fibula
7. Lateral process of calcaneus
8. Lateral tubercle of talus
9. Neck of talus
10. Medial malleolus of tibia
11. Medial process of calcaneus
12. Medial tubercle of talus
13. Navicular
14. Region of inferior tibiofibular joint
15. Sustentaculum tali of calcaneus
16. Talus
17. Tibia
18. Tuberosity of base of fifth metatarsal

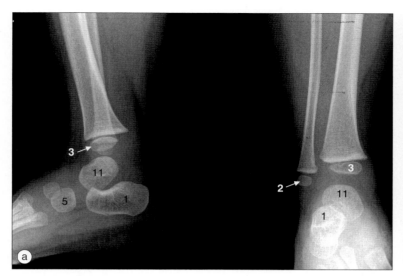

(a) Ankle of a 3-year-old girl.

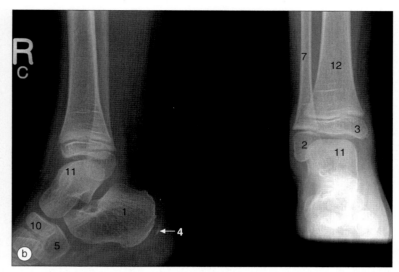

(b) Ankle of a 5-year-old girl.

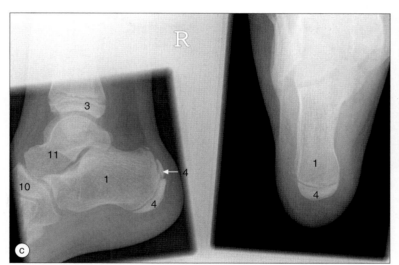

(c) Ankle of a 13-year-old girl.

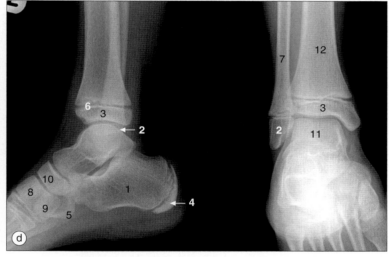

(d) Calcaneus of a 10-year-old girl.

1.	Calcaneus
2.	Centre for distal fibula
3.	Centre for distal tibia
4.	Centre for posterior aspect of calcaneus
5.	Cuboid
6.	Epiphyseal line
7.	Fibula
8.	Intermediate cuneiform
9.	Lateral cuneiform
10.	Navicular
11.	Talus
12.	Tibia

Tarsal bones (c)	Appears	Fused
Calcaneus	3 miu	14–16 yrs
Talus	6 miu	
Navicular	3 yrs	
Cuneiform lateral	6 mths–1 yr	
Cuneiform intermediate	2–3 yrs	
Cuneiform medial	1–2 yrs	
Cuboid	9 miu	

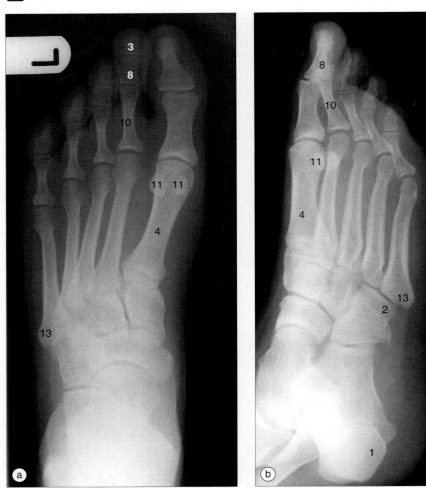

Foot, **(a)** dorsoplantar film, **(b)** dorsoplantar oblique film, **(c)** and **(d)** os naviculare.

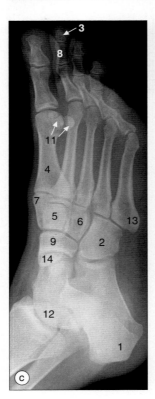

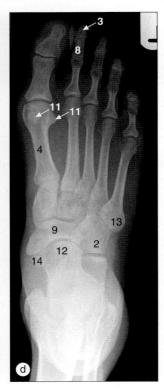

1. Calcaneus
2. Cuboid
3. Distal phalanx of second toe
4. First metatarsal
5. Intermediate cuneiform
6. Lateral cuneiform
7. Medial cuneiform
8. Middle phalanx of second toe
9. Navicular
10. Proximal phalanx of second toe
11. Sesamoid bones in flexor hallucis brevis muscle
12. Talus
13. Tuberosity of base of fifth metatarsal
14. Os naviculare

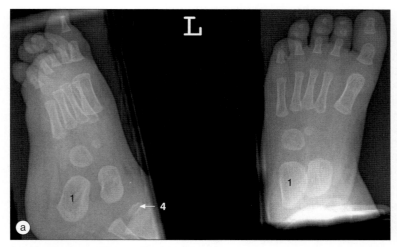

(a) Foot of an 11-month-old girl.

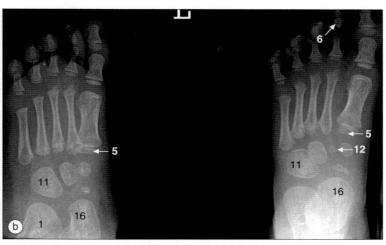

(b) Foot of a 3-year-old girl.

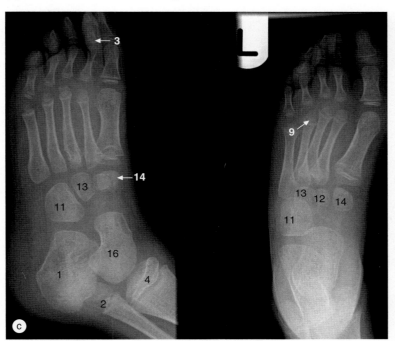

(c) Foot of a 6-year-old girl.

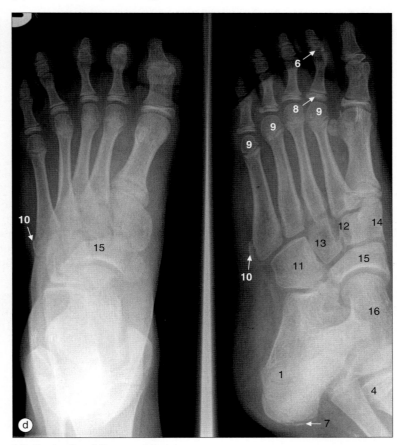

(d) Foot of a 12-year-old girl.

1. Calcaneus
2. Centre for distal fibula
3. Centre for middle phalanx of second toe
4. Centre for distal tibia
5. Centre for first metatarsal
6. Centre for middle phalanx of second toe
7. Centre for posterior aspect of calcaneus
8. Centre for proximal phalanx of second toe
9. Centre for second metatarsals (applies to second to fifth metatarsal)
10. Centre for tuberosity of base of fifth metatarsal
11. Cuboid
12. Intermediate cuneiform
13. Lateral cuneiform
14. Medial cuneiform
15. Navicular
16. Talus

Metatarsals (c)	Appears	Fused
Shafts	9 wiu	
Heads (2–5) or base (1)	3–4 yrs	17–20 yrs
Tuberosity of 5	10–12 yrs	13–15 yrs
Phalanges (c)		
Shaft	9–12 wiu	
Bases (variable)	1–6 yrs	14–18 yrs

Tarsal bones (c)	Appears	Fused
Calcaneus	3 miu	14–16 yrs
Talus	6 miu	
Navicular	3 yrs	
Cuneiform lateral	6 mths–1 yr	
Cuneiform intermediate	2–3 yrs	
Cuneiform medial	1–2 yrs	
Cuboid	9 miu	

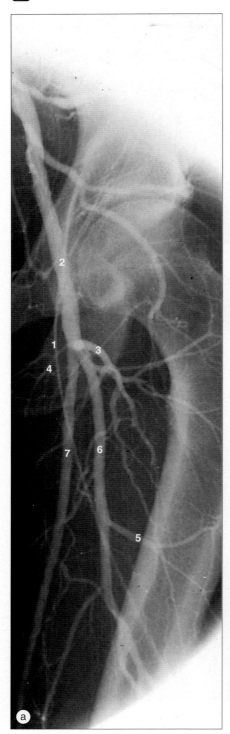

(a) Femoral arteriogram.

The femoropopliteal and tibial arteries are imaged by catheterising the distal abdominal aorta and injecting contrast medium. The column of contrast is then followed as it passes down the legs. If only one leg is to be imaged, an injection into the ipsilateral femoral artery suffices. The external iliac artery continues as the common femoral artery, which originates deep to the inguinal ligament, dividing into the superficial and deep (profunda) femoral arteries. An oblique view is often useful to image the femoral bifurcation and to identify atheroma at the origins of these vessels.

1. Catheter introduced into distal abdominal aorta via left femoral artery
2. Common femoral artery
3. Lateral circumflex femoral artery
4. Medial circumflex femoral artery
5. Perforating artery
6. Profunda femoris artery
7. Superficial femoral artery

(b) Popliteal arteriogram.

The superficial femoral artery becomes the popliteal artery as it passes through the hiatus in the adductor magnus muscle. The popliteal artery terminates at the lower border of the popliteus muscle, dividing into the anterior and posterior tibial arteries.

1. Anterior tibial artery
2. Inferior lateral genicular artery
3. Inferior medial genicular artery
4. Muscular branches of anterior tibial artery
5. Muscular branches of posterior tibial artery
6. Peroneal artery
7. Popliteal artery
8. Posterior tibial artery
9. Superior lateral genicular artery
10. Superior medial genicular artery
11. Tibio-peroneal trunk

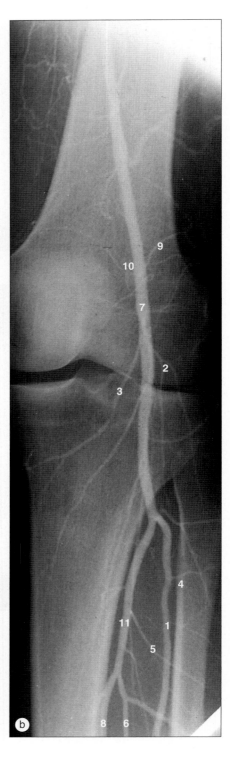

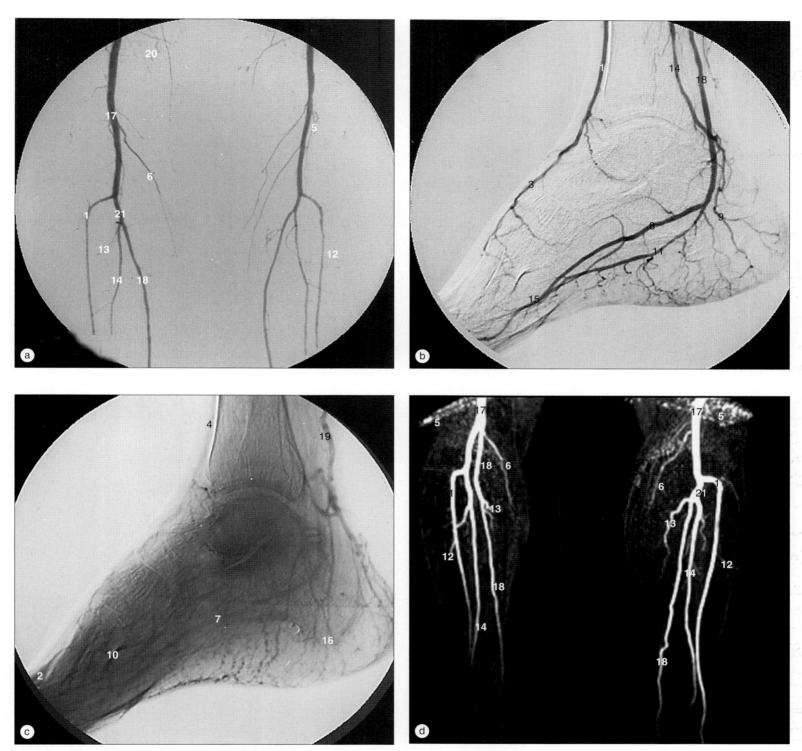

(a) Popliteal arteriogram, (b) foot arteriogram, lateral image, (c) foot venogram, (d) MR angiogram of calf arteries.

1. Anterior tibial artery
2. Dorsal venous arch
3. Dorsalis pedis artery
4. Great saphenous vein
5. Inferior lateral genicular artery
6. Inferior medial genicular artery
7. Lateral marginal vein
8. Lateral plantar artery
9. Medial calcaneal artery
10. Medial marginal vein
11. Medial plantar artery
12. Muscular branches of anterior tibial artery
13. Muscular branches of posterior tibial artery
14. Peroneal artery
15. Plantar arch
16. Plantar cutaneous venous plexus
17. Popliteal artery
18. Posterior tibial artery
19. Small saphenous vein
20. Superior medial genicular artery
21. Tibio-peroneal trunk

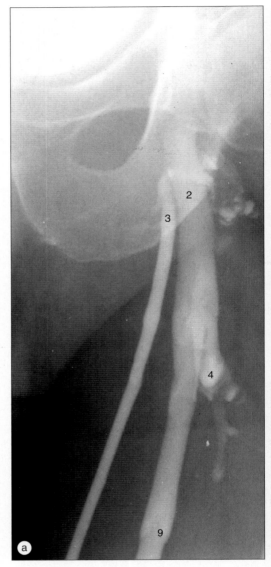

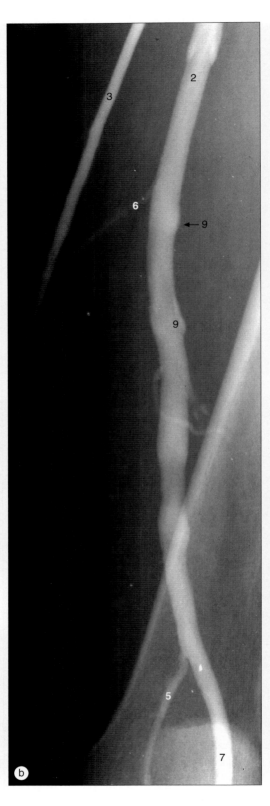

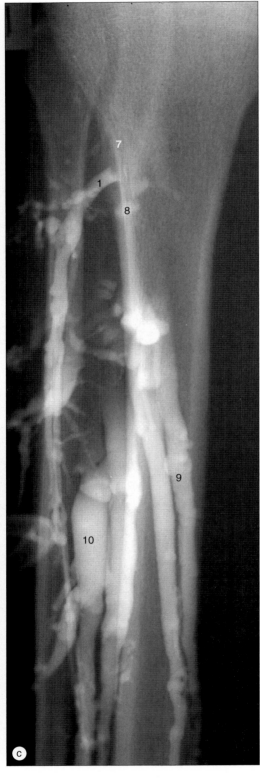

(a)–(c) Lower limb venograms.

1. Anterior tibial vein
2. Femoral vein
3. Great (long) saphenous vein
4. Lateral circumflex vein
5. Muscular tributary of femoral vein
6. Perforating vein
7. Popliteal vein
8. Posterior tibial veins
9. Venous valves
10. Venous calf plexus

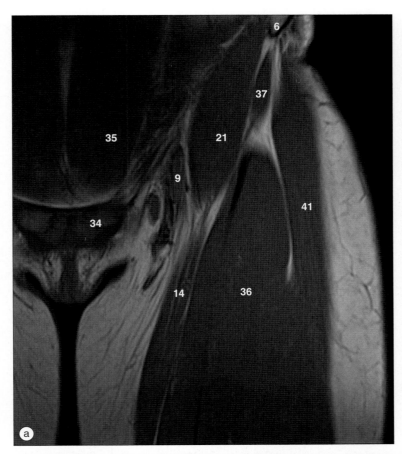

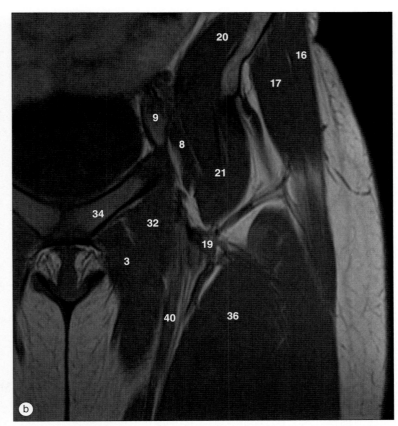

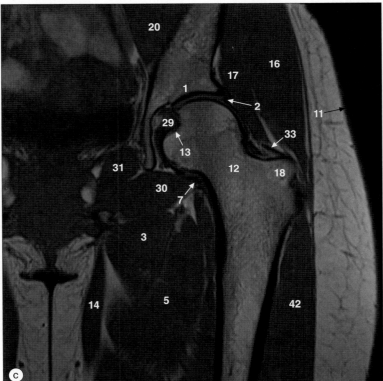

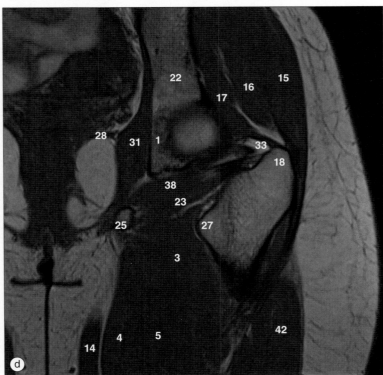

(a)-(f) Hip and upper thigh, coronal MR images, from anterior to posterior.

For label key see page 220.

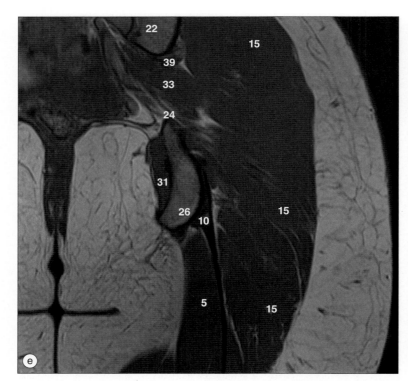 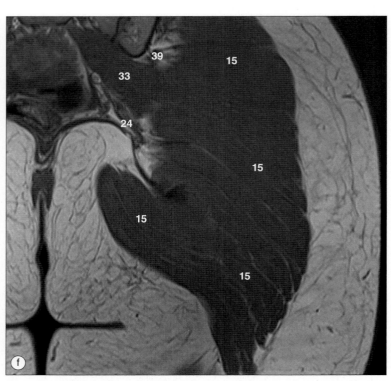

(a)-(f) Hip and upper thigh, coronal MR images, from anterior to posterior.

1. Acetabulum	15. Gluteus maximus muscle	29. Ligamentum teres
2. Acetabular labrum	16. Gluteus medius muscle	30. Obturator externus muscle
3. Adductor brevis muscle	17. Gluteus minimus muscle	31. Obturator internus muscle
4. Adductor longus muscle	18. Greater trochanter of femur	32. Pectineus muscle
5. Adductor magnus muscle	19. Great saphenous vein	33. Piriformis
6. Anterior superior iliac spine	20. Iliacus muscle	34. Pubis
7. Capsule of hip joint (zona orbicularis)	21. Iliopsoas muscle	35. Rectus abdominis muscle
8. Common femoral artery	22. Ilium	36. Rectus femoris muscle
9. Common femoral vein	23. Inferior gemellus muscle	37. Sartorius muscle
10. Common hamstring origin	24. Inferior gluteal vessels	38. Superior gemellus muscle
11. Fascia lata	25. Inferior pubic ramus	39. Superior gluteal vessels
12. Femoral neck	26. Ischial tuberosity	40. Superficial femoral vein
13. Fovea capitis	27. Lesser trochanter of femur	41. Tensor fascia lata muscle
14. Gracilis muscle	28. Levator ani muscle	42. Vastus lateralis muscle

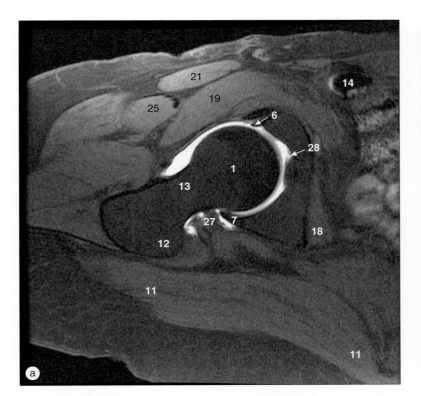

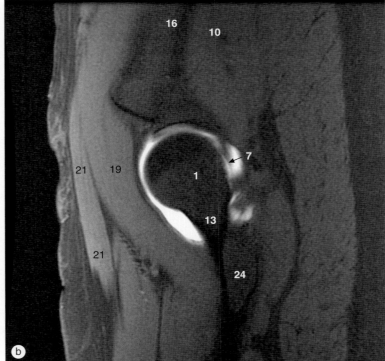

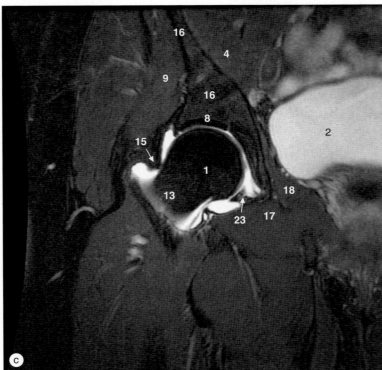

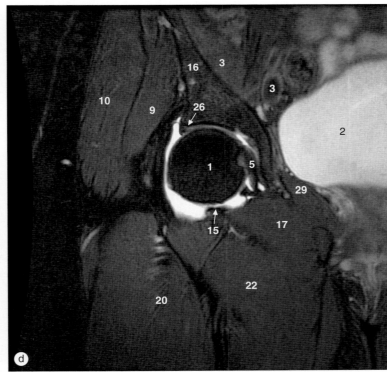

Hip, MR arthrogram images, (a) axial, (b) sagittal, (c) and (d) coronal.

1. Femoral head	11. Gluteus maximus muscle	21. Sartorius muscle
2. Bladder	12. Greater trochanter	22. Adductor longus muscle
3. External iliac artery	13. Femoral neck	23. Transverse acetabular ligament
4. Iliacus muscle	14. Femoral artery	24. Quadratus femoris muscle
5. Ligamentum teres	15. Zona orbicularis (circular fibrous capsule)	25. Rectus femoris muscle
6. Anterior acetabular labrum	16. Iliac bone	26. Superior acetabular labrum
7. Posterior acetabular labrum	17. Obturator externus muscle	27. Gemellus muscle
8. Acetabular roof	18. Obturator internus muscle	28. Acetabular notch (pulvinar)
9. Gluteus minimus muscle	19. Iliopsoas muscle	29. Pectineus muscle
10. Gluteus medius muscle	20. Vastus intermedius muscle	

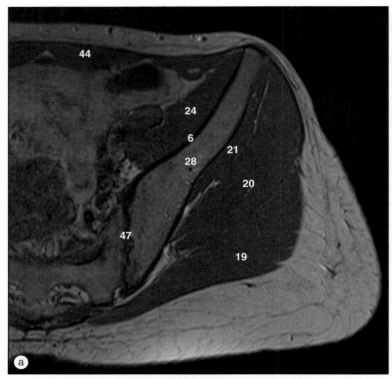

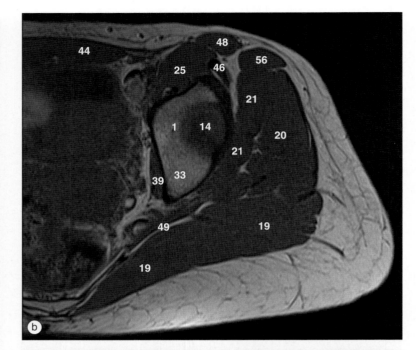

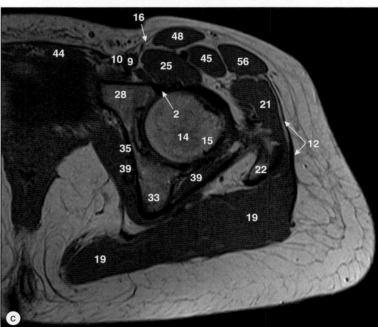

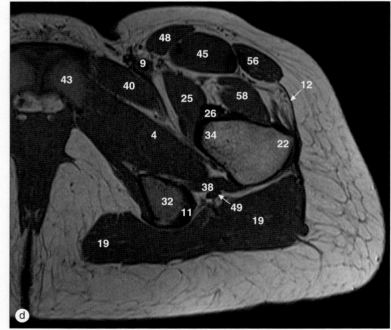

(a)-(g) Hip and upper thigh, axial MR images, from superior to inferior.

1. Acetabulum	**11.** Common hamstring origin	**21.** Gluteus minimus muscle
2. Acetabular labrum	**12.** Fascia lata	**22.** Greater trochanter of femur
3. Adductor brevis muscle	**13.** Femur	**23.** Great saphenous vein
4. Adductor longus muscle	**14.** Femoral head	**24.** Iliacus muscle
5. Adductor magnus muscle	**15.** Femoral neck	**25.** Iliopsoas muscle
6. Anterior superior iliac spine	**16.** Femoral nerve	**26.** Iliopsoas tendon
7. Biceps femoris muscle	**17.** Fovea capitis	**27.** Iliotibial tract
8. Capsule of hip joint (zona orbicularis)	**18.** Gracilis muscle	**28.** Ilium
9. Common femoral artery	**19.** Gluteus maximus muscle	**29.** Inferior gemellus muscle
10. Common femoral vein	**20.** Gluteus medius muscle	**30.** Inferior gluteal vessels

Numbers 1–59 are common to pages 222–223.

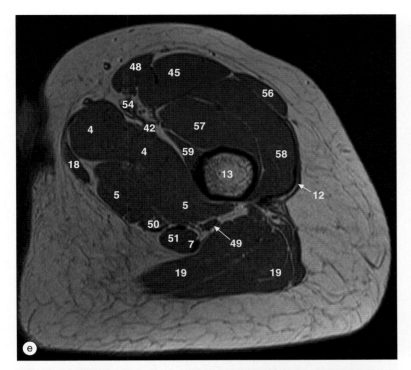

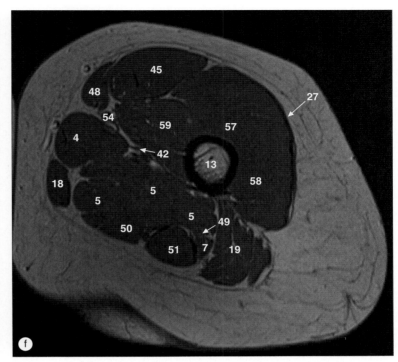

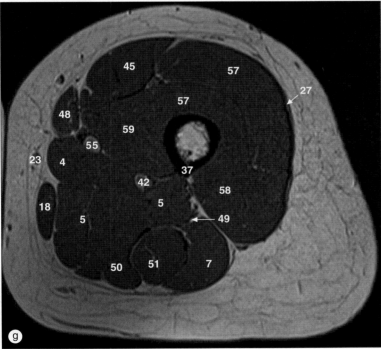

(a)-(g) Hip and upper thigh, axial MR images, from superior to inferior.

31. Inferior pubic ramus	**41.** Piriformis muscle	**51.** Semitendinosus muscle
32. Ischial tuberosity	**42.** Profunda femoris vessels	**52.** Superior gemellus muscle
33. Ischium	**43.** Pubis	**53.** Superior gluteal vessels
34. Lesser trochanter of femur	**44.** Rectus abdominis muscle	**54.** Superficial femoral artery
35. Levator ani muscle	**45.** Rectus femoris muscle	**55.** Superficial femoral vein
36. Ligamentum teres	**46.** Rectus femoris tendon	**56.** Tensor fascia lata muscle
37. Linea aspera of femur	**47.** Sacroiliac joint	**57.** Vastus intermedius muscle
38. Obturator externus muscle	**48.** Sartorius muscle	**58.** Vastus lateralis muscle
39. Obturator internus muscle	**49.** Sciatic nerve	**59.** Vastus medialis muscle
40. Pectineus muscle	**50.** Semimembranosus muscle	

Numbers 1–59 are common to pages 222–223.

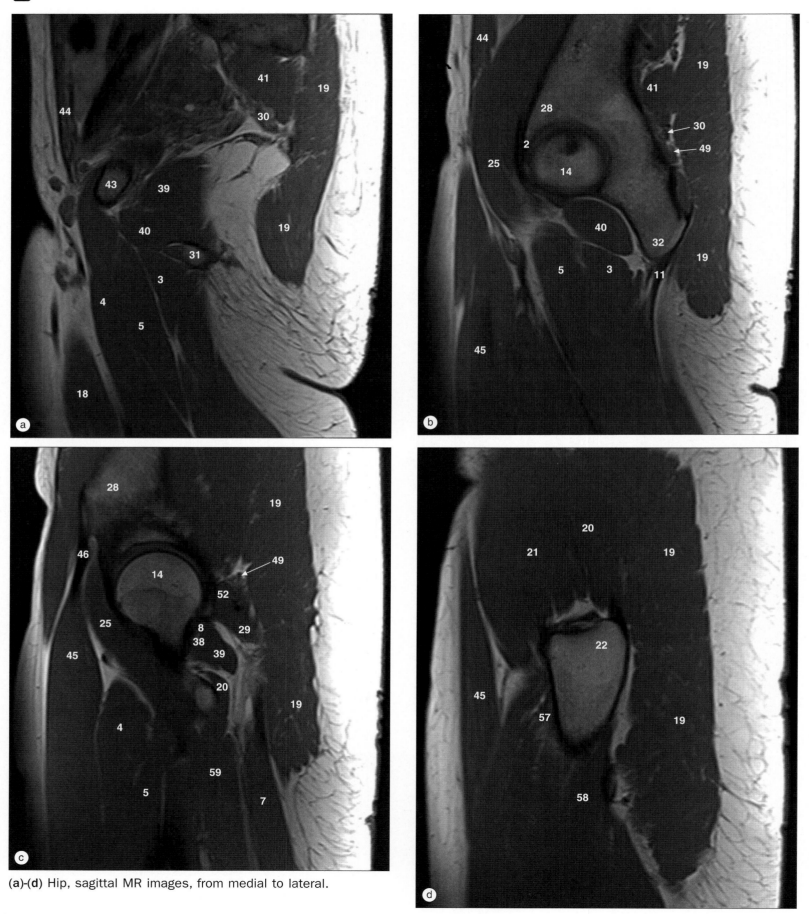

(a)-(d) Hip, sagittal MR images, from medial to lateral.

For label key see pages 222–223.

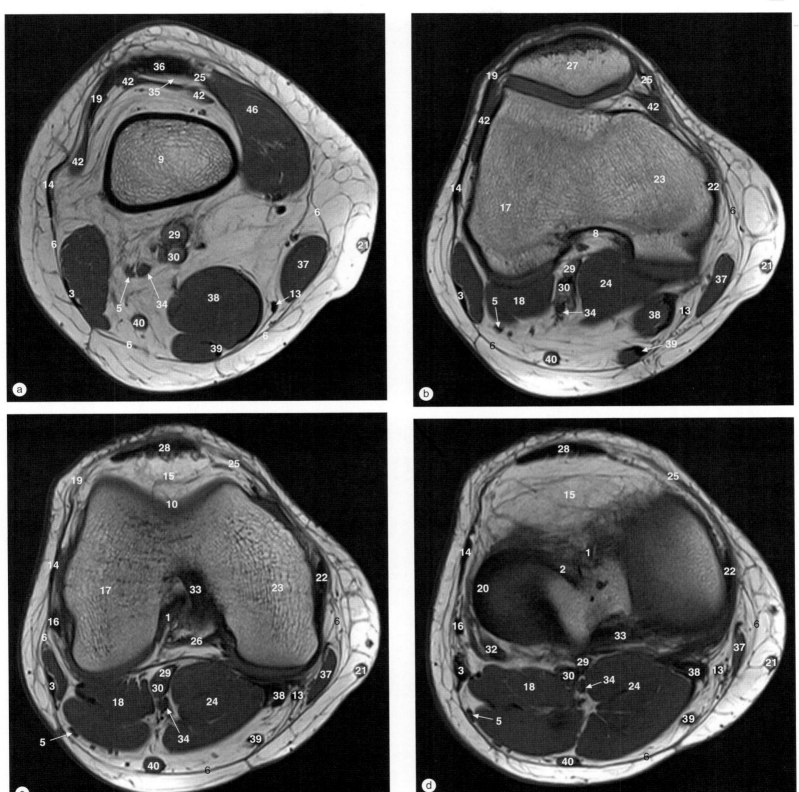

(a)–(f) Knee, axial MR images, from superior to inferior.

For label key see page 226.

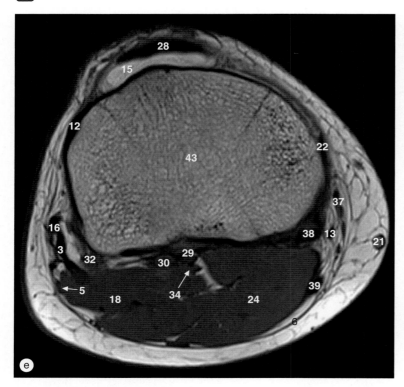

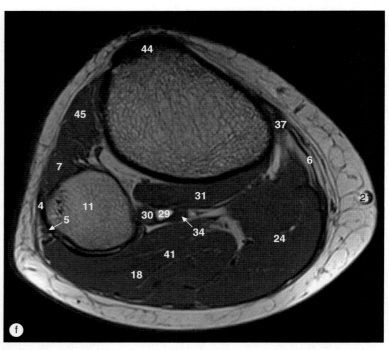

(a)-(f) Knee, axial MR images, from superior to inferior.

1. Anterior cruciate ligament	**17.** Lateral femoral condyle	**33.** Posterior cruciate ligament
2. Anterior root of lateral meniscus	**18.** Lateral head of gastrocnemius muscle	**34.** Posterior tibial nerve
3. Biceps femoris tendon	**19.** Lateral patella retinaculum	**35.** Quadriceps fat pad
4. Conjoint tendon	**20.** Lateral meniscus (body)	**36.** Quadriceps tendon
5. Common peroneal nerve	**21.** Long (great) saphenous vein	**37.** Sartorius muscle
6. Deep fascia (fascia lata)	**22.** Medial collateral ligament	**38.** Semimembranosus muscle/tendon
7. Extensor digitorum longus muscle	**23.** Medial femoral condyle	**39.** Semitendinosus tendon
8. Femoral intercondylar notch	**24.** Medial head of gastrocnemius muscle	**40.** Short (lesser) saphenous vein
9. Femoral metaphysis	**25.** Medial patella retinaculum	**41.** Soleus muscle
10. Femoral trochlear groove	**26.** Meniscofemoral ligament	**42.** Suprapatellar bursa
11. Fibula	**27.** Patella	**43.** Tibia
12. Gerdy's tubercle of tibia	**28.** Patellar tendon	**44.** Tibial tuberosity
13. Gracilis tendon	**29.** Popliteal artery	**45.** Tibialis anterior muscle
14. Iliotibial tract	**30.** Popliteal vein	**46.** Vastus medialis muscle
15. Infrapatellar (Hoffa's) fat pad	**31.** Popliteus muscle	
16. Lateral collateral ligament	**32.** Popliteus tendon	

Numbers 1–46 are common to pages 225–226.

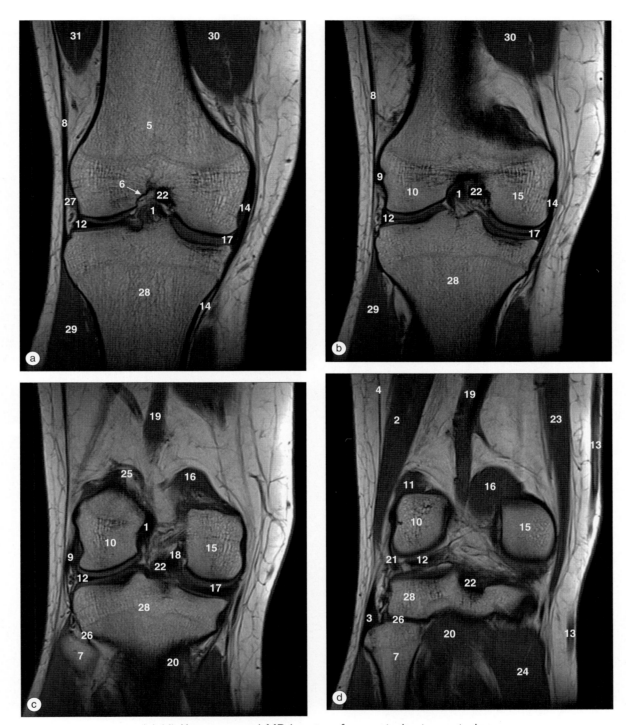

(a)-(d) Knee, coronal MR images, from anterior to posterior.

1. Anterior cruciate ligament
2. Biceps femoris muscle
3. Conjoint tendon
4. Deep fascia (fascia lata)
5. Femur
6. Femoral intercondylar notch
7. Fibula
8. Iliotibial tract
9. Lateral collateral ligament
10. Lateral femoral condyle
11. Lateral head of gastrocnemius muscle
12. Lateral meniscus
13. Long (great) saphenous vein
14. Medial collateral ligament
15. Medial femoral condyle
16. Medial head of gastrocnemius muscle
17. Medial meniscus
18. Meniscofemoral ligament (posterior, of Wrisberg)
19. Popliteal vessel
20. Popliteus muscle
21. Popliteus tendon
22. Posterior cruciate ligament
23. Semimembranosus muscle
24. Soleus muscle
25. Superior lateral genicular vessels
26. Superior tibiofibular joint
27. Synovial recess (superolateral)
28. Tibia
29. Tibialis anterior muscle
30. Vastus medialis muscle
31. Vastus lateralis muscle

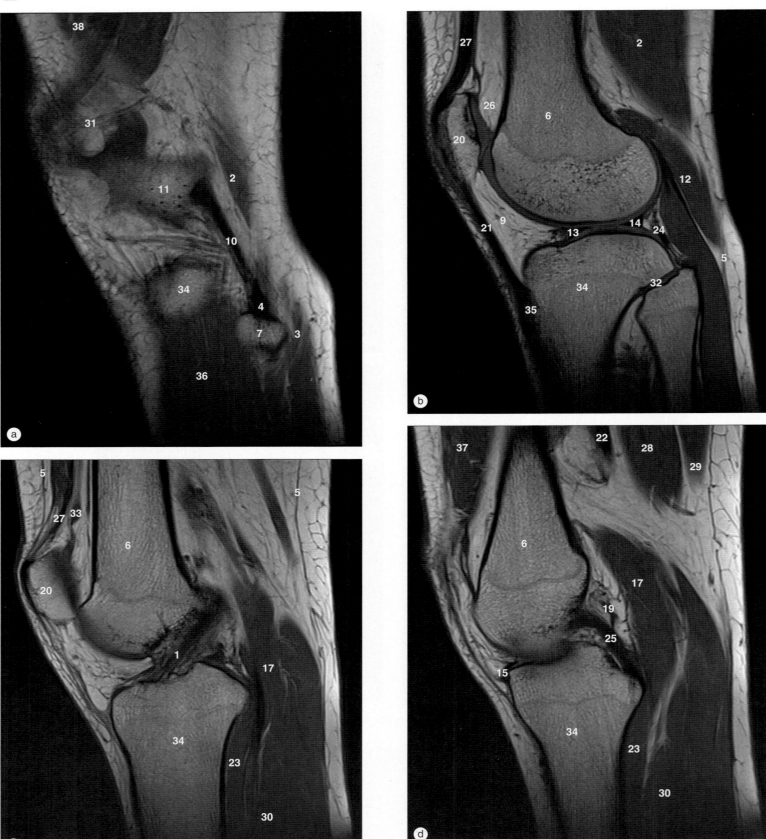

(a)-(f) Knee, sagittal MR images, from lateral to medial.

For label key see page 229.

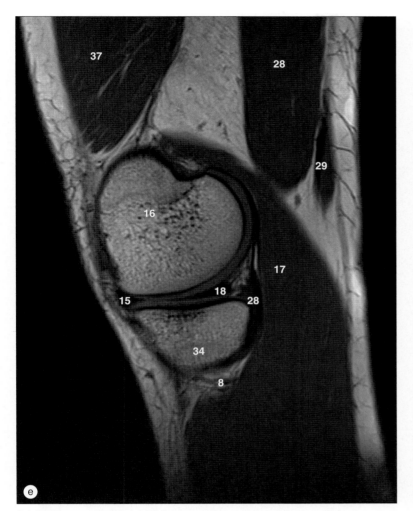

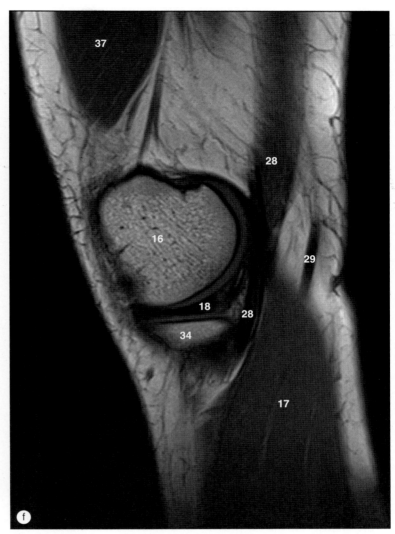

(a)-(f) Knee, sagittal MR images, from lateral to medial.

1. Anterior cruciate ligament	**14.** Lateral meniscus posterior horn	**26.** Quadriceps fat pad
2. Biceps femoris muscle	**15.** Medial meniscus anterior horn	**27.** Quadriceps tendon
3. Common peroneal (fibular) nerve	**16.** Medial femoral condyle	**28.** Semimembranosus tendon
4. Conjoint tendon	**17.** Medial head of gastrocnemius muscle	**29.** Semitendinosus tendon
5. Deep fascia (fascia lata)	**18.** Medial meniscus posterior horn	**30.** Soleus muscle
6. Femur	**19.** Meniscofemoral ligament (posterior, of	**31.** Superior lateral geniculate vessels
7. Fibular head	Wrisberg)	**32.** Superior tibiofibular joint
8. Inferior genicular vessels	**20.** Patella	**33.** Suprapatellar bursa
9. Infrapatellar (Hoffa's) fat pad	**21.** Patellar tendon	**34.** Tibia
10. Lateral collateral ligament	**22.** Popliteal vessel	**35.** Tibial tuberosity
11. Lateral femoral condyle	**23.** Popliteus muscle	**36.** Tibialis anterior muscle
12. Lateral head of gastrocnemius muscle	**24.** Popliteus tendon	**37.** Vastus medialis muscle
13. Lateral meniscus anterior horn	**25.** Posterior cruciate ligament	**38.** Vastus lateralis muscle

Numbers 1–38 are common to pages 228–229.

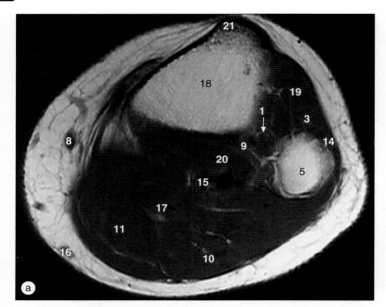

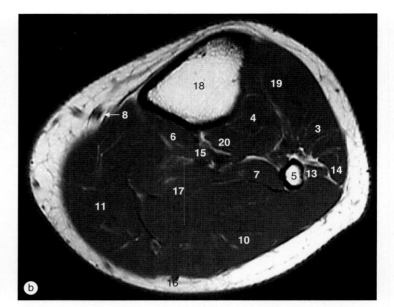

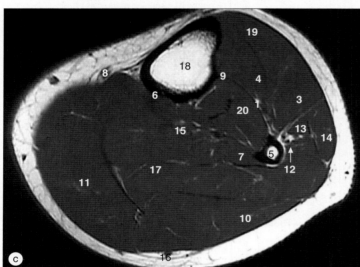

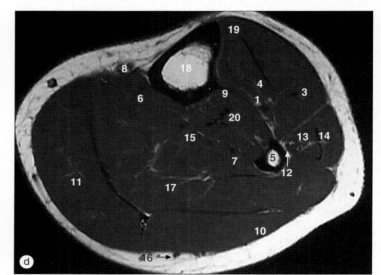

(a)–(e) Calf, axial MR images, from superior to inferior.

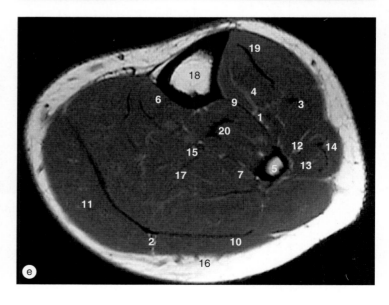

1. Anterior tibial artery
2. Aponeurosis of gastrocnemius muscle
3. Extensor digitorum longus muscle
4. Extensor hallucis longus muscle
5. Fibula
6. Flexor digitorum longus muscle
7. Flexor hallucis longus muscle
8. Great (long) saphenous vein
9. Interosseous membrane
10. Lateral head of gastrocnemius muscle
11. Medial head of gastrocnemius muscle
12. Peroneal artery
13. Peroneus brevis muscle
14. Peroneus longus muscle
15. Posterior tibial artery
16. Small saphenous vein
17. Soleus muscle
18. Tibia
19. Tibialis anterior muscle
20. Tibialis posterior muscle
21. Tuberosity of tibia

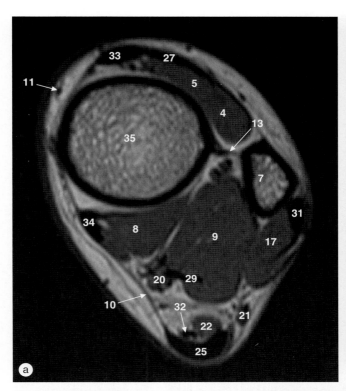

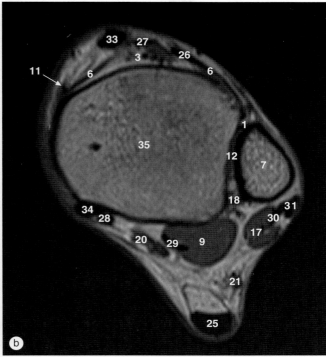

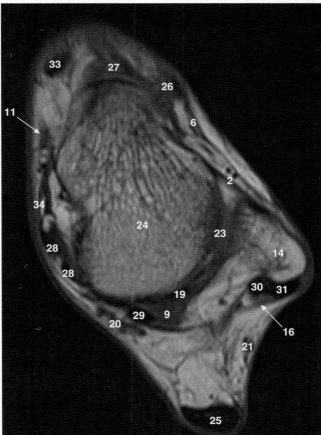

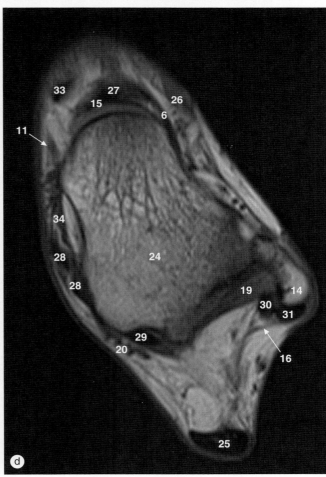

(a)-(d) Ankle, axial MR images, from superior to inferior.

1. Anterior inferior tibiofibular ligament
2. Anterior talofibular ligament
3. Anterior tibial vessels
4. Extensor digitorum longus muscle
5. Extensor hallucis longus muscle
6. Extensor retinaculum
7. Fibula
8. Flexor digitorum longus muscle
9. Flexor hallucis longus muscle
10. Flexor retinaculum
11. Great (long) saphenous vein
12. Inferior tibiofibular joint
13. Interosseous membrane
14. Lateral malleolus
15. Navicular
16. Peroneal (fibular) retinaculum
17. Peroneus brevis muscle
18. Posterior inferior tibiofibular ligament
19. Posterior talofibular ligament
20. Posterior tibial neurovascular bundle
21. Small (short) saphenous vein
22. Soleus muscle
23. Talofibular joint
24. Talus
25. Tendo calcaneus (Achilles' tendon)
26. Tendon of extensor digitorum muscle
27. Tendon of extensor hallucis longus muscle
28. Tendon of flexor digitorum longus muscle (high division)
29. Tendon of flexor hallucis longus muscle
30. Tendon of peroneus (fibularis) brevis muscle
31. Tendon of peroneus (fibularis) longus muscle
32. Tendon of plantaris muscle
33. Tendon of tibialis anterior muscle
34. Tendon of tibialis posterior muscle
35. Tibia

(a)-(f) Forefoot, axial MR images, from superior to inferior.

1. Abductor digiti minimi muscle
2. Abductor hallucis muscle
3. Calcaneofibular ligament
4. Calcaneus
5. Cuboid
6. Extensor digitorum brevis muscle
7. Fifth metatarsal base (tuberosity)
8. Flexor digitorum brevis muscle
9. Flexor accessorius (quadratus plantae) muscle
10. Fourth metatarsal base
11. Flexor retinaculum
12. Great (long) saphenous vein
13. Intermediate cuneiform
14. Lateral bundle of plantar aponeurosis (fascia)
15. Lateral cuneiform
16. Lateral plantar neurovascular bundle
17. Medial bundle of plantar aponeurosis (fascia)
18. Medial plantar neurovascular bundle
19. Medial cuneiform
20. Navicular
21. Peroneal (fibular) retinaculum
22. Posterior tibial neurovascular bundle
23. Second metatarsal
24. Small (short) saphenous vein

25. Sustentaculum tali
26. Talar head
27. Talocalcaneal (cervical) ligament
28. Talocalcaneonavicular (spring) ligament
29. Talonavicular joint
30. Tendo calcaneus (Achilles' tendon)

31. Tendon of abductor hallucis muscle
32. Tendon of flexor digitorum longus muscle (high division)
33. Tendon of flexor hallucis longus muscle
34. Tendon of peroneus (fibularis) brevis muscle

35. Tendon of peroneus (fibularis) longus muscle
36. Tendon of tibialis posterior muscle
37. Third metatarsal

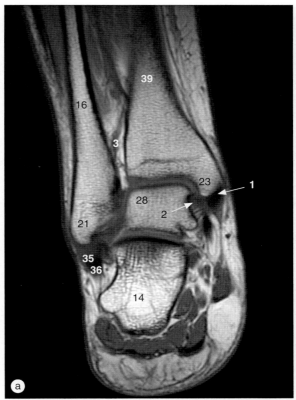

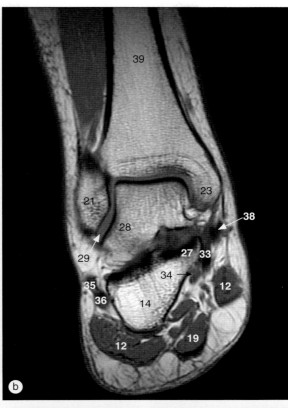

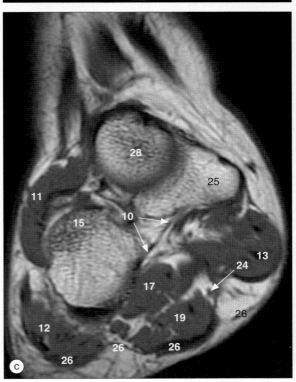

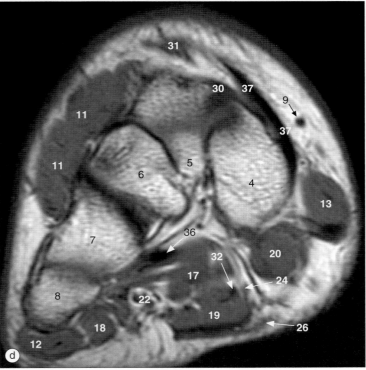

(a)–(d) Ankle and foot, coronal MR images, from posterior to anterior.

1. Deltoid ligament, superficial portion
2. Deltoid ligament, deep portion
3. Tibiofibular ligament
4. First metatarsal
5. Second metatarsal
6. Third metatarsal
7. Fourth metatarsal
8. Fifth metatarsal
9. Great (long) saphenous vein
10. Plantar calcaneonavicular (spring) ligament
11. Extensor digitorum brevis muscle
12. Abductor digiti minimi muscle
13. Abductor hallucis muscle
14. Calcaneus
15. Cuboid
16. Fibula

17. Flexor accessorius muscle
18. Flexor digiti minimi muscle
19. Flexor digitorum brevis muscle
20. Flexor hallucis brevis muscle
21. Lateral malleolus
22. Lateral plantar nerve and vessels
23. Medial malleolus
24. Medial plantar nerve and artery
25. Navicular

26. Plantar aponeurosis
27. Sustentaculum tali
28. Talus
29. Talofibular joint
30. Tendon of extensor digitorum longus muscle
31. Tendon of extensor hallucis longus muscle
32. Tendon of flexor digitorum brevis muscle
33. Tendon of flexor digitorum longus muscle

34. Tendon of flexor hallucis longus muscle
35. Tendon of peroneus (fibularis) brevis muscle
36. Tendon of peroneus (fibularis) longus muscle
37. Tendon of tibialis anterior muscle
38. Tendon of tibialis posterior muscle
39. Tibia

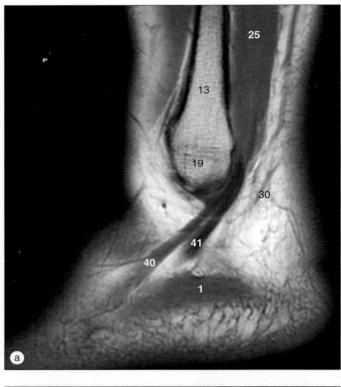

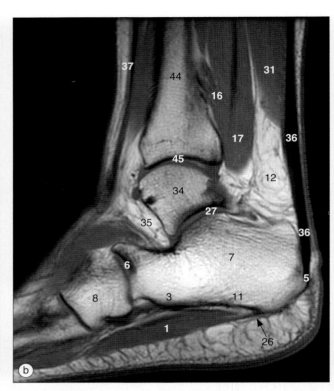

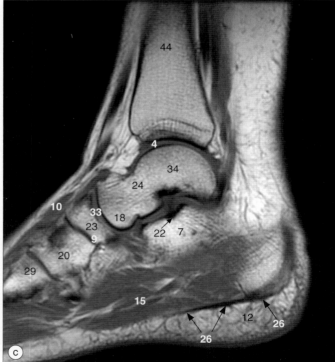

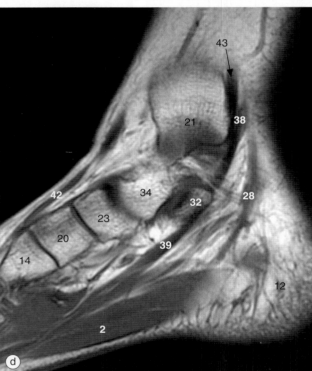

1. Abductor digiti minimi muscle
2. Abductor hallucis muscle
3. Anterior tubercle of calcaneus
4. Articular cartilage
5. Insertion of Achilles' tendon
6. Calcaneocuboid joint
7. Calcaneus
8. Cuboid
9. Cuneonavicular joint
10. Extensor digitorum brevis muscle
11. Lateral calcaneal process
12. Fat pad
13. Fibula
14. First metatarsal
15. Flexor digitorum brevis muscle
16. Flexor digitorum longus muscle
17. Flexor hallucis longus muscle
18. Head of talus
19. Lateral malleolus
20. Medial cuneiform
21. Medial malleolus
22. Middle facet, subtalar joint
23. Navicular
24. Neck of talus
25. Peroneus brevis muscle
26. Plantar aponeurosis
27. Posterior subtalar joint
28. Posterior tibial artery and vein
29. Metatarsal base
30. Small (short) saphenous vein
31. Soleus muscle
32. Sustentaculum tali

(a)–(d) Ankle, sagittal MR images, from lateral to medial.

33. Talonavicular joint
34. Talus
35. Tarsal sinus
36. Tendocalcaneus (Achilles' tendon)
37. Tendon of extensor digitorum muscle
38. Tendon of flexor digitorum longus muscle
39. Tendon of flexor hallucis longus muscle
40. Tendon of peroneus brevis muscle
41. Tendon of peroneus longus muscle
42. Tendon of tibialis anterior muscle
43. Tendon of tibialis posterior muscle
44. Tibia
45. Tibiotalar part of ankle joint

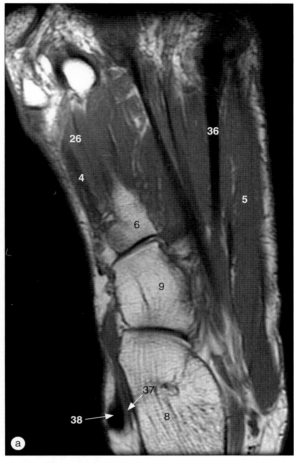

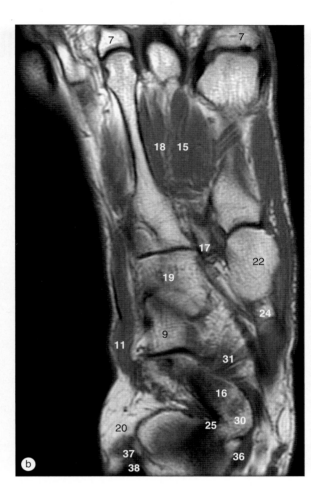

1. Head of first metatarsal
2. Sesamoid bones in flexor hallucis brevis
3. Flexor digitorum longus
4. Abductor digiti minimi muscle
5. Abductor hallucis muscle and tendon
6. Base of metatarsal
7. Base of proximal phalanx
8. Calcaneus
9. Cuboid
10. Dorsal interosseous muscle
11. Extensor digitorum brevis muscle
12. Flexor accessorius muscle (quadratus plantae)
13. Flexor digiti minimi muscle
14. Flexor digitorum brevis muscle
15. Flexor hallucis brevis muscle
16. Head of talus
17. Intermediate cuneiform
18. Interossei muscles
19. Lateral cuneiform
20. Lateral malleolus

(a)–(b) Foot, axial MR images.

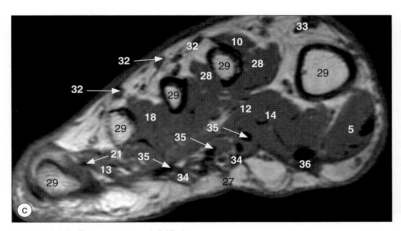

(c) and **(d)** Foot, coronal MR images.

21. Lateral plantar nerve
22. Medial cuneiform
23. Medial plantar nerve and artery
24. Navicular
25. Neck of talus
26. Opponens digiti minimi muscle
27. Plantar aponeurosis
28. Plantar interossei muscle
29. Shafts of first to fifth metatarsals
30. Talus
31. Tarsal sinus
32. Tendon of extensor digitorum longus muscle
33. Tendon of extensor hallucis longus muscle
34. Tendon of flexor digitorum brevis muscle
35. Tendon of flexor digitorum longus muscle
36. Tendon of flexor hallucis longus muscle
37. Tendon of peroneus brevis muscle
38. Tendon of peroneus longus muscle

Bonus e-materials

Slidelines for radiograph features: Anteroposterior radiograph of the pelvis (female), AP radiograph of the right knee, Lateral radiograph of the knee, Lateral view radiograph of the left ankle, Mortise view radiograph of the left ankle

Cross-sectional image stack slideshows: Sagittal T2-weighted gradient echo sequence MRI of the right knee

Selected pages from Imaging Atlas 4e

Tutorials: Tutorial 8

Ultrasound videos: Video 11.1 Dynamic ultrasound of the common peroneal (fibular) nerve (transverse), Video 11.2 Dynamic ultrasound of the flexor compartment from the ankle to mid-calf (transverse)

Single best answer (SBA) self-assessment questions

Table of Variations

Variant	Frequency	Clinical implications
Peroneus tertius	63%	Can cause painful snapping over talus (originates from the anterior leg compartment inserting into dorsum of base of 5th metatarsal).
Profunda femoris arterial divisions	42%	18% medial circumflex femoral artery originates from SFA; 15% LFCA originates from SFA, 4% both originate from SFA, 3% duplicated LCFA from SFA/profunda. Knowledge of these conditions can prevent unexpected iatrogenic injury in surgery and intervention, e.g. muscle flaps, arterial bypass (profunda rarely involved in atherosclerosis), angioplasty.
Femoral vein duplication	33%	Missed thrombosis in duplicant on Doppler US for deep vein thrombosis (duplication associated with increased risk of thrombosis).
Fabella	20%	Posterolateral pain and tenderness exacerbated in knee extension from fabella syndrome due to chondromalacia.
Peroneus quartus	10% (MRI) to 20% (ultrasound)	Can cause lateral ankle pain and instability in athletes from hypertrophy of its calcaneal attachment and peroneal tenosynovitis due to anterior subluxation from crowding other peroneal tendons. Its tendon can mimic longitudinal tears of adjacent peroneal tendons. If identified may be used to repair peroneal retinacular injuries.
Peroneal arterial major foot contribution	7–12%	Posterior tibial artery originates from distal peroneal artery in 5.6% of cases.
Flexor digitorum accessorius longus	6–8%	Causes 12% of tarsal tunnel syndrome from fleshy fibres within the tunnel superficial to the posterior tibial neurovascular bundle.
Discoid lateral meniscus	3–6% (Western), 20% (Asian)	Irregular meniscocapsular ligamentous connection confers instability; disorganised circumferential collagen predisposes to tear. Younger children may present with painless clunking and lack of terminal extension; older children with pain and locking. More recently, the approach to treatment is conservative.
Small saphenous vein duplication	3–5%	Failure to recognise on Doppler US or at surgery results in early recurrence of varicose veins.
Bipartite patella	2%	Occasionally symptomatic, 9× commoner in males.
Great saphenous vein duplication	1%	Failure to recognise on Doppler US or at surgery results in early recurrence of varicose veins.

LFCA, Lateral femoral circumflex artery; *MRI*, magnetic resonance imaging; *SFA*, superficial femoral artery; *US*, ultrasound.

12 | Functional imaging

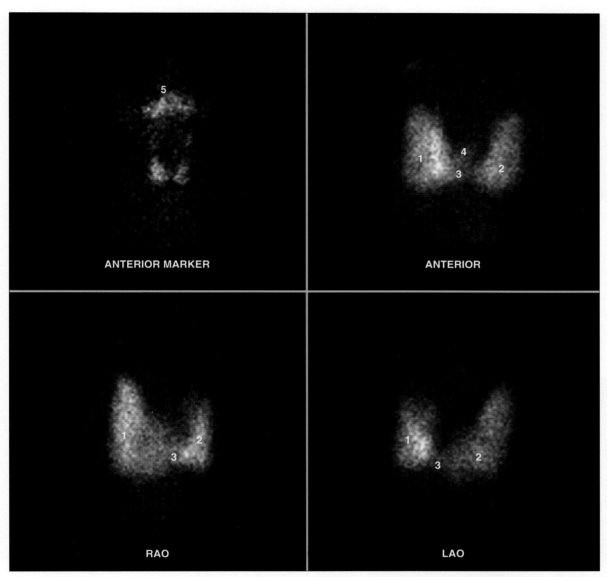

Normal thyroid scan (imaging agent is Tc-99m pertechnetate). These are four standard imaging views of the thyroid. The anterior marker image is a landscape image showing most of the head and upper thorax. In the middle of the image the thyroid gland is seen and above that are the salivary glands. The three additional images are close up images over the thyroid in the anterior, right anterior oblique (RAO) and left anterior oblique (LAO) projections.

1. Right lobe of thyroid
2. Left lobe of thyroid
3. Isthmus
4. Pyramidal lobe
5. Salivary glands

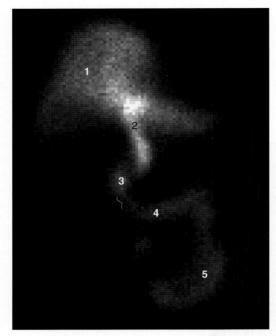

Hepatobiliary scan. The hepatocytes of the liver extract most of the injected dose and excrete it into the intrahepatic ducts. From there, the tracer flows into the common hepatic and common bile ducts. The agent passively fills the gallbladder with visualization within one hour of isotope injection. The gallbladder is not seen in this example. Reasons for nonvisulaization of the gallbladder may be due to surgically removal, gallbladder distention or active contraction during imaging, or the patient has had a prolonged fast prior to imaging). The agent then will enter into the duodenum through the ampulla of Vater, and eventually into the small bowel.

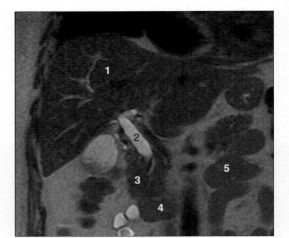

Coronal MRCP.

1. Liver
2. Bile duct
3. Descending (second) part of duodenum
4. Horizontal (third) part of duodenum
5. Jejunum

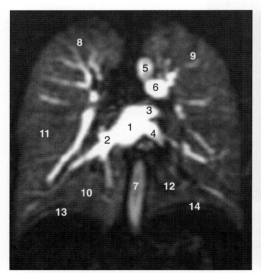

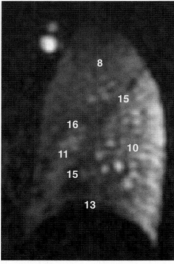

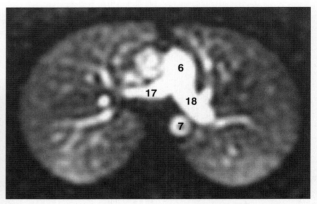

- MR functional perfusion imaging of the lungs during injection of intravenous gadolinium contrast. These images demonstrate dynamic contrast-enhanced perfusion images at peak enhancement with 1 second temporal resolution and 4mm isotropic spatial resolution.
- The sagittal image demonstrates the gravitational dependence in perfusion (whiter posterior compared to less white anterior). The sagittal and coronal images also reveal the fissures of the lungs.

1. Left atrium	7. Descending thoracic aorta	13. Right hemidiaphragm
2. Right inferior pulmonary vein	8. Right upper lobe	14. Left hemidiaphragm
3. Left superior pulmonary vein	9. Left upper lobe	15. Right major fissure
4. Left inferior pulmonary vein	10. Right lower lobe	16. Right minor fissure
5. Aortic arch	11. Right middle lobe	17. Right main pulmonary artery
6. Pulmonary trunk	12. left lower lobe	18. Left main pulmonary artery

MR images of the lungs are courtesy of Scott Nagle, PhD MD, Sean Fain, PhD, and Robert Cadman, PhD, from the University of Wisconsin, Madison, Wisconsin.

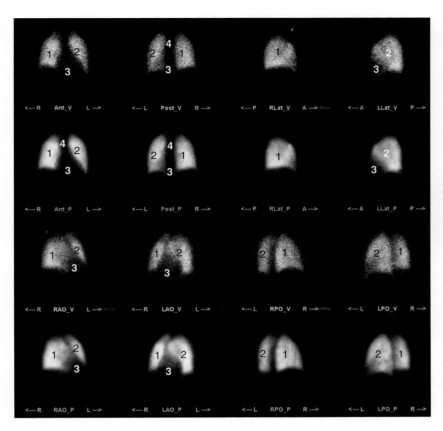

Lung Scan. Imaging of the lungs involves both ventilation and perfusion. In a normal scan, the ventilation and perfusion images should appear the same and match. The order of imaging the ventilation and perfusion depends on the agents used. Both ventilation and perfusion imaging evaluate the lungs in eight projections (anterior, posterior, right lateral, left lateral, right anterior oblique (RAO), left anterior oblique (LAO), right posterior oblique (RPO) and left posterior oblique (LPO)). The first and third rows are ventilation and the second and fourth rows are the matching perfusion.

1. Right lung
2. Left lung
3. Cardiac silhouette
4. Mediastinum

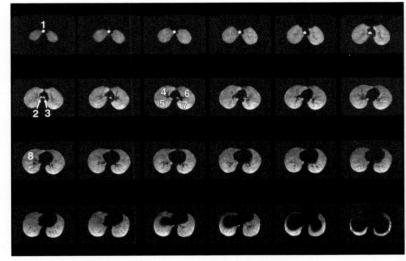

Consecutive axial images of the lungs (superior to inferior) demonstrating the normal ventilation of the lungs during a breath-hold of ³He gas using MRI.

1. Trachea
2. Right mainstem bronchus
3. Left mainstem bronchus
4. Right upper lobe
5. Right lower lobe
6. Left upper lobe
7. Left lower lobe
8. Right middle lobe

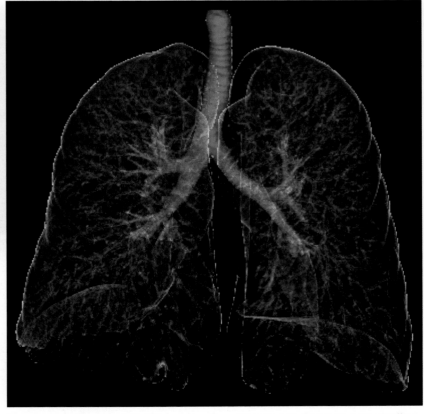

Lungs and airways, 3D CT image. See Chapter 7, Thorax: non-cardiac, p.118.

MR images of the lungs are courtesy of Scott Nagle, PhD MD, Sean Fain, PhD, and Robert Cadman, PhD, from the University of Wisconsin, Madison, Wisconsin.

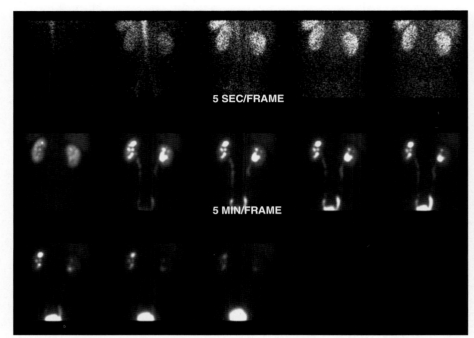

5 SEC/FRAME

5 MIN/FRAME

Renogram: Serial images acquired after venous injection of the radiopharmaceuticals Tc-99m DTPA or Tc-99m MAG3. Initial image (top left) reveals the agent in the aorta, with subsequent images demonstrating cortical and then medullary activity in the kidney and, finally, excretion into ureters and bladder. DTPA: DiethyleneTriaminePentAcetate; MAG3: mercaptoacetyltriglycine

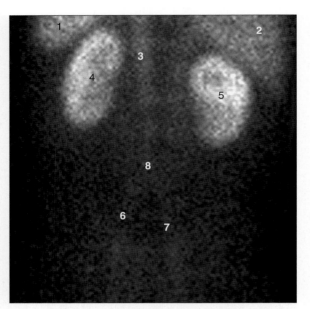

Renal imaging is generally performed with the camera closest to the kidneys and often with the patient supine. In a MAG3 renal study, perfusion, uptake, excretion and drainage can be assessed. In the perfusion phase, some of the agent remains in the blood pool allowing visualization of the aorta and iliac branches, liver and spleen.

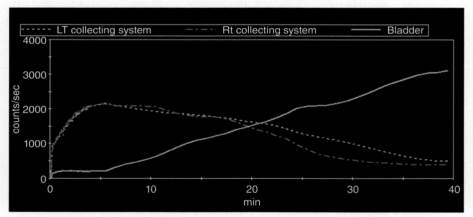

Normal time-activity renogram curve. The activity in the renal collecting systems increases, then reaches a maximum; as the collecting system activity decreases, the bladder activity increases.

1. Spleen
2. Liver
3. Abdominal aorta
4. Left kidney
5. Right kidney
6. Left common iliac artery
7. Right common iliac artery
8. Abdominal aortic bifurcation

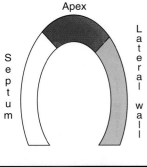
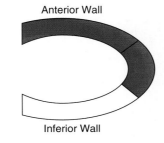
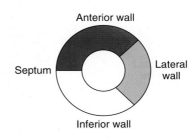

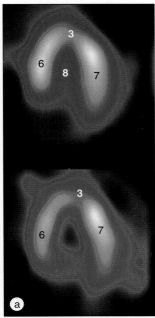
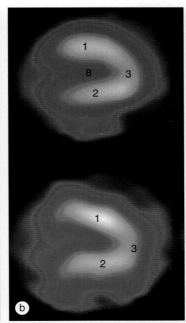
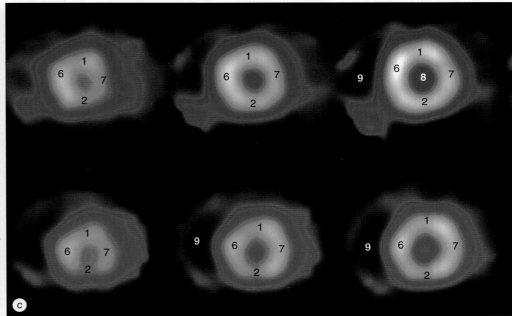

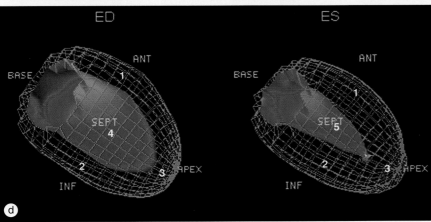

Cardiac scans. (a)–(c) Images obtained during stress (exercise or pharmaceutical) are represented by the top row of images; those obtained during rest are represented by the bottom row of images. A defect which is fixed (its decreased perfusion appears the same rest and stress) indicates infarction or chronic ischemia whereas reversible (its perfusion is decreased during stress and is improved at rest) defect suggests inducible ischemia. After imaging, the is imaged in different planes to evaluate the specific walls and circulation that supplies them. The left ventricle appears as a 'horseshoe' shape on the vertical long axis (a) and horizontal long axis (b), and as a 'doughnut' on the short axis (a) views. The anterior wall, apex and part of the septum are supplied by the anterior descending artery. The right coronary artery supplies inferior wall and part of the septum, and the circumflex artery supplies the lateral wall.

Cardiac scans. (d) 3D reconstructions of the left ventricle at end diastole (ED) and end systole (ES). Subtracting the ventricular volume at ES from ED represents the ejection volume during systole.

1. Anterior wall of left ventricle
2. Inferior wall of left ventricle
3. Apical portion of left ventricle
4. Blood pool volume within the left ventricle at end diastole
5. Blood pool volume within the left ventricle at end systole
6. Interventricular septum
7. Lateral wall of left ventricle
8. Left ventricle cavity
9. Right ventricle cavity

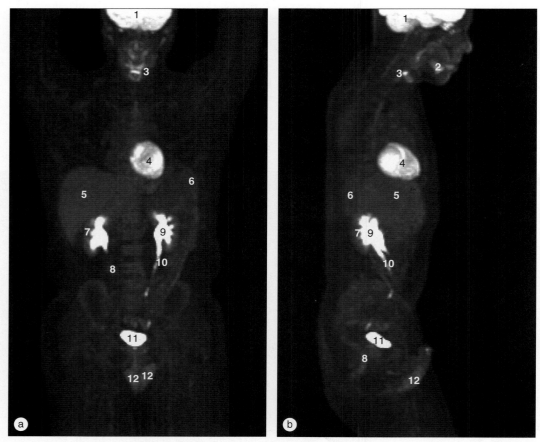

Maximal intensity projection (MIP) images; frontal and lateral.

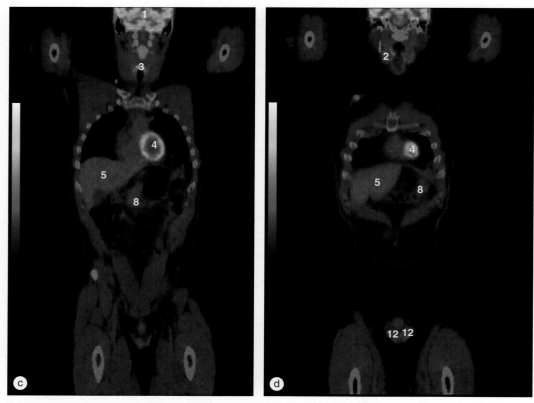

Coronal fused (CT with PET) images.

For labels see page 243.

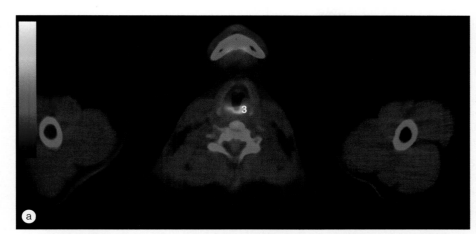

The most common radioisotope used in PET imaging is fluorodeoxyglucose (FDG). FDG is a glucose analogue and to optimize scanning, patients should be fasted, with a blood glucose less than 100 mg/dL. Extensive exercise should be avoided the day before the scan to minimize normal muscle uptake of the radiotracer. Following injection, the patient must rest quietly for 1 hour before scanning. Most PET imaging is performed to evaluate for cancer, but it can also be used to evaluate for infection, vasculitis, cardiac viability, and in brain imaging. This is a normal scan of male patient demonstrating physiologic activity in the following structures.

1. Brain
2. Salivary glands (submandibular)
3. Vocal cords
4. Heart
5. Liver
6. Spleen
7. Kidney
8. Bowel loops
9. Renal collecting system
10. Ureters
11. Bladder
12. Testes

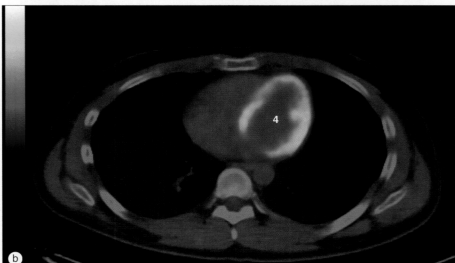

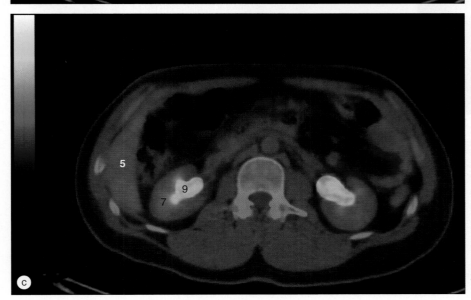

Axial fused (CT with PET) images.

Functional MR imaging (fMRI) is performed to assess motor, sensory and association processing regions of the brain in patients with epilepsy or brain tumors. In these patients who may benefit from surgical intervention it is helpful to know how close these functional regions of the brain are prior to surgical resection.

The foundation of fMRI relies on the changes of oxygen in hemoglobin. Oxygen is delivered to neurons by hemoglobin in capillary red blood cells. When neuronal activity increases there is an increased demand for oxygen and the local response is an increase blood flow to regions of increased neural activity. Hemoglobin is diamagnetic when oxygenated but paramagnetic when deoxygenated. This difference in magnetic properties leads to small differences in the MR signal of blood depending on the degree of oxygenation. Since blood oxygenation varies according to the levels of neural activity these differences can be used to detect brain activity. This form of MRI is known as blood oxygenation level dependent (BOLD) imaging.

Some functional tests that can be performed can localize language and motor function. The patient is imaged during these tests, with breaks between imaging sets. Tests used to localize language cortex include silent word generation (Broca's area for expressive language), text reading contrasted with symbol discrimination, and true-false statements contrasted with symbol matching (Wernicke's area for receptive language). Motor tests include finger or foot tapping, tongue movements, and lip pursing from visual cues.

Diffusion tensor imaging (DTI) occurs with the patient at rest. MR imaging allows the measurement of microscopic water diffusion the brain. Water in white mater diffuses more rapidly in the direction aligned with the internal structure (i.e. along the neural fibers), and more slowly perpendicular to the preferred direction. Thus DTI is a probe in vivo of the 3D diffusion properties of water in tissues. DTI can be used to evaluate the integrity of the white matter in the brain or to map the neural fiber connections from one region to another.

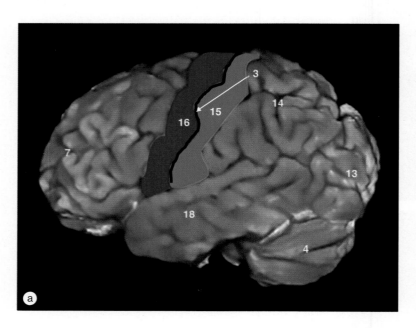

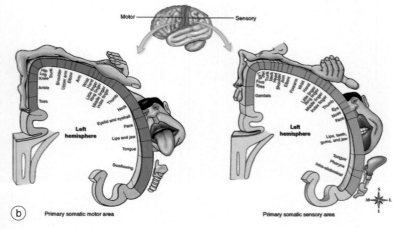

1. Broca's area	8. Interhemispheric fissure	16a. Movement of right foot
1a. Text symbol processing	9. Internal capsule, anterior limb	16b. Movement of right finger
1b. True/false processing	10. Internal capsule, genu	16c. Movement of tongue side to side
1c. Antonym and silent word	11. Internal capsule, posterior limb	with mouth closed
processing	12. Lateral ventricles	16d. Movement of lips (pursing)
2. Caudate head	13. Occipital lobe	17. Putamen
3. Central sulcus	13a. Visual cortex (looking at text)	18. Temporal lobe
4. Cerebellum	14. Parietal lobe	19. Thalamus
5. Corona radiata	15. Postcentral gyrus (somatosensory	20. Wernicke's area
6. Corpus callosum	cortex)	20a. Text symbol processing
7. Frontal lobe	16. Precentral gyrus (primary motor cortex)	20b. True/false processing

Numbers 1–20 are common to pages 244–248.

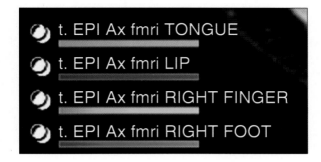

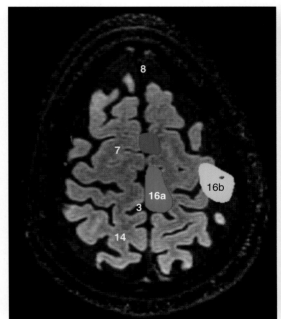
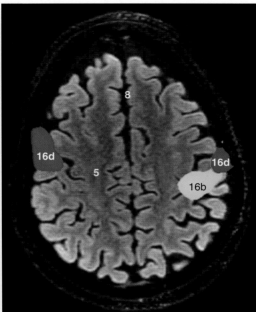
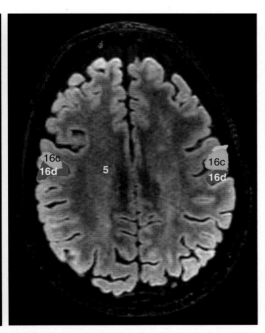

fMRI and DTI images are courtesy of Aaron Field, MD, PhD, Vivek Prabhakaran, MD, PhD, and Tammy Heydle, RT from the University of Wisconsin, Madison, Wisconsin.

1. Broca's area
   1a. Text symbol processing
   1b. True/false processing
   1c. Antonym and silent word processing
2. Caudate head
3. Central sulcus
4. Cerebellum
5. Corona radiata
6. Corpus callosum
7. Frontal lobe

8. Interhemispheric fissure
9. Internal capsule, anterior limb
10. Internal capsule, genu
11. Internal capsule, posterior limb
12. Lateral ventricles
13. Occipital lobe
    13a. Visual cortex (looking at text)
14. Parietal lobe
15. Postcentral gyrus (somatosensory cortex)
16. Precentral gyrus (primary motor cortex)

16a. Movement of right foot
16b. Movement of right finger
16c. Movement of tongue side to side with mouth closed
16d. Movement of lips (pursing)
17. Putamen
18. Temporal lobe
19. Thalamus
20. Wernicke's area
    20a. Text symbol processing
    20b. True/false processing

Numbers 1–20 are common to pages 244–248.

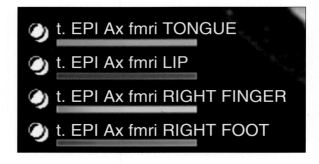

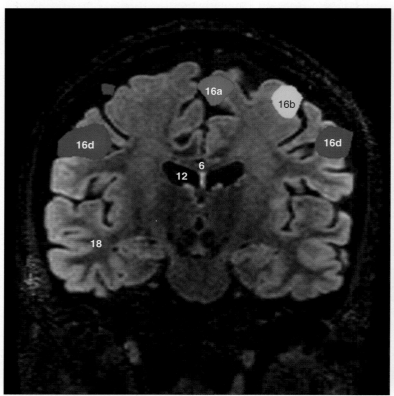

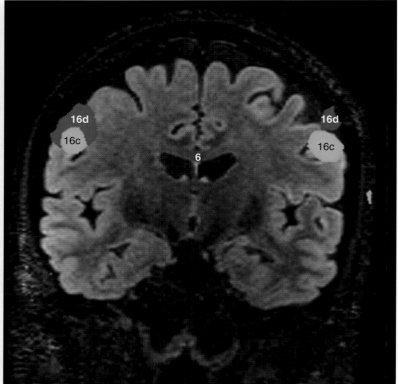

1. Broca's area	**8.** Interhemispheric fissure	**16a.** Movement of right foot
1a. Text symbol processing	**9.** Internal capsule, anterior limb	**16b.** Movement of right finger
1b. True/false processing	**10.** Internal capsule, genu	**16c.** Movement of tongue side to side
1c. Antonym and silent word	**11.** Internal capsule, posterior limb	with mouth closed
processing	**12.** Lateral ventricles	**16d.** Movement of lips (pursing)
2. Caudate head	**13.** Occipital lobe	**17.** Putamen
3. Central sulcus	**13a.** Visual cortex (looking at text)	**18.** Temporal lobe
4. Cerebellum	**14.** Parietal lobe	**19.** Thalamus
5. Corona radiata	**15.** Postcentral gyrus (somatosensory	**20.** Wernicke's area
6. Corpus callosum	cortex)	**20a.** Text symbol processing
7. Frontal lobe	**16.** Precentral gyrus (primary motor cortex)	**20b.** True/false processing

Numbers 1–20 are common to pages 244–248.

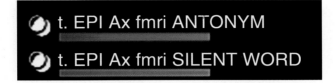

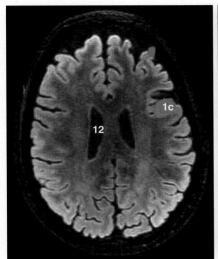

Broca and Wernicke's testing.

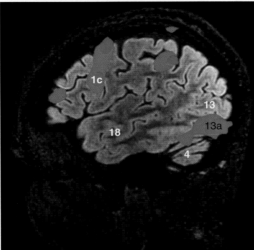

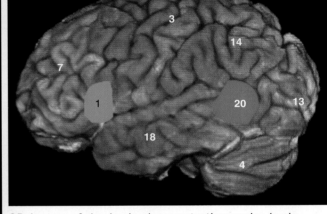

3D image of the brain demonstrating major brain segments and general locations of the Broca's and Wernicke's areas as demonstrated on the accompanying functional MR images.

1. Broca's area
   1a. Text symbol processing
   1b. True/false processing
   1c. Antonym and silent word processing
2. Caudate head
3. Central sulcus
4. Cerebellum
5. Corona radiata
6. Corpus callosum
7. Frontal lobe
8. Interhemispheric fissure
9. Internal capsule, anterior limb
10. Internal capsule, genu
11. Internal capsule, posterior limb
12. Lateral ventricles
13. Occipital lobe
   13a. Visual cortex (looking at text)
14. Parietal lobe
15. Postcentral gyrus (somatosensory cortex)
16. Precentral gyrus (primary motor cortex)
16a. Movement of right foot
16b. Movement of right finger
16c. Movement of tongue side to side with mouth closed
16d. Movement of lips (pursing)
17. Putamen
18. Temporal lobe
19. Thalamus
20. Wernicke's area
   20a. Text symbol processing
   20b. True/false processing

Numbers 1–20 are common to pages 244–248.

EPI Ax fmri TEXT SYMBOL

EPI Ax fmri TRUE FALSE

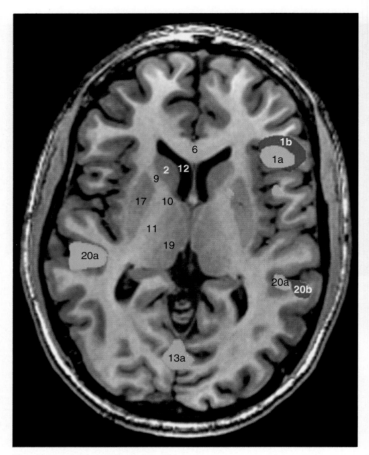

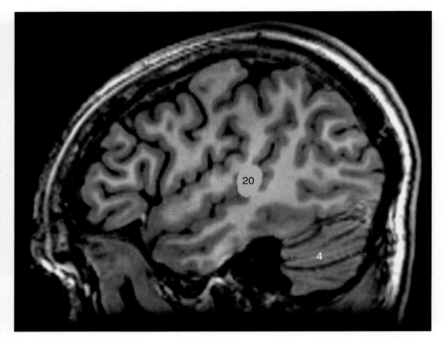

Broca and Wernicke's testing.

1. Broca's area	**8.** Interhemispheric fissure	**16a.** Movement of right foot
1a. Text symbol processing	**9.** Internal capsule, anterior limb	**16b.** Movement of right finger
1b. True/false processing	**10.** Internal capsule, genu	**16c.** Movement of tongue side to side
1c. Antonym and silent word processing	**11.** Internal capsule, posterior limb	with mouth closed
	12. Lateral ventricles	**16d.** Movement of lips (pursing)
2. Caudate head	**13.** Occipital lobe	**17.** Putamen
3. Central sulcus	**13a.** Visual cortex (looking at text)	**18.** Temporal lobe
4. Cerebellum	**14.** Parietal lobe	**19.** Thalamus
5. Corona radiata	**15.** Postcentral gyrus (somatosensory cortex)	**20.** Wernicke's area
6. Corpus callosum		**20a.** Text symbol processing
7. Frontal lobe	**16.** Precentral gyrus (primary motor cortex)	**20b.** True/false processing

Numbers 1–20 are common to pages 244–248.

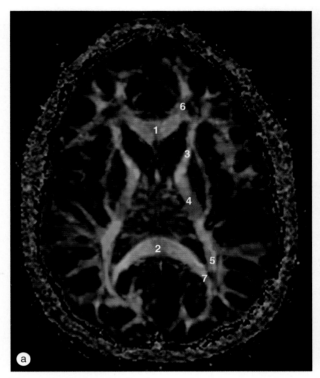

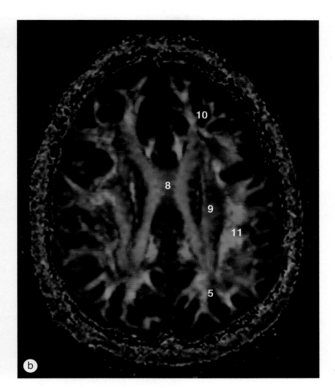

Tractography of the brain.

1. Corpus callosum, genu	8. Corpus callosum
2. Corpus callosum, splenium	9. Superior region of the corona radiata
3. Anterior limb of internal capsule	10. Anterior region of the corona radiata
4. Posterior limb of internal capsule	11. Superior longitudinal fasciculus
5. Posterior region of corona radiata	12. Fornix
6. Forceps minor	13. Corticospinal tract
7. Forceps major	14. Corona radiata

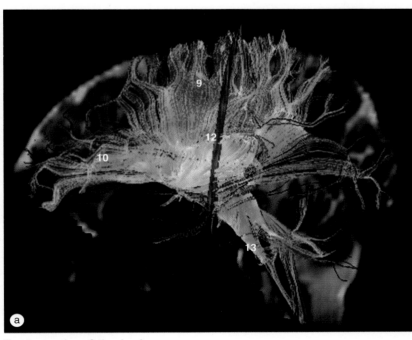

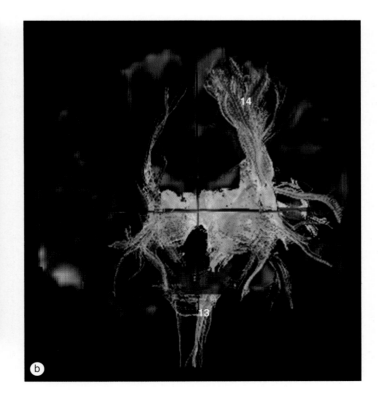

Tractography of the brain.

Bonus e-materials

Tutorials: Tutorial 9

Table of Variations

Variant	Frequency	Clinical implications
Heart ventricular uptake		Irregular uptake is common. Focal areas of increased or decreased uptake should not be considered evidence of disease without the appropriate supporting cardiac history.
Diffuse thyroid uptake of FDG		Normal thyroid tissue has an SUV of 1.3. Higher levels of uptake may be seen in Graves' disease and chronic thyroiditis. In general the SUV cutoff between benign and malignant is 2.0–2.5. Lower SUVs are benign; higher ones are more likely to be malignant.
Breast uptake of FDG		Low-grade uptake is normal in premenopausal women, with amount of uptake decreasing with age. Lactation can cause diffuse increase in uptake. Focal uptake can be sign of both benign and malignant conditions.
Bowel uptake of FDG		Small bowel has less uptake than large bowel. Right colon is also most prominent. Focal or segmental areas of uptake often represent disease.
Genitourinary tract uptake		Kidneys excrete any filtered FDG. Activity can be seen in renal collecting systems, ureters and bladder. Can lead to false positives and false negatives.
Draining of sentinel node to internal mammary lymph node or contralateral axilla		
Aberrant intrahepatic duct	5–13%	Ducts may join the common hepatic duct, common bile duct, cystic duct, right hepatic duct and gallbladder. Can result in a bile leak if severed during interventional procedures.
Agenesis of gallbladder	<1%	Failure to visualise gallbladder on HIDA scan can result in false positive scan.
Congenital biliary atresia	1 in 10,000–15,000 newborns	Absence or severe deficiency of the extrahepatic biliary tree. Most common reason for liver transplantation in children. More common in males. Presents within the first 3 months of life; most are normal at birth.
Bronchial atresia		Obliteration of the proximal lumen of a segmental bronchus. Emphysematous due to air trapping; may appear similar to pneumothorax or bolus changes. Results in abnormal ventilation on a lung scan with normal perfusion.

FDG, *Fluorodeoxyglucose*; HIDA, *hepatobiliary iminodiacetic acid*; SUV, *standard uptake value.*

Index

Page numbers followed by "*f*" indicate figures, "*t*" indicate tables, "*b*" indicate boxes, and "*e*" indicate online content.